WHEN CHINA SNEEZES

WHEN CHINA SNEEZES

From the Coronavirus Lockdown to the
Global Politico-Eonomic Crisis

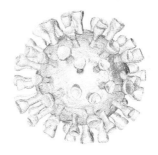

Edited by
Cynthia McKinney, Ph.D.

Clarity Press, Inc.

© 2020 Cynthia McKinney
ISBN: 978-1-949762-24-2
EBOOK ISBN: 978-1-949762-25-9

In-house editor: Diana G. Collier
Cover design: R. Jordan Santos
Cover photo credit: Jeanne Lemlin

Library of Congress Control Number: 2020942750

Clarity Press, Inc.
2625 Piedmont Rd. NE, Ste. 56
Atlanta, GA 30324, USA
https://www.claritypress.com

TABLE OF CONTENTS

Introduction

Cynthia McKinney

BEWARE: This book goes where you dare not tread—but must, if you are to fully understand the importance of SARS-CoV-2 and COVID-19 as not just menaces to global health, but also as delivery systems for global population control: physical, political, and economic. Be sure to buckle your seatbelt, because by the time you've completed these pages, your outlook on health, wealth, and global governance won't be the same.

I worked very hard to assemble a team of *avant-garde* thinkers, with thinkers being the operative word, who have never allowed themselves to be pigeonholed into any special-interest, Deep State boxes. And, in an age when our present reality of lived experiences is being rewritten, before our very eyes, into prosaic snippets that bear no resemblance to our real lives, the contributors to *When China Sneezes* have preserved snapshots of what we know today as real because it seems, from the propaganda that separates us from what we experience and what we know, that this critical point in time will not be remembered as we have lived it.

This book dares to put in writing what has been on the minds of many people in the U.S., the U.K., and Western Europe who are currently being subjected to a brutal barrage of anti-China and anti-Russia hysteria while, at the same time, being victimized by an eerily similar set of seemingly disconnected policies that strikingly all result in incalculable transfers of wealth out of the pockets of those who have the least and into the pockets of the m/billionaire class. The propaganda and hysteria have the effect of obfuscating this very real global theft taking place by the same forces that financed the seafarers of old who set out to colonize their world. At the same time, the world's increasingly dispossessed populations are witnessing governments introduce population surveillance and control techniques with the stated purpose of promoting health and security. Frighteningly, the human bloodstream has become a 21st Century battlefield.

These official narratives are deliberately deceptive efforts to explain the profound changes now taking place in our daily lives. Our contributors cut through all of that deception and deliver a sobering call to arms to wake up or else "We are all Palestinians, now; We are all Black now; We are all slaves now" will be quickly consolidated into a global reality for billions of humanity.

Brown, Romanoff, our Anonymous "Lockdown Diarists," Rasmus, Hudson, Koenig, Robinson, Webb, Peretti, Barnett, Buyniski and Skouras, and de Zayas deliver a powerful message to all of the truth seekers out there, that now is our time! With a foundation of truth, I do believe that one day, we will be able to live together as a global community rooted in justice, peace, and Earth and human dignity. This book sets us on our way.

PART I
COVID-19: The Disease and Its Virus

CHAPTER ONE

EVERYTHING YOU WANTED TO KNOW ABOUT CORONAVIRUSES (CoV), BUT WERE AFRAID TO ASK

Jeff J. Brown

MICROBIOLOGY 101

In order to appreciate and understand where coronaviruses (CoV) fit into your life and future, it is important to put them into proper perspective. Microbiology is one of the most misunderstood sciences, yet one that has such a powerful impact on our existence, for better and for worse.

It reminds me of a comment from a friend who successfully worked all his professional life with his Master of Public Health (MPH) degree. He told me numerous times that an MPH is a recession-proof career, since agriculture, poultry, livestock, food processing, quality control, government inspections, medicine and research and development (R&D) all have a big microbiology component.

As you read this chapter, two good questions to ponder are,

Do we control all these micro-critters, or do they control us? Do we live in their world, or do they live in ours?

THE GOOD GUYS

Coronaviruses are the focus of this book, but they are only a handful of the estimated one trillion (1,000,000,000,000) species of microbes that exist on Earth.[1] These include:

- Bacteria (they are everywhere)
- Archaea (thermal vent bacteria)
- Protozoa (single cell animals)

---

1 Jay T. Lennon and Kenneth J. Locey, "There are more microbial species on Earth than stars in the galaxy," *Aeon,* September 10, 2018, https://aeon.co/ideas/there-are-more-microbial-species-on-earth-than-stars-in-the-sky.

- Fungi (molds and mushrooms)
- Algae (seaweed, kelp and diatoms)
- Viruses (the living dead)[2]

While China and the United States spar over where SARS-Cov-2 *patient zero* came from, our origins are in no doubt. Around 3.5 billion years ago, in the hot soup that was Earth's primordial, protein-filled seas, the first microbe formed. From it evolved all extinct and extant species to this day. So much so that 30% of your human DNA originated from bacteria and yes, eight percent evolved from viruses.[3] Yikes, maybe Franz Kafka's novella *The Metamorphosis* is more truth than fiction!

While being 38% of microbial origin, your body harbors 1,000 of these species. You carry around—24/7—100 trillion (100,000,000,000,000) unseen critters, weighing a total of 1.5 kilograms. That's ten times as many microbes as there are cells in your entire body (muscle, bone, brain, heart, etc.). Collectively, this system is called the *human microbiota* or *human microbiome*. It is an unseen multiple universe in and on your solar system body.

Your skin is your largest organ, 1.8 square meters for an adult. It is covered with 1.5 trillion (1,500,000,000,000) microbes, as well as a billion (1,000,000,000) microscopic skin mites, mostly demodex. All these critters act as your first line of defense against invading, pathogenic (harmful) microbes, like a Star Trek deflector shield keeping you safe. Take them away and you can start counting the hours before you die a grizzly death from massive infections throughout your body. Not to mention, they keep your skin clean and smooth, since they eat all your dead skin and excess oil (sebum). Otherwise, you'd look like a greaseball Elephant Man. Your skin has about 20 unique microbiomes (scalp, ears, armpits, groin, hands, feet, etc.) and although it has not been used in court yet, it is thought that the profiles of each person's local dermal microbiomes are as unique as fingerprints.

However, all this exterior stuff is just scratching the surface, if you'll pardon the pun. Where your microbial world gets *deeply* interesting is inside you. One place in your body that is close to sterile (meaning free of microbes) is your bladder. This is why some people drink their own urine and do not get sick, while apparently offering a number of health benefits. It is also why bladder infections are taken so seriously.

---

2 "On and in you: Your body full of microbes," *ARTIS Microbia,* accessed April 23, 2020, https://www.micropia.nl/en/discover/stories/on-and-in-you/.

3 "How did so much microbial DNA got incorporated in human chromosomes?" question asked Dec. 12, 2016 in the Project Evolution of Human, *ResearchGate,* accessed April 23, 2020, https://www.researchgate.net/post/How_did_so_much_microbial_DNA_got_incorporated_in_human_chromosomes.

Other parts of your body have plenty of microbes, starting with your mouth, which has 700 different healthy species. Your throat, sinuses and lungs are like pullulating Petri culture dishes, veritable micro-critter plantations. A woman's vagina has 300 healthy bacterial species. After years of assuming "sterility," a beneficial blood microbiota is being more and more accepted as fact.[4] So, wherever blood circulates in your body, there are apparently helpful microbes along for the ride, including in the brain and other organs.

But, bug central is your digestive tract. With 1,200 healthy microbial species, it contains the vast majority of that 1.5kg of microbes in your body. In fact, there are so many micro-critters in your gut, which are responsible for helping digest your food, that 50% of the feces you leave in the toilet is microbes.

FOOD BUGS MAKE YOUR KITCHENS COME ALIVE

It is hard to imagine cooking around the world, without the benefit of bacteria and fungi. Fermentation to make many foods and beverages would all be impossible without microbes. Internationally famous Chinese tofu, Korean kimchee, Japanese miso soup, German sauerkraut, Belgian beer, French wine, Russian vodka and pancultural thousands of bread products, cheeses, yogurts, butters, meats, vegetables, beverages, desserts and sauces all depend on specific bacteria and fungi to make them yummy and unique. Did I forget to mention thousands of varieties of mushrooms and dried seaweed to dice and slice? A day without microbes on the plate and in the glass is a dull one indeed.

NOW FOR THE BAD BOYS

Louis Pasteur practically invented the modern, global, multi-billion dollar/euro food processing industry, by making it possible to preserve foods for extended lengths of time, with his invention of *pasteurization*, a well-deserved moniker. This is heating a food above 60 degrees Celsius for about 15 seconds to kill pathogenic microbes like tuberculosis, brucellosis, staphylococcus, salmonella and listeria. Before his invention, millions of uncounted people died every year from food poisoning and food borne deadly diseases. Merci beaucoup, Doctor Pasteur!

For us humans, all the good critters described in the above section keep microbes that can sicken or kill us at bay, as long as our immune systems are healthy and robust. Nevertheless, if we abuse alcohol, tobacco and other drugs, get mentally or physically stressed out, depressed, lack sleep or adequate (good)

---

4 Diego J. Castillo, Riaan F. Rifkin, Don A. Cowan, and Marnie Potgieter, "The Healthy Human Blood Microbiome: Fact or Fiction?" *Frontiers in Cellular and Infection Microbiology,* May 8, 2019, https://www.frontiersin.org/articles/10.3389/fcimb.2019.00148/full.

nutrition, don't exercise, have a serious injury or eat tainted food, our shield of 100 trillion protective microbes can weaken, and this is when invaders like coronaviruses can overwhelm, say, the healthy microbiome in your sinuses and lungs, to make you sick. Our bodies always harbor a certain number of bad microbes, especially our dermal, respiratory and digestive systems, because they receive the most constant outside exposure, but as long as we limit all those aforementioned harmful lifestyle choices, our micro-good guys can keep the bad boys down in numbers, so that the latter don't make us ill.

Not always, but most of the time. Food poisoning is a good example. If you eat enough of a dish that has a high harmful microbial count, such a huge influx is going to sicken even the hardiest iron-gut world travelers. It's a battle of numbers. Getting eaten up with malarial mosquitoes will likely conquer the strongest of immune systems.

Bacteria versus Viruses

When I took university microbiology courses in the early seventies, it was fashionable to say that viruses really weren't "alive," since they are nothing more than a strand of genetic code, called ribonucleic acid (RNA) or deoxyribonucleic acid (DNA), with a protective cover of protein, called the *capsid*. Some, like coronaviruses, also have an outer covering called the *envelope*. There's something to be said about that "zombie" claim. Like deciding whether Pluto is a planet or not, biologists still debate how to classify viruses on the tree of life.

Bacteria, archaea, protozoa, fungi and algae all have a DNA-filled nucleus inside a cellular wall, reproducing by simple division. Many of them are motile, with tails and pilli (hairs) that they can beat to move around.

Ebola virus, on the other hand, looks like a small, thin piece of kinky wire. Its RNA code is only 19 kilobases (kb) long. Polio is a viral runt, with only 7 kb, influenza has 14 kb. Coronaviruses are some of the biggest known. SARS-CoV-2 tips the scales at 30 kb, which is the upper limit that a viral strand of RNA can function, without imploding. This is compared to the smallest bacteria with 130 kb, up to 14 megabases.[5]

All cellular microbes eat like we do, taking in nutrients like sugars, proteins, fats, vitamins and minerals, which are absorbed through their cell walls. Viruses don't eat anything. They have a special place on their strip of RNA/DNA that can attach to your body's cells, cleave a hole in them and inject themselves or their genetic code inside. Once there, they trick the host cells into using their own DNA to replicate the virus' genetic code.

---

5 Rupert Beale, "Wash Your Hands," *London Review of Books,* Vol. 42 No. 6, March 19, 2020, https://www.lrb.co.uk/the-paper/v42/n06/rupert-beale/short-cuts.

How do they do that? There are two possibilities. Drum roll, please.

Either the host cell divides normally while also producing the invading viral RNA/DNA to multiply together, or the host cell gets killed and out pops new viruses to continue to multiply. If that sounds like a gross out scene from an *Alien* movie, you're not far off the mark. Pathogenic viruses are clever parasites that live off of host cells: your sinuses, lungs, (other) organs, skin and the good microbes living on and inside you.

VIRUSES UP CLOSE

The genetic code in viruses is like an old telex or telegraph message, but instead of words, dots and dashes, respectively, it is a long series of five possible nucleotides, abbreviated A, C, G, T and U. There are twelve other letters to show where more than one of the first five can stake a claim, which you will see in later visuals. This long chain of letters, that numbers in the thousands (kilobases), is called a *nucleotide sequence.*

Virologists, those microbiologists who study viruses, focus their research on the part of a virus' code that attaches to host cells, to create an opening for entry. This is sometimes called the binding or attachment point. If a virus does a poor job of penetrating host cells, it will multiply slower and be less infectious. Conversely, if one has a very efficient binding point, then it can rapidly expand in numbers to make its host animal or plant sicker and possibly kill it.

This attachment point is where natural or bioengineered mutations can dramatically increase the pathogenicity of the virus, or in the case of making vaccines, to attenuate them, meaning to make them weaker. These mutations usually consist of slight changes in the genetic code letter sequence, or an insertion can occur, where a few nucleotide letters are added in the genetic strand's binding point. As you will see below, just switching or inserting four letters can completely change the pathogenicity of a virus.

CORONAVIRUSES: THE STARS OF THE SHOW

While SARS-CoV-2 has turned the world upside down since December 2019, coronaviruses have been around for a long time in human history. The most recent common ancestor (MRCA) of coronaviruses was with us around 8,000 BCE, the dawn of organized civilization. Coronaviruses love to live in warm-blooded flying animals, bats and birds, but over the millennia, evolved in domesticated poultry, cattle, dogs, cats and pigs—all which have lived closely with humans going back

10,000 years ago. The earliest known human coronavirus, NL63, can be traced back to the Middle Ages.[6]

Coronaviruses are so ubiquitous in human sinus and respiratory systems that you are probably home to some right now, but they are being kept in check by all your aforementioned good microbes. Many common colds and good old-fashioned seasonal influenza are caused by four human coronaviruses (HCoV), HCoV-229E, -NL63, -OC43 and -HKU1. Additionally, you are probably carrying around the most common flu- and cold- causing critters, influenzaviruses A, B and C. Do you have a clogged-up nose, sore throat and/or bronchitis? You can likely thank an army of coronaviruses or influenzaviruses overwhelming your immune system.

If you are in poor health, old and/or have co-morbidities, like heart disease, cancer, diabetes, tuberculosis, hepatitis, etc., these common coronaviruses can completely overrun your human biota, causing pneumonia and/or death.

Three coronaviruses are bad boys:

1. The 2002-03 severe acute respiratory syndrome coronavirus (SARS-CoV);
2. 2012–15's Middle East respiratory syndrome-related coronavirus (MERS-CoV); and
3. Today's 2019–20 severe acute respiratory syndrome coronavirus 2 (SARS-CoV-2).

Number three was earlier called *COVID-19* and *novel coronavirus 2019*. The new, correct name says volumes about the origins of this new virus. It's SARS Junior.

Coronaviruses get their name from Latin, *corona*, which means crown or wreath. Poor Mexican Corona beer has found this out the hard way, as its sales have purportedly fallen through the floor.

This family of viruses has such a huge, global, deleterious economic impact on livestock, poultry and humans, that there is a specialized field of study called *coronavirology*, but I'm not sure telling someone you are a *coronavirologist* would be a very good pick-up line, especially during these days of *social distancing*.

Coronaviruses look like some science fiction death star, round shaped and covered in spikes. These spikes are not just for looks. They are the binding points they use to penetrate host cells, like the epithelial tissue lining your sinuses, throat, bronchial tubes and lungs. Coronaviruses play for keeps. They don't live

---

6 "Coronavirus," *Wikipedia,* accessed April 23, 2020, https://en.wikipedia.org/wiki/Coronavirus.

cooperatively in host cells to replicate nicey-nicey. They go full *Alien* and destroy them to reproduce.

Needless to say, these spikes are the fascination and obsession of coronavirologists, along with their replicating genes, which we will see below. Much of their research involves studying every nucleotide A, C, G, T, U +12, in what they call the *CoV spike glycoprotein*. Change just a few of its letters and we can get a MERS-CoV, which has a very high 35% mortality rate,[7] yet since 2012 it has only infected about 2,500 people worldwide. Given its lethality, we are lucky it is not very infectious. This could be due to a weak envelope that can't survive in the air, after sneezing or coughing, or its attachment point is not very effective.

SARS Senior[8] has a death rate of almost 10%. It has infected about 8,100 and killed 774 worldwide. The fact that it spread to 29 countries in North America, Africa, Europe, the Middle East, Asia and 96% of the fatalities were ethnic Chinese is telling, when investigating bioweapon engineering.[9] Like MERS, SARS-CoV is not very infectious. However, its 10% mortality rate is similar to 1918's global "Spanish" flu (in reality it started in the US).[10]

On the other hand, SARS Junior, today's headline grabber, seems to spread like wildfire, but as of this writing, has a lower mortality rate, about four percent.[11] This is lower than humanity's annual seasonal influenza, in which the aforementioned common coronaviruses play a part. Every year, tens of millions of people catch the flu, of which 3–5 million cases are considered serious.[12] About 290,000-650,000 deaths in this serious group are attributed to seasonal influenza. This calculates to a mortality rate of 6-13%.

---

7 "Middle East respiratory syndrome coronavirus (MERS-CoV)," World Health Organization, accessed April 23, 2020, https://www.who.int/emergencies/mers-cov/en/

8 "Severe acute respiratory syndrome," *Wikipedia,* accessed April 23, 2020, https://en.wikipedia.org/wiki/Severe_acute_respiratory_syndrome.

9 "Almost 100% of all Covid-19 deaths around the world are ethnic Chinese. SARS was 96%. Why almost no Whites, Blacks, Browns, Reds and other Yellows? What does this tell us? You need to know the truth," *China Rising Radio Sinoland,* March 4, 2020, https://chinarising.puntopress.com/2020/03/04/almost-100-of-all-covid-19-deaths-around-the-world-are-ethnic-chinese-sars-was-96-why-almost-no-whites-blacks-browns-reds-and-other-yellows-what-does-this-tell-us-you-need-to-know-the-truth-ch/.

10 "How the US Army infected the World with Spanish Flu," *Limpia por dentro,* accessed April 23, 2020 http://limpia.centroeu.com/how-the-us-army-infected-the-world-with-spanish-flu/.

11 "Coronavirus (COVID-19)," World Health Organization, updated April 26, 2020, https://covid19.who.int/.

12 "Influenza (Seasonal)" fact sheet, World Health Organization, November 6, 2018, accessed April 23, 2020, https://www.who.int/news-room/fact-sheets/detail/influenza-(seasonal).

However, all SARS-CoV-2 death statistics prove one salient point: sick and old people die disproportionately from all kinds of serious flus. Below are statistics from China on SARS-CoV-2 for age groups and co-morbidities:[13]

AGE	DEATH RATE*
80+ years old	14.8%
70-79 years old	8.0%
60-69 years old	3.6%
50-59 years old	1.3%
40-49 years old	0.4%
30-39 years old	0.2%
20-29 years old	0.2%
10-19 years old	0.2%
0-9 years old	no fatalities

Italy's statistics show the same phenomenon:[14] The median age of the infected is 63 but most of those who die are older.

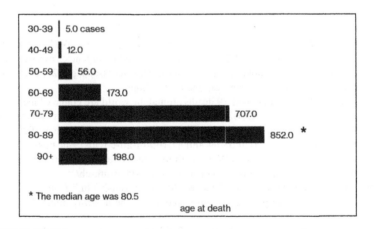

13 Brian Wang, "Coronavirus Fatality Statistics By Age, Gender and Conditions," *Next Big Future,* February 25, 2020, https://www.nextbigfuture.com/2020/02/coronavirus-fatality-statistics-by-age-gender-and-conditions.html.

14 ISS Italy National Health Institute, March 17, 2020 sample.

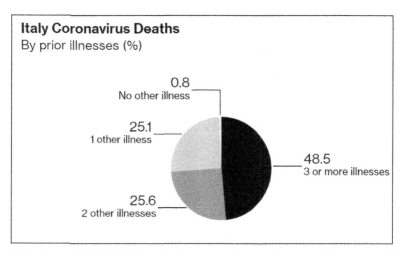

Italy Coronavirus Deaths
By prior illnesses (%)

0.8
No other illness

25.1
1 other illness

48.5
3 or more illnesses

25.6
2 other illnesses

The above SARS-CoV-2 statistics are mundane and expected for seasonal flu.

One obvious point in all this number crunching, which is often overlooked, is that if you don't test for SARS-CoV-2, then you don't have a SARS-CoV-2 problem. Your number of cases is *zero* and zero percent of the population. In a well-organized, well-governed country like China, which is treating this epidemic like an act of war,[15] millions of citizens were and are being tested. That level of confirmation may not be as high in many other countries and there are some that surely only have the money and resources to do limited tests, or none at all.

The truth of the matter is we will never know how many people have caught SARS-CoV-2. The same can be said for serious cases of seasonal flu. Patients may or may not get tested, in order to select the best treatment. With billions of people's lives being completely overturned, self-confined or mandated to do so by various levels of government, and the global economy at risk of being driven into Great Depression II, the sad and bitter irony is that compared to our annual seasonal flu cases and deaths, SARS-CoV-2 is barely registering on the epidemiological radar, especially knowing that peak flu season, December–February has already passed.

Given its infection rate, all this could change, but it also means that like HCoV-229E, -NL63, -OC43 and -HKU1, if Planet Earth keeps testing for SARS-CoV-2, there will probably always be positive results. With a mortality rate lower than serious seasonal influenza, while attacking the same old/ill groups of people, when will the hysteria and panic end? Will it ever? Is it even merited? Why not

---

15   "Is "Uriah Heep" speaking Wuhan coronavirus truth to power or just blowing Sino-sci-fi out his backside?" *China Rising Radio Sinoland,* Feb. 12, 2020, https://chinarising. puntopress.com/2020/02/12/is-uriah-heep-speaking-wuhan-coronavirus-truth-to-power-or-just-blowing-sino-sci-fi-out-his-backside-china-rising-radio-sinoland-200212/.

the same concern and response for common seasonal flu bugs, which kill many times more people?

SARS-CoV and MERS-CoV have very low infection rates and eventually ran their course. However, SARS-CoV-2 could end up as another general seasonal flu virus that infects millions, with almost all people having nothing more than the usual sinus infection, sore throat and/or bronchitis. About one-third of people who have influenza don't even know it, they are asymptomatic.[16] This may be the case for SARS-CoV-2 in the years to come.

*   *   *

BIOWEAPONS AND BIOWARFARE ARE A FACT OF 20TH–21ST CENTURY GEOPOLITICS

What is so strange about coronaviruses is that they have been around for centuries, but it has only been since 2002 that (now) three human newcomers have suddenly appeared on the world stage. This brings up research into coronaviruses and the possibility that this infamous trio was engineered in bioweapon laboratories.

Proving this conclusively is difficult to do, since there is severe censorship on this subject in established scientific research journals, which you will see below. Bioweapons are like the "pedophilia" of microbiological research. Everybody knows it is happening, but all are forbidden to talk about it. Better to just look the other way. Otherwise you may lose all that grant money.

It also goes without saying that the West's multibillion dollar/euro biowarfare industry, is being secretly developed inside Biosafety Level 3 and 4 laboratories around the world, of which there are thousands,[17] 200 in the United States alone, in all 50 states and Washington, D.C..[18] The whole point of bioweapon research by Defense Advanced Research Projects Agency (DARPA), Medical Research Institute of Infectious Diseases, U.S. Army Medical Research Institute of Infectious Diseases (USAMRIID) and the rest of this poisonous alphabet soup

---

16 "Influenza: Types of Virus," *Wikipedia,* accessed April 23, 2020, https://en.wikipedia.org/wiki/Influenza#Types_of_virus.

17 "Biosafety Level 4 Labs and BSL Information," Federation of American Scientists, https://fas.org/programs/bio/biosafetylevels.html.

18 Alison Young and Nick Penzenstadler, "Inside America's secretive biolabs," *USA Today,* updated May 28, 2016, https://www.usatoday.com/story/news/2015/05/28/biolabs-pathogens-location-incidents/26587505/.

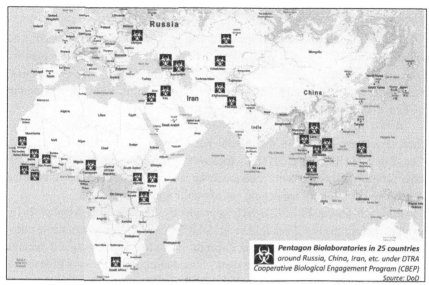

Just a few of the Pentagon's estimated 400 bioweapon laboratories around the world. Is it a coincidence that many of them are near the United States' geopolitical enemies Russia, Iran and China?

is to work in absolute secrecy, invisible on the global scene, to produce germ warfare that kills the West's perceived global enemies.[19]

Business is booming. The number of BSL-4 centers increased from five in 2001 to 15 in 2009.[20] Justifications for more bioweapon capacity will surely grow with the ongoing global SARS-CoV-2 hysteria. Given the long history of the United States, Britain, Europe and Israel in using chemical, biological and nuclear weapons since the end World War II, all public and official statements that they aren't creating biological weapons takes us back the pedophilia analogy: why, your governments would *never* do something like that!

---

19 Jeff J. Brown, "The Face of Western Imperialism Exposed by Ebola, from 'China Rising-Capitalist Roads, Socialist Destinations,'" *China Rising,* March 31, 2018, https://chinarising.puntopress.com/2018/03/31/the-face-of-western-imperialism-exposed-by-ebola-from-china-rising-capitalist-roads-socialist-destinations/

20 "Experts on Iranian TV: COVID-19 May Be an American "Ethnic Weapon" Targeting the Genome of Iranians, Chinese," MEMRI TV video, 7:13, March 10, 2020, https://www.memri.org/tv/iranian-discussion-coronavirus-ethnic-bioterrorism-weapon-america-target-iranians-chinese; and "Biosafety Level—List of BSL-4 Facilities," *Liquisearch,* accessed April 23, 2020, https://www.liquisearch.com/biosafety_level/list_of_bsl_4_facilities.

RESEARCH INTO CORONAVIRUSES

The lie about bioweapon research is that it is to "protect the citizens and soldiers," by producing vaccines. This gives bioweapon laboratories carte blanche to create Frankenbugs, so that they can supposedly then develop vaccines against them. How convenient. They create monsters that have the capacity to wipe out the human race, so that they can then try to save you.

A case in point is patents on pathogenic microbes under a careful reading. There are many patents in this global hall of horrors: coronaviruses, Ebola, Zika, Dengue, HIV, Lyme, H1N1, African swine fever, avian influenza, etc., all have various patents on them. There is even a scientific research journal called *Bioengineered.*[21] It is all happening out of public sight, out of mind.

European Patent EP3172319B1, coincidentally filed on 20 November 2019, just days before the headlines filled with SARS-CoV-2, is a patent to make coronavirus vaccines. It is owned by the Pirbright Institute,[22] which is said to receive funding from the Bill and Melinda Gates Foundation. Pirbright says it develops poultry and livestock vaccines and *Pirbright does not currently work with human coronaviruses.* Yet, on page 27 of Pirbright's patent, it states (emphasis mine):

> [0176] The disease may be any disease caused by a coronavirus, such as *a respiratory disease and and/or gastro-enteritis in humans* and hepatitis, gastroenteritis, encephalitis, or a respiratory disease in other animals.
>
> [0177] The disease may be infectious bronchitis (IB); Porcine epidemic diarrhoea; Transmissible gastroenteritis; Mouse hepatitis virus; Porcine haemagglutinating encephalomyelitis; *Severe acute respiratory syndrome (SARS)*; or Bluecomb disease.
>
> [0186] The vaccine or vaccine composition of the invention may be used *to treat a human,* animal or avian subject. For example, the subject may be a chick, chicken or mouse (such as a laboratory mouse, e.g. transgenic mouse).
>
> [0187] Typically, *a physician* or veterinarian will determine the actual dosage which will be most suitable for an individual subject or group of subjects and it will vary with the age, weight and response of the particular subject(s).

---

21   "Bioengineered," *Taylor & Francis Online,* accessed April 23, 2020, https://www.tandfonline.com/toc/kbie20/current.

22   Home page, The Pirbright Institute, accessed April 23, 2020, www.pirbright.ac.uk/.

Thus, this coronavirus patent said to be for chickens against avian infectious bronchitis (IBV) can also be used on you for SARS, which target only humans and bats. You just need to ask your physician what proper bird vaccine dosage is needed to protect us against SARS, any human respiratory disease and/or gastro-enteritis. All the other diseases listed for this same vaccine are for pigs, poultry and mice. Egad!

On page 6 is the list of how coronaviruses are divided, based on their genetic similarity and differences (emphasis mine):

[0044] Coronaviruses are divided into four groups, as shown below:

Alpha
- Canine coronavirus (CCoV)
- Feline coronavirus (FeCoV)
- Human coronavirus 229E (HCoV-229E)
- Porcine epidemic diarrhoea virus (PEDV)
- *Transmissible gastroenteritis virus* (TGEV) [pigs]
- Human Coronavirus NL63 (NL or New Haven)

Beta
- Bovine coronavirus (BCoV)
- Canine respiratory coronavirus (CRCoV)—Common in SE Asia and Micronesia
- Human coronavirus OC43 (HCoV-OC43)
- *Mouse hepatitis virus* (MHV)
- Porcine haemagglutinating encephalomyelitis virus (HEV)
- Rat coronavirus (RCV). Rat Coronavirus is quite prevalent in Eastern Australia where, as of March/April 2008, it has been found among native and feral rodent colonies.
- (No common name as of yet) (HCoV-HKU1)
- *Severe acute respiratory syndrome coronavirus* (SARS-CoV)
- *Middle East respiratory syndrome coronavirus* (MERS-CoV)
- *Severe respiratory syndrome coronavirus-2* (SARS-CoV-2) [added here, as it was classified as a Beta coronavirus right after this patent was filed]

Gamma
- *Infectious bronchitis virus (IBV)* [this patent is to create a vaccine for this disease]
- Turkey coronavirus (Bluecomb disease virus)
- Pheasant coronavirus
- Guinea fowl coronavirus

Delta
- Bulbul coronavirus (BuCoV)
- Thrush coronavirus (ThCoV)
- Munia coronavirus (MuCoV)
- Porcine coronavirus (PorCov) HKU15

On the next page, it says that this vaccine's viral *variant* (mutant) *replicase gene* (the gene that produces the replicase enzyme, which catalyzes the virus' RNA for reproduction) (emphasis mine):

> [0045] The variant replicase gene of the coronavirus of the present invention may be derived from an alphacoronavirus such as *TGEV*; a betacoronavirus such as *MHV*; or a gammacoronavirus such as IBV.

Thus, the replicating gene of this patent's Gamma avian (respiratory) coronavirus can be replaced by an Alpha porcine gastroenteritic version (TGEV) or a Beta mouse hepatitis one. Notice it uses the conjunction *such as*, which means *not limited to*. Thus, this patent's virus could use any of the Alpha, Beta or Gamma replicase genes, and it is a list to give anyone serious pause. Alpha coronaviruses include ones that infect dogs, cats, pigs and humans. Beta coronaviruses include cows, cats, mice, rats, humans and the three infamous late generation coronaviruses, the two SARS and MERS. Gamma coronaviruses include other avian species, besides chickens, turkeys, pheasants and Guinea fowl.

In sum, this means that this "avian" patent is approved to "jump" to completely different species, from completely different coronavirus groups, non-respiratory viruses, as well as human viruses, including three that are considered highly pathogenic and lethal to humans!

Other interesting observations about this patent are the references cited (emphasis mine):

- V. D. MENACHERY ET AL: "Attenuation and *Restoration of Severe Acute Respiratory Syndrome Coronavirus Mutant* Lacking 2'-O-Methyltransferase Activity," JOURNAL OF VIROLOGY, vol. 88, no. 8, 29 January 2014 (2014-01-29), pages 4251-4264, XP055215583, ISSN: 0022-538X, DOI: 0.1128/JVI.03571-13

- *Anonymous:* "EM_STD:KF377577," 30 October 2013 (2013-10-30), *XP55216202,* Retrieved from

- the Internet: URL:http://ibis/exam/dbfetch.jsp?id=EM_STD :KF377577 [retrieved on 2015-09-25]

- WANG ET AL: "Attenuation of porcine reproductive and respiratory syndrome virus strain MN184 *using chimeric construction* with vaccine sequence," VIROLOGY, ELSEVIER, AMSTERDAM, NL, vol. 371, no. 2, 31 October 2007 (2007-10-31), pages 418-429, XP022439793, ISSN: 0042-6822, DOI: 10.1016/J.VIROL.2007.09.032

Observations:

Restoration of Severe Acute Respiratory Syndrome Coronavirus Mutant: it is interesting that a purported bird vaccine patent uses research on the infamous, 2002-2003 human SARS-CoV, this one a mutant.

Anonymous: just as curious is an Anonymous' research, which cannot be found on the internet. Who might they be? Good question. Why the mystery? Is it DARPA or Fort Detrick? They clearly do not want anybody to know. Web searching *XP55216202* takes you to another Pirbright Institute coronavirus patent, WO2016/012793Al, from 2013.

...using chimeric construction: In Greek mythology, a chimera is a female monster that breathes fire. She is put together with a goat's body, lion's head and serpent's tail. Thus, in bioweapon research, chimeric construction is another way of saying that a microbe was created that never existed in nature before. In other words, a Frankenbug.

This coronavirus patent created one four-nucleotide substitution, as shown here:

[0016] The replicase gene may comprise one or more nucleotide substitutions selected from the list of:
C to T at nucleotide position 12137;
G to C at nucleotide position 18114;
T to A at nucleotide position 19047; and
G to A at nucleotide position 20139;
compared to the sequence shown as SEQ ID NO: 1.

[0017] The coronavirus may be an infectious bronchitis virus (IBV).

[0018] The coronavirus may be IBV M41.

[0019] The coronavirus may comprise an S protein at least part of which is from an IBV serotype other than M41.

[0020] For example, the S1 subunit or the entire S protein may be from an IBV serotype other than M41.

Notice that it only takes changing four nucleotides [0016] to make this mutated virus attenuated, or weakened for vaccine use. Please hang on to that number "four" for later.

They also changed four amino acids in the replicase gene:

> [0100] The variant replicase gene of the coronavirus of the present invention may encode a protein which comprises the amino acid mutations:
> Pro to Leu at position 85 of SEQ ID NO: 6,
> Val to Leu at position 393 of SEQ ID NO: 7;
> Leu to Ile at position 183 of SEQ ID NO: 8; and
> Val to Ile at position 209 of SEQ ID NO: 9.

In another section, they state that their mutations may be:

> [0141] The nucleotide sequence may be natural, synthetic or recombinant.

> [0142] The nucleotide sequence may be codon optimised for production in the host/host cell of choice.

A synthetic nucleotide sequence is one that is completely fabricated in the laboratory and does not exist in nature, in other words, completely bioengineered in the test tube, in other words, a chimera. A recombinant one can be a mixture of natural and synthetic genetic codes. A reversed engineered virus is one that they make an exact copy of one, like when they dug up Inuit cadavers, extracted dead extinct viruses to recreate the "Spanish" flu of 1918.[23] Life imitating *Jurassic Park*.

Codon-optimized viruses have mutated genes to increase protein production. For vaccines, that means more attenuated viruses produced, to make more doses.

Further on, they report:

> [0166] Thus the present invention also provides a method for producing a coronavirus as defined in the claims which comprises the following steps:
> (i) infection of a cell with a coronavirus according to the invention;
> (ii) allowing the virus to replicate in the cell; and
> (iii) harvesting the progeny virus.

In other words, they have created a system to produce large quantities of hopefully *nice* Frankenbugs, to sell lots of vaccines.

---

23   J. van Aken, "Is it wise to resurrect a deadly virus?" *Heredity* (2007) 98, 1–2, published online October 11, 2006, https://www.nature.com/articles/6800911.pdf.

Throughout this patent, the word *mutation* is used 89 times, *variant* (meaning mutant) 69 times *recombinant,* 53 times, *substitution* (= mutation) 27 times, (nucleotide) *insertion* eight times, *synthetic* six times and *deletion* (= mutation) four times.

What does all this tells us? First, I'll never get another vaccine for the rest of my life, except if I get bitten by a stray dog and do not want to risk lethal rabies. Otherwise, this patent study should scare the bejeezus out of everyone, since these microbiologists can mutate dangerous animal viruses, mix human and non-human mutated genetic material together, and then have the right to give them to both farm animals and people. They always talk about microbes jumping from animals to humans. Earth's micro-critters don't need to wait centuries for natural evolution to make it happen. It is clearly being done on a massive scale in laboratories to make vaccines, with open-ended uses. I don't know about you, but I find this more than just creepy. I think it is shocking, disgusting and unethical. But, it is apparently legal.

Is SARS-Cov-2 a Bioengineered Germ Weapon?

The aforementioned study of a coronavirus patent doesn't even take into consideration bioweapon labs doing the same thing, to engineer microbes to kill millions of people who are considered the Western empire's economic and/or geopolitical enemies.

Vaccine makers want to attenuate microbes, lessening their pathogenicity. This, so that they can be injected live into you, to elicit an immune response to create an immunity against the same wild-type bug found in nature that is considered dangerous. If vaccine makers can play around with only four nucleotide mutations insertions and four replicase gene amino acids to weaken a microbe, is it logical that biowarfare labs can use the exact same methods, mixing and matching human and animal genetics, to make killer Frankenbugs? Can bioweapon scientists use mutations, variants, recombinants, chimeras, substitutions, insertions, synthetics and deletions to produce highly pathogenic, lethal microbes?

I'll give you three guesses and the first two don't count.

Two scientific research papers on SARS-CoV-2 caused a bit of a stir in these circles, as well as briefly in the alternative media.

The spike glycoprotein of the new coronavirus 2019-nCoV contains a furin-like cleavage site absent in CoV of the same clade was published in February 2020 in the journal *Antiviral Research*. The reason that *furin* is so meaningful is because this enzyme protein is only found naturally in humans, not microbes. Furin, like all enzymes, acts like a catalyst to break down or connect two or more biological molecules to be useful in the body. When you see a word ending in -*ase*, in the context of living things, it is likely an enzyme. When I was in graduate school taking biochemistry classes, studying all of life's many pathways (vitamins, minerals, oxygen, carbon, sugars, fats, proteins, amino acids, etc.), hundreds of "-ases" danced in my head, as I memorized each step. A good example is alcohol dehydrogenase, the enzyme that removes hydrogen from the ethanol in your wine or beer, so that it can be oxygenated and metabolized into a sugar for energy.

In humans, furin activates proteins that would otherwise remain dormant or unused, by cleaving them into smaller chunks. This paper says,

> For instance, the pathogenesis of some CoV has been previously related to the presence of a furin-like cleavage site in the S-protein sequence. For example, the insertion of a similar cleavage site in the infectious bronchitis virus (IBV) S-protein results in higher pathogenicity, pronounced neural symptoms and neurotropism in infected chickens (Cheng et al., 2019).

> … highly pathogenic forms of influenza have a furin-like cleavage site cleaved by different cellular proteases, including furin, which are expressed in a wide variety of cell types allowing a widening of the cell tropism of thevirus (Kido et al., 2012).

In plain language, when a coronavirologist mutates the binding point spike protein to add a furin-like cleavage, this makes the virus more infectious and potentially more deadly, since it can enter host cells more easily. In bioengineering, the opposite of attenuation is called *gain of function*, meaning increasing the pathogenicity of microbes. Adding a furin-like cleavage to a coronavirus is gain of function.

SARS Senior from 2002-2003 was already mutated to jump species. The paper says,

> The SARS-CoV binds to both bat and human cells, and the virus can infect both organisms (Ge et al., 2013; Kuhn et al., 2004).

These researchers also mention the similarities between SARS-CoV-2 with SARS Senior:

> Notably, the IFPs [internal fusion peptides] of the 2019-nCoV and SARS-CoV are identical, displaying characteristics of viral fusion peptides (Fig. 2).

Since SARS Senior and Junior are not in the same coronavirus clade, this suggests that genetic sequences were taken from Senior to make a mutation in Junior.

They go onto say that (emphasis mine),

Since *furin is highly expressed in lungs,* an enveloped virus that infects the respiratory tract may successfully exploit this convertase to activate its surface glycoprotein (Bassi et al., 2017; Mbikay et al., 1997). *Before the emergence of the 2019-nCoV, this important feature was not observed in the lineage b of betacoronaviruses.* However, it is shared by other CoV (HCoV-OC43, MERS-CoV, MHV-A59) harbouring furin-like cleavage sites in their S-protein (Fig. 2; Table 1), which were shown to be processed by furin experimentally (Le Coupanec et al., 2015; Mille and Whittaker, 2014). *Strikingly, the 2019-nCoV S-protein sequence contains 12 additional nucleotides upstream of the single*

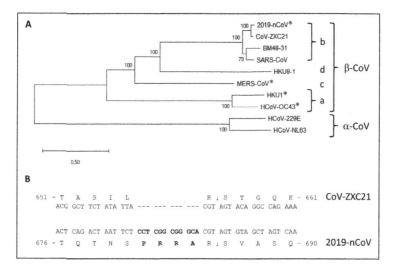

Fig. 1. Characterization of an nCoV-peculiar sequence at the S1/S2 cleavage site in the S-protein sequence, compared SARS-like CoV. (A) Phylogenetic tree of selected coronaviruses from genera alphacoronavirus (α-Cov) and betacoronavirus (β-CoV), lineages a, b, c and d: 2019-nCoV (NC_045512.2), CoV-ZXC21 (MG772934), SARS-CoV (NC_004718.3), SARS-like BM4821 (MG772934), HCoV-OC43 (AY391777), HKU9-1 (EF065513), HCoV-NL63 (KF530114.1), HCoV229E (KF514433.1), MERS-CoV (NC019843.3), HKU1 (NC_006577.2). The phylogenetic tree was obtained on the Orf1ab amino acid sequence using the Maximum Likelihood method by Mega X software. **Asterisks indicate the presence of a canonical furin-like cleavage motif at site 1;** *(B) Alignment of the coding and amino acid sequences of the S-protein from CoV-ZXC21 and 2019-nCoV at the S1/S2 site. The 2019-nCoV-specific sequence is in bold. The sequence of CoV-ZXC21 S-protein at this position is representative of the sequence of the other betacoronaviruses belonging to lineage b, except the one of 2019-nCoV.*

Arg↓cleavage site 1 (Figs. 1B and 2) leading to a predictively solvent-exposed PRRAR↓SV sequence, which corresponds to a canonical furin-like cleavage site (Braun and Sauter, 2019; Izaguirre, 2019; Seidah and Prat, 2012). This furin-like cleavage site, is supposed to be cleaved during virus egress (Mille and Whittaker, 2014) for S-protein "priming" and may provide a gain-of-function to the 2019-nCoV for efficient spreading in the human population compared to other lineage b beta-coronaviruses.

Having a strikingly extra 12 nucleotides (clearly seen in Part B) in the S-protein (binding point) is significant. We saw in the study of the aforementioned coronavirus patent, that it only takes four of these to be changed to completely alter its pathogenicity. How did they get there? Writing that (surprisingly) *a gain-of-function to the 2019-nCoV for efficient spreading in the human population* is tacitly suggesting that SARS-CoV-2 is a bioengineered bug.

Below is an extract from the same paper, showing key envelope protein cleavage sequences for SARS Senior and Junior, plus a sister bat coronavirus.

Comparative sequences of envelope protein cleavage site(s) in coronaviruses (above) and in other RNA viruses			
Coronavirus	S1/S2, site 1	S1/S2, site 2	S2'
SARS-CoV-2	SPRRAR↓SVAS	IAY↓TMS	SKPSKR↓SF
Bat-AC45	TASILR↓STGQ	IAY↓TMS	SKPSKR↓SF
SARS-CoV	TVSLLR↓STGQ	IAY↓TMS	LKPTKR↓SF

This S1/S2 locus is the attachment point that coronaviruses use to cleave open their host cells, to inject themselves and/or their genetic material to replicate. The similarities, with only miniscule differences in the nucleotides is *uncanny*, a word will see more of below.

The above paper has not been censored, as well as hundreds of others that have not yet been peer-reviewed, due the huge influx of SARS-CoV-2 papers flooding scientific journals. Its wording was more oblique about the *gain-of-function* findings, so it seems to have made it through the establishment censorship gauntlet.

These kinds of research papers are called *preprints*. As I write this chapter, there are already 868 papers studying SARS-CoV-2.[24]

---

24 "COVID-19 SARS-CoV-2 preprints from medRxiv and bioRxiv," bioRxiv, Cold Spring Harbor Laboratory, [2114 articles as of April 23, 2020], https://connect.biorxiv.org/relate/content/181.

While the above *furin-cleavage* paper was more diplomatic, a recent Indian research entitled, *Uncanny similarity of unique inserts in the 2019-nCoV spike protein to HIV-1 gp120 and Gag* hit the bioweapon bullseye, so much so that it was withdrawn from *bioRxiv* in a matter of days. Using the adjective *uncanny* in the title, which means *unnatural* or *abnormal*, was provocative language. It takes us back to my earlier analogy about avoiding talking about pedophilia. This title dares to suggest to other microbiology researchers that 2019-nCoV (SARS-CoV-2) is abnormal or unnatural.

In their study, they analyzed 55 SARS-CoV-2 samples, narrowing them down to 28, which is highly statistically significant. Analyzing them and lining them up against SARS Senior, it shows that the latter is the closest relative, which has also been reported by other researchers. They then cut to the chase:

> On careful examination of the sequence alignment we found that the 2019-nCoV spike glycoprotein contains 4 insertions [Fig.2].

> We found that these 4 insertions [inserts 1, 2, 3 and 4] are unique to 2019-nCoV and are not present in other coronaviruses analyzed. Another group from China had documented three insertions comparing fewer spike glycoprotein sequences of coronaviruses. Another group from China had documented three insertions comparing fewer spike glycoprotein sequences of coronaviruses (Zhou et al., 2020).

In plain language, these insertions are *uncanny*, indeed. Two other research teams in China found the same thing, but with only three insertions. However, they did not test as many spike glycoprotein sequences of coronaviruses as this Indian team did.

Like the coronavirus patent and the furin-like cleavage study, the number of nucleotides in the four unexpected insertions is not big. While explaining this, these scientists deliver the knockout punch (emphasis mine),

> *Surprisingly, each of the four inserts aligned with short segments of the Human immunodeficiency Virus-1 (HIV-1) proteins. The amino acid positions of the inserts in 2019-nCoV and the corresponding residues in HIV-1 gp120 and HIV-1 Gag are shown in Table 1. The first 3 inserts (insert 1, 2 and 3) aligned to short segments of amino acid residues in HIV-1 gp120. The insert 4 aligned to HIV-1 Gag. The insert 1 (6 amino acid residues) and insert 2 (6 amino acid residues) in the spike glycoprotein of 2019-nCoV are 100% identical to the residues mapped to HIV-1 gp120. The insert 3 (12 amino acid residues) in 2019-nCoV maps to HIV-1 gp120 with gaps [see Table 1]. The insert 4 (8 amino acid residues) maps to HIV-1 Gag with gaps.*

Although, the 4 inserts represent discontiguous short stretches of amino acids in spike glycoprotein of 2019-nCoV, *the fact that all three of them share amino acid identity or similarity with HIV-1 gp120 and HIV-1 Gag (among all annotated virus proteins) suggests that this is not a random fortuitous finding. In other words, one may sporadically expect a fortuitous match for a stretch of 6-12 contiguous amino acid residues in an unrelated protein. However, it is unlikely that all 4 inserts in the 2019-nCoV spike glycoprotein fortuitously match with 2 key structural proteins of an unrelated virus (HIV-1).*

This uncanny similarity of novel inserts in the 2019- nCoV spike protein to HIV-1 gp120 and Gag is unlikely to be fortuitous.

Of course, *fortuitous* means *darned lucky.*

Under the discussion section at the end, they lay it all out (emphasis mine):

We found four new insertions in the S protein of 2019-nCoV when compared to its nearest relative, SARS CoV. The genome sequence from the recent 28 clinical isolates showed that the sequence coding for these insertions are conserved amongst all these isolates. This indicates that *these insertions have been preferably acquired by the 2019-nCoV, providing it with additional survival and infectivity advantage. Delving deeper we found that these insertions were similar to HIV-1. Our results highlight an astonishing relation between the gp120 and Gag protein of HIV, with 2019-nCoV spike glycoprotein.* These proteins are critical for the viruses to identify and latch on to their host cells and for viral assembly (Beniac et al., 2006). Since surface proteins are responsible for host tropism, changes in these proteins imply a change in host specificity of the virus. According to reports from China, there has been *a gain of host specificity in case 2019-nCoV as the virus was originally known to infect animals and not humans but after the mutations, it has gained tropism to humans as well.*

Phrases like *preferably acquired* and *gain of host specificity* tacitly suggest a bioengineered microbe.

All of this very concrete, detailed information was not necessary to get this paper withdrawn. In microbiology research circles, alarm bells were already going off in the first paragraph. In this paper's abstract at the very beginning, the bioweapon cannon was clearly shot across the industry's bow (emphasis mine),

The finding of 4 unique inserts in the 2019-nCoV, all of which have identity /similarity to amino acid residues in key structural proteins of HIV-1 is unlikely to be fortuitous in nature.

The justification for pulling their paper was that the HIV lengths of the genetic code they found in SARS-CoV-2 were not long enough to be significant. They found sequence matches of 6, 6, 8 and 12. Nevertheless, we saw very clearly in the study of the aforementioned coronavirus patent, it mutated only 4 nucleotides or 4 amino acids in the lab, which reduced its pathogenicity enough to inject it live into animals or humans, plus they can effortlessly mix, match and synthesize viral animal and human genetics.

This strongly suggests that the reason given for withdrawing this paper is not about the number of nucleotide/amino acid SARS-CoV-2 matches with HIV. It was more likely removed because it got too close to the bioweapon fire. Only censoring editors who want to avoid the pedophilia paradigm can have it both ways. I tip my hat to the courageous members of this Indian research team. Scientists thrive, struggle or starve, depending on how much grant money they get from NGOs, institutes, schools, governments, etc. Telling the truth could cost them fundraising in the future.

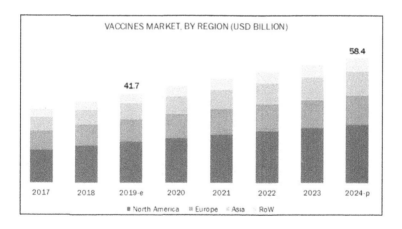

CONCLUSION

The final salient point of everything presented in this chapter is the incestuous, closed loop relationship between "good" vaccine research and the development of biowarfare. They are two sides of a very disturbing, dare I say *uncanny* industry. Bioengineers who make weapons to kill millions of perceived global enemies need the fig leaf of, "we are developing dangerous, lethal microbes, in order to make vaccines to protect you." Vaccine makers in turn make tens of billions of dollars/euros injecting people and animals to hopefully immunize them from same-said dangerous, lethal Frankenbugs. Before SARS-CoV-2 exploded on the world scene in the final weeks of 2019, the global vaccine market was already projected to hit $41.7 billion, with continuous growth to $58.4 billion by 2024.[25]

Business is booming. You are given Frankenbugs on the one hand. On the other, you are expected to take vaccines against them that are supposed to keep you "safe."

---

25   "Vaccines Market," *Markets and Markets,* accessed April 23, 2020, https://www. marketsandmarkets.com/Market-Reports/vaccine-technologies-market-1155.html.

PART II
The Lockdown

CHAPTER TWO

DEALING WITH DEMONS

Larry Romanoff

THE LOCKDOWN

At the outbreak of the COVID-19 epidemic, China implemented the most comprehensive and rigorous measures ever taken. Wuhan was locked down on January 23, 2020 as were several other cities in Hubei Province quickly thereafter, then the entire province.[1] All public transportation was suspended. Airports, train stations, bus depots, subways, boat and ferry docks were closed, all toll highways shut down and most roads blocked. All the subways and buses stopped running, and all people were instructed to remain in their homes. The initial lockdown involved about 20 million people, extending to about 60 million within a month, this at a time when China had only about 500 infections. The move, unprecedented in modern times and undoubtedly a difficult decision, spoke volumes about the gravity of the situation and the seriousness with which the government viewed the public health threat. China's President Xi issued a rather stern warning at the time, that "Governments of all levels are obliged to resolutely take all preemptive measures to rein in the fast spread of the virus and be completely transparent about their local situation so that the country can unite to fight the pandemic together, and ensure that the world has a true picture of the situation. As Xi made clear, the mistakes of the past must not be repeated." All the evidence suggests the Chinese authorities acted effectively as soon as they realized the danger they might be facing.

Remembering the SARS troubles, the Chinese did much more. In most large centers in the country, all sports venues, theaters, museums, tourist attractions, all locations that attract crowds, were closed, as were all schools. All group tours were cancelled. Not only the city of Wuhan but virtually the entire province of Hubei was locked down, with thousands of flights and train trips cancelled until further notice. Some cities like Shanghai and Beijing were conducting

---

1 Wang Xiaodong, Xin Wen and Zhou Lihua, "Wuhan sealed to contain virus; isolated cases seen elsewhere," *China Daily,* January 24, 2020, https://www.chinadaily.com.cn/a/202001/24/WS5e2a0374a310128217273141.html.

temperature tests on all roadways leading into the cities. In addition, Wuhan was building two portable hospitals of 25,000 square meters each to handle infected patients. As well, Wuhan asked citizens to neither leave nor enter the city without a compelling reason. All were wearing face masks.

The scale of the challenge was immense, comparable to closing down all transport links for a city five times the size of Toronto or Chicago, two days before Christmas. These decisions were unprecedented, but testified to the determination of the authorities to limit the spread and damage of this new pathogen. They took into account not only the gravity of the situation but also with serious consideration for public health, facing up to unfortunate and difficult decisions since the Chinese New Year's holiday was destroyed for hundreds of millions of people. Most public entertainment was cancelled, as were tours, and many weddings as well. The damage to the economy during this most festive of all periods was enormous. Hong Kong would suffer severely in addition to all its other troubles, since visits from Mainland Chinese typically support much of its retail economy during this period.

Yet already the Western media was in full China-bashing mode,[2] some claiming that lockdowns and quarantines were "a violation of human rights" and were in any case ineffective, with Mr. Pompeo of the U.S. State Department already lamenting the "lack of transparency" in the Chinese government, and London's Imperial College claiming infections in China were understated by a factor of ten.[3] And of course China's friends in Langley, Virginia, were busy making posts on Weibo claiming this was "the end of the world" with everyone "on the verge of tears," while the UK *Guardian* claimed "panic was spreading" in China.[4]

Within a week of Wuhan being locked down, virtually all rail and air traffic in all of China had been suspended to deny the virus a means of travel. This was the most awkward time imaginable to have to do so, with much of the population on the verge of traveling home for the Chinese New Year holiday. All mass-gathering areas were closed. Restaurants, shopping malls, cinemas, museums, markets, tourist resorts and many similar places were shut down to prevent gatherings, and many factories were seriously challenged by unexpected difficulties in

---

2 AFP, "China locks down two cities to curb virus outbreak," *The Guardian,* January 23, 2020, https://guardian.ng/news/china-locks-down-two-cities-to-curb-virus-outbreak/.

3 AFP, "China warns virus could mutate, spread as death toll rises," *Yahoo! News,* January 21, 2020, https://news.yahoo.com/china-warns-virus-could-mutate-spread-death-toll-061915563.html.

4 Lily Kuo, "China virus: ten cities locked down and Beijing festivities scrapped," *The Guardian,* January 23, 2020, https://www.theguardian.com/world/2020/jan/23/coronavirus-panic-spreads-in-china-with-three-cities-in-lockdown.

operation due to the quarantines. The strong measures, effective though they were, inevitably inflicted pain on some parts of the Chinese economy as well as causing inconvenience and some hardship in people's daily lives. But the unprecedented moves yielded positive results, with new infections quickly dropping.

Using Shanghai as an example, by the end of February the city was subjecting all travelers from severely-affected countries to medical examination at the city's airports to prevent imported infections. All incoming passengers who had lived or traveled in the hardest-hit countries were automatically subjected to a 14-day quarantine at home or at designated hotels.[5,6] These passengers were not permitted to take taxis or public transport but instead were driven to designated quarantine locations by customs authorities, where community workers would be waiting for them with a team of neighborhood officials, and a doctor and a police officer would guide them to home quarantine. This large group consisted of volunteers who lived temporarily in nearby hotels, avoiding their own homes due to the risk of spreading the virus.[7]

Foreign nationals were considered in advance, and offered necessary assistance from the communities where they lived to solve their difficulties after entering the city.[8] By early March China put major restrictions on inbound air travel and effectively closed off the borders. Those without a place of residence and a permanent job in Shanghai were not permitted to enter the city by road, except for medical reasons.[9] The Central Government temporarily suspended entry into the country of foreign passport holders even those with valid visas or residence permits, which was an unprecedented but necessary step to prevent imported infections.[10,11]

---

5 Zhou Wenting, "Shanghai airports strengthen measures," *China Daily,* March 10, 2020, https://www.chinadaily.com.cn/a/202003/10/WS5e66fd23a31012821727dcaf.html.

6 "Quarantine for all arrivals from badly hit nations," *Shine,* March 4, 2020, https://www.shine.cn/news/nation/2003043372/.

7 Cai Wenjun, "All people from key areas to be quarantined," *Shine,* January 26, 2020, https://www.shine.cn/news/metro/2001260649/.

8 Xu Qing Zhong Youyang Zhou Shengjie, "How Shanghai controls the influx of coronavirus cases from overseas," *Shine,* March 12, 2020, https://www.shine.cn/news/metro/2003124131/.

9 Chen Huizhi, "Police detail who can enter city by road," *Shine,* February 19, 2020, https://www.shine.cn/news/metro/2002192363.

10 Mo Jingxi and Wang Keju, "China puts major restrictions on inbound air travel," *China Daily,* March 28, 2020, http://www.chinadaily.com.cn/a/202003/28/WS5e7e9310a310128217282a28.html.

11 Zhao Yusha and Chen Qingqing, "China temporarily bans entry of foreigners in response to surging imported infections," *Global Times,* March 27, 2020, https://www.globaltimes.cn/content/1183923.shtml.

Residential areas in most Chinese cities are comprised of communities that are largely self-contained, similar in some ways to gated communities in the West, making isolation and quarantine easier and more effective than in the sprawling suburbs of North America. In my community in Shanghai, as an example, the road leading to the community was blocked, meaning no one left and no one entered. Special permits were available for some kinds of official travel or medical needs, but in practice these were few. All businesses in the community were temporarily shuttered as were schools and gathering places. Everyone mostly remained in their homes and, when brief excursions were necessary, masks were always worn and proximity to other persons avoided.

But there was much more leadership and planning that were not visible. Immediately upon executing the community quarantine, local officials contracted with a major food supplier to continue provisions. An online mobile phone APP was designed overnight, which was used to place orders for all foods, fresh vegetables and meat. Every two or three days a delivery truck would clear the barriers and enter the community, with the drivers prohibited from human contact. Each order was bagged and sealed separately and set out at the community center office where residents could collect them and pay online after delivery. A similar system was arranged for the regular supply of medications. Courier deliveries were deposited at the road barrier where residents could come one by one to collect their packages. Nothing was overlooked, and dutiful participation was more or less total. It was seen as a civic duty for community residents to remain at home, protect each other, and prevent any spreading of the virus. The local security guards proved extremely helpful. They were well-informed on all procedures, competent to take temperatures and able to make decisions. We had not a single infection.

With most residents remaining secluded in their homes, online ordering and delivery demands surged by a factor of perhaps ten, Shanghai's supermarkets and e-commerce platforms working intensely to ensure adequate food supplies during the lockdown.[12] The surge in demand posed challenges because many food suppliers and logistics firms had already halted work during the Spring Festival, but China's domestic supply chains are exceptional, far beyond those existing in any other nation. Each of the large suppliers quickly arranged distribution of between five and ten times their normal daily amounts, each bringing in hundreds of tons of food and organising community distributions. At the same time, many e-commerce platforms quickly arranged programs with manufacturers to source urgent medical supplies including masks, disinfectant and protective clothing.

---

12 Huang Yixuan, "Suppliers work hard to satisfy surging demand," *Shine,* January 30, 2020, https://www.shine.cn/biz/economy/2001300922/.

Most created special areas on their mobile phone APPs to enable residents to easily purchase all necessary items.

LEADERSHIP

One reason the Chinese were able to deal with the epidemic while the UK and USA floundered in the dark is that the Chinese think, with considerable justification, that they have been under biological attack, on and off since c.1950, and were therefore prepared with well-laid plans and competent organisers to respond to such an event. As soon as the central government learned the specific nature of the outbreak, it responded massively and to a very large extent the population understood the necessity of what was asked of them and cooperated.

Chinese President Xi Jinping said "The Coronavirus is a Demon, and we cannot let this demon hide."[13] He said China was "faced with the grave situation of an accelerating spread" of the virus, that "The Chinese people are engaging in a serious battle against the outbreak of the new coronavirus pneumonia. People's lives and health are always the first priority for the Chinese government, and the prevention and control of the epidemic is the most important task at present, so I have been directing and deploying the works myself."

Mr. Xi gave this battle the highest priority, personally chairing a meeting of the Standing Committee where he listened to all the reports and decided immediately to set up a CPC Central Committee group to oversee the national effort, and also to send a high-level planning group to Hubei to direct the work on the ground.[14] Soon after the outbreak occurred and the pathogen identified, a Central Guiding Group appeared in Wuhan to oversee all COVID-19 efforts, to free the medical staff from administration and planning responsibilities and to ensure they were provided with all necessities.[15]

It was due to this leadership that Wuhan's available hospital beds increased from 5,000 to about 25,000 within ten days, that hundreds of medical teams and about 50,000 physicians were dispatched from all across China to Hubei Province, and that the lockdowns and quarantines were put in place. And due to this leadership China's fatalities were limited to little more than 4,000, most of those in Wuhan with the entire rest of the nation of 1.4 billion people being spared.

---

13 "Coronavirus is a DEMON, and we cannot let this demon hide – Chinese president to World Health Organization chief," *RT,* January 28, 2020, updated May 6, 2020, https://www.rt.com/news/479403-china-xi-coronavirus-demon/.

14 *QS Theory,* April 28, 2020, http://www.qstheory.cn/zhuanqu/bkjx/2020-04/28/c_1125917119.htm.

15 Xinhua, "Xi chairs leadership meeting on regular epidemic control, supporting Hubei development," *Shine,* April 29, 2020, https://www.shine.cn/news/nation/2004297248/.

How did China do it? It wasn't "China." It was the Chinese people, their civilization and culture. All of Chinese society was mobilised, not only the Central Government and the medical officials in Hubei, but all citizens, corporations, SOEs, foundations, instantly assessed their abilities to assist, and then acted.[16] The city of Wuhan received timely full-scale support from the entire nation, not only to fight the battle but to recover from the effects of the war. It wasn't only that lockdowns and quarantines cut off channels of escape for the virus. Hundreds of millions of Chinese sacrificed something of their normal lives to contain the spread of the virus, acting in unison and working together in a collective response. Westerners will never understand this.

The U.S. media were busily trashing China for a "sluggish response" to the virus (while conveniently ignoring the first three wasted months in their own country). Americans understand only dimly (if at all) the Chinese ability for rapid execution which, to the chagrin of all Americans everywhere, is due primarily to two things—China's political system and the socialism embedded in Chinese cultural DNA. While the English-speaking West is very much an "every man for himself" culture, the Chinese are a civilization, and despite the vast scope that the term implies, act in unison as such, with the result that virtually everyone is onside in things of importance to the nation. Thus, despite the fact that there can be competing private and selfish interests, a nationwide plan can be conceived, examined, discussed, approved, and executed in a much shorter time than in a country like the U.S.—and with full public cooperation and approval. Such interests still accept the overall plan and authority and are onside. For example, when the new Beijing-Shanghai high-speed rail was built, the airlines had to severely curtail their flights because the train was faster and cheaper. They may not have liked it, but it was in the best interests of the nation and all went along without objection.

China's political system is much more unified than in the West, making local governments accountable to the central government whereas in Western nations the local authorities are largely autonomous, making unanimity and even cooperation almost impossible. Thus, in times of emergency in China, bureaucratic blockage simply evaporates, and the country's massive labor force makes speed of execution possible with no sacrifice in quality. And, with the general population widely sharing the nation's objectives, courses of action which might be resisted in the West are widely approved in China. Due to China's systemic organization, the central government has the ability to rapidly mobilise any resources the country needs. Building a new hospital in ten days or a new high-speed railway in one or two years is possible due to a government-led mobilization of Chinese

---

16 "COVID-19: How China fought the war," People's Daily Online, April 20, 2020, http://en.people.cn/n3/2020/0420/c90000-9681452.html.

society. Because China has only one political party there is a complete absence of partisan infighting, enabling the government to act as a unit with the population and, once a clear and resolute course of action is determined, virtually the entire Chinese civilization is not only eager to participate but willing to sacrifice in order to do so, something very difficult for Western populations as a whole to replicate. Many workers interviewed on CGTN were proud to say they slept only two hours in three days on construction of the new hospitals.[17]

As Martin Jacques, a senior fellow at the Department of Politics and International Studies at Cambridge University, noted, "The capacity of China to deal with emergencies of this kind is far more developed and far more capable than could be achieved by any Western government. The Chinese system, the Chinese government, is superior to other governments in handling big challenges like this. And there are two reasons: First of all, the Chinese state is a very effective institution, able to think strategically and mobilise society. And the other reason is that the Chinese expect the government to take leadership on these kinds of questions and they will follow that leadership."[18]

As the numbers of infections rose beyond the capacity of local hospitals, reaching 15,000 new patients per day at the peak, the planning group directed their attention first to the provision of additional hospital capacity.[19] They planned, designed, and built two large new hospitals. These were not "flimsy bare-bones barracks" as described in the Western media; viewed from the interior, their appearance was identical to any fully-equipped modern hospitals.[20,21] They were modular concrete units designed for rapid assembly, in a manner similar to setting shipping containers side by side, with full accommodation for A/C, heating, ventilation, negative pressure, abundant electricity, and more. Once assembled, these units function as a whole, with all the equipment and facilities one would

17 "Wuhan to build special hospital in six days to receive patients," *CGTN,* January 23, 2020, https://news.cgtn.com/news/2020-01-23/Wuhan-to-build-special-hospital-in-six-days-to-receive-patients-NuQ9ulvAo8/index.html.

18 Global Times, "Capacity of state in China to deal with epidemic far more developed than Western govt: Martin Jacques," *China Daily,* updated March 19, 2020, http://www.chinadaily.com.cn/a/202003/19/WS5e72d148a31012821728052b.html.

19 Zhao Lei, "Medical leader calls makeshift hospitals a success," *China Daily,* May 5, 2020, https://www.chinadailyhk.com/article/129477#Medical-leader-calls-makeshift-hospitals-a-success.

20 Haroon Saddique, "Chinese city plans to build coronavirus hospital in days," *The Guardian,* January 24, 2020, https://www.theguardian.com/science/2020/jan/24/chinese-city-wuhan-plans-to-build-coronavirus-hospital-in-six-days.

21 Yuliya Talmazan, "China's coronavirus hospital built in 10 days opens its doors, state media says," *NBC News,* February 3, 2020, https://www.nbcnews.com/news/world/china-s-coronavirus-hospital-built-10-days-opens-its-doors-n1128531.

normally see in any regular hospital. The first was built in ten days by 16,000 men, the shifts working 24 hours a day. The second hospital was larger, and completed in only 6 days.[22] To clear and level the site and lay the substructure, there were 240 pieces of construction equipment working on the same site at the same time—also 24 hours per day. The Chinese media posted time-lapse videos of the construction process, which were astonishing to watch. Such hospitals were built in several cities in Hubei Province.

Immediately upon completion of the first hospital, more than 3,000 doctors and nurses from about 300 hospitals around the country were sent to staff it. The group did much more than build regular hospitals. A total of 16 temporary hospitals were created by converting public venues, several existing hospitals were renovated to cater exclusively to COVID-19 patients, and more than 500 hotels, training centers and sanitaria were converted into quarantine sites.[23] One makeshift hospital in Wuhan was created from a sports center transformed into a Traditional Chinese Medicine (TCM) treatment clinic, while many exhibition centers and gymnasiums were converted into temporary hospitals for those with mild symptoms but still requiring quarantine.[24] This Central Guiding Group played an irreplaceable role in Wuhan's anti-virus battle.

What the world apparently fails to notice is that of China's total deaths of 4,600, 4,500 of those (98%) were in Hubei Province. If China's leaders had not immediately locked down the city of Wuhan and then quarantined the entire province, the death toll might well have been in the hundreds of thousands. According to a paper published in late March in the journal *Science*,[25] co-author Christopher Dye said, "Our analysis suggests that without the Wuhan travel ban and the national emergency response there would have been more than 700,000 confirmed COVID-19 cases outside of Wuhan by [February]. China's

---

22 Jessica Wang, Ellie Zhu and Taylor Umlauf, "How China Built Two Coronavirus Hospitals in Just Over a Week," *The Wall Street Journal,* updated February 6, 2020, https://www.wsj.com/articles/how-china-can-build-a-coronavirus-hospital-in-10-days-11580397751.

23 Xinhua, "Makeshift hospitals play 'irreplaceable' role in Wuhan's anti-virus battle: official," Shine, April 28, 2020, https://www.shine.cn/news/nation/2004287119/.

24 Xinhua, "All 16 temporary hospitals in Wuhan closed," *People's Daily,* March 11, 2020, http://en.people.cn/n3/2020/0311/c90000-9666866.html.

25 Penn State, "China's control measures may have prevented 700,000 COVID-19 cases," *EurekaAlert!,* March 31, 2020, https://www.eurekalert.org/pub_releases/2020-03/ps-ccm033120.php.

control measures appear to have worked by successfully breaking the chain of transmission."[26]

Most Asian countries followed China's example, with similar results. The U.S. refused to do so, permitting the virus to spread freely by avoiding lockdowns and quarantines and, at the time of writing, appears headed for at least 100,000 (mostly) unnecessary deaths. The American way of dealing with the epidemic was to do next to nothing, while throwing stones at China.[27] Canada was the same: Shanghai is only two hours from Wuhan and had no time to prepare or plan, yet it had only a few hundred infections and only 7 deaths. Canada, with a population similar to Shanghai, 10,000 kms from Wuhan and with months to prepare, had more infections and fatalities (6,028 by May 20) than all of China combined.

That said, China's response wasn't perfect. In the beginning, a few local officials in Wuhan were reluctant to face the possibility of a major epidemic at such a crucial time and were hesitant to publicize the fact that deaths were already occurring. While that was indeed an embarrassment for China, it can be easily demonstrated that the net effect was zero because the medical detective work continued unabated and, as soon as the new pathogen was discovered, that information was made public to China and to the world. The reluctance of a few local officials to publicize a new illness caused no significant delay either in China or internationally, because until that point there was no information to communicate other than the fact that a few dozen people had become ill with an unusual respiratory infection. All the accusations of China causing the U.S. to lose two or three months of preparation time were merely juvenile political smoke, because the Chinese authorities communicated everything they knew as soon as they knew it.

For the West, this brief hesitation was a propaganda plus, because it provided unlimited (and apparently interminable) opportunities for gleeful China-bashing, demonstrating political opportunism at its finest. By contrast, the displeasure inside China at its initial shortcomings was real, for both the public and the central government, which immediately fired or replaced those same local officials, facing its mistakes openly with the public and taking immediate action. Compare this to the discovery in the U.S. of the CIA operating the largest network of torture prisons in the history of the world. What happened? Much media whining, a fraudulent Congressional hearing, most information classified and suppressed, and the entire

---

26 Xinhua, "Xinhua Headlines: What makes a difference on COVID-19 death rate? Lessons beyond math," *Xinhua Net,* April 25, 2020, http://www.xinhuanet.com/english/2020-04/25/c_139005866.htm.

27 Zamir Ahmed Awan, "Why the U.S. has become the country worst hit by COVID-19," *People's Daily,* April 28, 2020, http://en.people.cn/n3/2020/0428/c90000-9684857.html.

matter swept under the rug, removed from the media radar, and quickly forgotten. The torture prisons are still open today and only one minor person paid a trivial penalty. All involved still retained their positions, and nothing changed.

To a foreigner such as myself watching from the inside, the Chinese government and the Chinese people were courageous as they took on this formidable task. From the very beginning they put people's lives and health first. The Central Government mobilized the entire nation, organized massive control and treatment mechanisms, and acted with openness and transparency, with most of the population making significant sacrifices without complaint.

National cohesion and coordination were admirable. All of the 50,000 front-line medical staff and many others who went to Wuhan were volunteers, 90% of them Party members who had sworn to "bear the people's burden first and enjoy their pleasures last." To a Western ear, that sounds suspiciously like idle propaganda, but many of these front-line staff died in that battle. It wasn't propaganda to them. Zhang Wenhong, a prominent Party member and Director of the Department of Infectious Diseases at Shanghai's Huashan Hospital, said, "When we joined the Party, we vowed that we would always prioritize people's interests and press forward in the face of difficulties. This is the moment we live up to the pledge. All CPC members must rush to the front line. I don't care what you were actually thinking when you joined the party. Now it's time to live up to what you promised. I don't care if you personally agree or not: it's non-negotiable."[28] That may sound harshly authoritarian to a Westerner, but there was much compassion behind the words. Zhang said later, "The first-aid team put themselves in great danger. They are tired and need to rest. We shouldn't take advantage of good people." At that point, he replaced almost all the front-line medics with members from different sectors.

We Westerners cannot understand that China's society and culture are much more compassionate than ours. The Chinese place a much higher value on the elderly than do we. In China (as in Italy), grandparents and the elderly live with the family, never tossed out into nursing homes to live and die more or less alone. When it was realized that the elderly primarily were threatened with premature and painful deaths, the Chinese put their entire economy on hold to save these people.

Dr. Bruce Aylward, head of the WHO International Mission, said, "In the face of a previously unknown disease, China has taken one of the most ancient approaches for infectious disease control and rolled out probably the most ambitious, and I would say, agile and aggressive disease containment effort in

---

28 Zhou Wenting, "Celebrity doctor hailed for frank speech style," *China Daily,* February 28, 2020, https://www.chinadaily.com.cn/a/202002/28/WS5e58664ca31012821727af1d.html.

history. China took old-fashioned measures like the national approach to hand-washing, the mask-wearing, the social distancing, the universal temperature monitoring. But then very quickly, as it started to evolve, the response started to change.... So they refined the strategy as they moved forward, and this is an important aspect as we look to how we might use this going forward. WHO has been here from the start of this crisis, an epidemic, working every single day with the government of China... WHO was here from the beginning and never left." He said further, "What struck me most was that every Chinese had a strong sense of responsibility and dedication to contribute to the fight against the epidemic." WHO Director-General Tan Desai commented, "China's speed and scale of action is rare ... This is the advantage of China's system, and the relevant experience is worthy of other countries to learn from."

The Global Times published an editorial titled: "China's miracles are beyond biased Western understanding":

The rhetoric accusing China of hiding the truth has already become a cliché. These so-called experts in the U.S. always presume that China is wrong or unreliable, and then try hard to prove the presupposed conclusion with ambiguous evidence and perverted logic. They are used to pinning their eyes on fictional stories about China, but few are willing to learn about what is really happening in the country. For a country which has let the epidemic spin out of control despite clear warnings sent by China, China's anti-virus fight is indeed a miracle. But for China itself, the outcome appears absolutely normal and deserved in view of the government's strong sense of responsibility for people's lives, the governing system's great ability of mobilization and the Chinese people's firm willingness to support all containment measures. Nowhere could this work as it works in China and so applying any country's models to China makes no sense. China has been working miracles over the past decades thanks to the tremendous efforts of both the government and the people. Since reform and opening-up, China has grown to become the world's second largest economy rapidly and lifted hundreds of millions of people out of extreme poverty.[29]

The Lancet published an article stating that "China deserves gratitude, not criticism over its handling of the COVID-19 pandemic." *Lancet's* editor, Richard Horton, said Chinese researchers were providing crucial information but no one in the West was listening, and they failed to prepare. In January, *The Lancet* published five papers that tell the story of what has unfolded in the Western world in the recent months. They showed a deadly virus had emerged that had no treatment and could be passed between people. We knew all of this in the last week of January but most Western countries and the United States of America wasted the

29 Shi Tian, "China's miracles beyond biased Western understanding," *Global Times,* April 12, 2020, https://www.globaltimes.cn/content/1185403.shtml.

whole of February and early March before they acted. That is the human tragedy of COVID-19. Thanks to the work of Chinese doctors and scientists working in international collaborations, all of this info was known in January but for reasons that are difficult to understand, the world did not pay attention. Thousands died unnecessarily as a result.[30]

Horton said further that the attacks on China made by [American] politicians were unwarranted. "I want to be on the record and thank my friends and colleagues who work in medicine and medical science in China for what they have done. As I have said, I think we owe them a great deal... they do not deserve criticism, they deserve our gratitude." And there was more: On May 15, 2020, *The Lancet* published a scathing assessment of the Trump administration's handling of the virus epidemic in which it urged all Americans to vote President Trump out of office [for his incompetence]. "Americans must put a president in the White House come January 2021, who will understand that public health should not be guided by partisan politics."[31]

The main objective of China's Government in the rejuvenation of China is in part demonstrably evidenced by its determined efforts made for the betterment and well-being of its population, which is reflected in the credibility and high level of trust the Chinese people place in their government. These sentiments don't exist in the West. In the U.S., the "world's model for everything," the people suspect a virus epidemic is seen as an opportunity for profiteering by large corporations, with sick people not being humans in need of assistance but merely a new lucrative "market" for those with money to pay. An American hospital is not a place for healing the sick but a kind of barnyard filled with cash cows being milked. This is a fundamental reason underlying America's chaotic and hopeless approach to dealing with the epidemic. The Trump administration failed to help itself, refused to help its friends, and even seized the opportunity to further imperil its enemies.

THE CHINESE PEOPLE'S RESPONSE

On April 4, China held a three-minute nationwide moment of reflection to honor those who died in the coronavirus outbreak, especially the medical staff now

---

30 "West suffering because it failed to listen to China on COVID-19, says Lancet editor," *CGTN,* May 2, 2020, https://newseu.cgtn.com/news/2020-05-02/West-suffering-because-it-failed-to-listen-to-China-Lancet-editor-Q9g3yHGFfq/index.html.

31 Josie Ensor, "The Lancet urges Americans to vote out Trump over coronavirus handling," *The Telegraph,* May 15, 2020, https://www.telegraph.co.uk/news/2020/05/15/medical-journal-lancet-urges-americans-vote-trump-coronavirus/.

seen as "martyrs" who fell while fighting what has become a global pandemic.[32] Commemorations took place in all major cities, but were particularly poignant in Wuhan, occurring on the traditional Qingming festival, when Chinese visit the graves of their ancestors. China's State Council ordered that national flags be flown at half-staff around the country and at Chinese embassies and consulates abroad.

It was heartwarming that during the epidemic, privately-owned Chinese hotels in Wuhan voluntarily provided free rooms for medical staff needing rest. Xiao Yaxing, the private owner of a four-star hotel in the city, opened a discussion group on WeChat where he appealed to his peers from more than 40 hotels to offer rooms for doctors and nurses who were working day and night to save lives. He said that since nearly all transportation had ceased in the large city, it was difficult for the medical staff to get to hospitals from home and needed rest places and, as he said, "Many hotels in Wuhan are shut down for travelers, leaving a lot of empty rooms that we can offer for free."[33] Yi Qingyan, a regional manager of Feizhu's hotel business in Central China's Hubei province, said when she heard about Xiao's group, she asked hotel managers she knew to provide rooms for medical staff.[34]

In March, the Communist Party of China donated 5.3 billion RMB (US$750 million) to be used to "extend solicitude" to the frontline medics, those serving the worst-hit Hubei Province to be favored.[35] The money was delivered to the Ministry of Finance which was entrusted with distribution, with a stipulation that families of medical workers who died on the front line would be eligible recipients, and also that some grassroots-level officials, public security officers, community workers, volunteers and frontline journalists could have access to the funds. Further, nearly 80 million Communist Party of China members across the country donated more than 8 billion RMB for the coronavirus effort, and donations were still arriving at the time of writing.

Being a socially-oriented society, China also has charities but these are very different animals than those existing in the West, most especially those in North

---

32 The Associated Press, "China honors virus victims with 3 minutes of reflection," *ABC News,* April 4, 2020, https://abcnews.go.com/International/wireStory/china-honors-virus-victims-minutes-reflection-69972806.

33 Wuhan hotels offer free lodging to outbreak medical workers," *People's Daily,* January 25, 2020, http://en.people.cn/n3/2020/0125/c90000-9651777.html.

34 Chen Jia, "Wuhan hotels offer free lodging to outbreak medical workers," *China Daily,* January 25, 2020, http://www.chinadaily.com.cn/a/202001/25/WS5e2bb430a310128217273341.html.

35 "CPC members donate $750 million to frontline medics, other workers," *Global Times,* March 28, 2020, https://www.globaltimes.cn/content/1184030.shtml.

America. Chinese charities don't spend 80% of collected funds on operating expenses and executive perquisites. In fact they normally don't collect money at all, but instead collect real goods that are distributed to the beneficiaries. As one example, when Wuhan hospitals put out a call for help, the Hubei Charity Federation received more than 1 million masks and other medical supplies which were immediately distributed to the hospitals.[36] In this case, they also raised 30 million RMB in cash from the community and from citizens in other provinces, which was immediately spent on the purchase of more supplies. Moreover, in China the public can supervise the distribution and usage of donated materials and, in the case of COVID-19, the provincial medical headquarters was available to unify the organization and allocation of the materials to hospitals and medical treatment centers, as well as guaranteeing speedy transportation and delivery.

All of China, in many ways we would never expect, strove to express their gratitude to the medical workers whom they feel saved their nation from catastrophe. As one example, more than 500 tourist areas in China announced free admission for all medical workers during the remainder of 2020, as a way to express local citizens' sincere gratitude to medical workers' commitment during the outbreak.[37] Given that the virus epidemic severely damaged China's internal tourism industry, at least for the short term, the Chinese Academy of Social Sciences conducted a poll asking citizens about their travel intentions for the remainder of 2020. According to their report, Wuhan was at the top of the list for Chinese travelers, all of whom said they wanted to contribute to the economic recovery of Wuhan and Hubei following the epidemic.[38]

From late January until April, the streets of Wuhan were deserted with the entire Province of Hubei not much better, but by late May the story was very different, with people around the country emptying supermarket shelves of everything Hubei had to offer—local delicacies, noodles, ducks, crayfish, fruits, manufactured goods of every kind—all with the intention of lifting Hubei's economy to its former level. "Buying Hubei" became a nationwide campaign with participation from ordinary citizens, officials, celebrities and corporations.[39] Hundreds of companies began live-streaming online broadcasts of Hubei

---

36 "Wuhan calls for more material help to deal with virus," *China Daily*, January 26, 2020, https://www.chinadailyhk.com/article/119530.

37 Yang Cheng and Yang Jun, "Chinese tourist spots offer free entrance to medical workers," February 17, 2020, http://www.chinadaily.com.cn/a/202002/17/WS5e4a3f38a3101282172781a9.html.

38 Cheng Si, "Wuhan tops travelers' wish lists in 2020," *China Daily*, April 29, 2020, https://www.chinadailyhk.com/article/129138#Wuhan-tops-travelers'-wish-lists-in-2020.

39 "'Buying Hubei' becomes nationwide campaign," *Global Times*, April 17, 2020, https://www.globaltimes.cn/content/1185879.shtml.

products and hundreds of millions of Chinese were spending money, "not for self-indulgence, but to extend a helping hand to their fellow countrymen in hardship. The result: Tens of millions of dollars were added to the local economy; tens of thousands of businesses and jobs were saved."

In one instance, a popular live-streaming hostess sold 150,000 lipstick sets within five minutes. In another, two TV celebrities attracted 122 million viewers and sold more than 40 million RMB of Hubei products in a two-hour program. In another session, two celebrities drew 127 million viewers and sold 61 million RMB of Hubei goods, the province's entire supply of popular duck snacks emptied within seconds. In another livestreaming instance, 6,000 tons of crayfish, worth 220 million yuan, disappeared within minutes, and one company manager said his daily production of 20,000 packages of crayfish snacks cleared out within seconds every day. He said, "The orders just exploded," adding that he'd never seen anything like it.[40] Alibaba has sold 20 million Kgs of Hubei agricultural products to date and reportedly procured 1 billion yuan worth of crayfish and 50 million yuan worth of local oranges to sell on its platforms.[41] JD.com sold 1,400 tons in the first week of April alone and vowed to sell 6 billion yuan worth of Hubei products. Boosting consumption became a primary cure to resurrect the virus-hit economy in Hubei.

Many Chinese citizens said they hadn't any medical skills to help Wuhan during the epidemic, but they could at least show their support by placing orders. That sentiment resonated so broadly across China that millions promised to "gain three jin (1.5 Kg.) of weight" for Hubei.[42] One online hostess said, "Many have described our cooperation as a show of our moral principles and sense of duty. But that is over the top. I am just doing what I'm good at to help Wuhan, to help local companies open the market with livestreaming promotion and to help them resume work quickly."

A local Party Chief in Hubei said, "I was completely moved and warmed by the active response from consumers all over the country in placing orders for Hubei products to support us, which fully reflects our valued Chinese tradition: When one falls into difficulty, all other parties come to help." Unfortunately, no other country could replicate this economic model since they haven't the infrastructure or the market for something of this magnitude, and few nations have the deep social and cultural cohesion which is the enabling force.

As well, many of China's state-owned enterprises (SOEs) mobilized to combat the epidemic, from emergency communications installations to providing funds

---

40 *Ibid.*

41 "Chinese 'gain weight' to support Hubei economic recovery," *Global Times,* April 14, 2020, http://www.globaltimes.cn/content/1185533.shtml.

42 "'Buying Hubei' becomes nationwide campaign," *op cit.*

to the hardest-hit areas.[43] These massive Chinese corporations are exemplary in their sense of social responsibility, some constructing low-cost housing apartment communities which they sell at cost or below, many building and supporting local schools and universities, and some providing cash to help eliminate the last traces of poverty in the country. In 2020, these firms are providing more than 3 billion RMB (about $500 million) to the poorest places and many have donated massive medical supplies and funds to these same areas.[44]

MEDICAL SUPPLIES

When China experiences a serious public health or similar emergency, the framework exists for immediate supply for all necessities that include personnel, goods and materials, transport vehicles, to be delivered to the site. The Ministry of Transport arranged an absolute prioritization of the transport of emergency supplies and medical staff to Wuhan, while national medical authorities coordinated the efforts of all medical supply manufacturers to identify and increase the supply of the most urgent and necessary items.[45] When Wuhan appealed to the central government for assistance and supplies, hundreds of tons of medical supplies were delivered each week, as were tens of thousands of additional medical staff during the crisis.[46]

At the same time, the Ministry of Commerce (MOC) was occupied in coordinating the production and supply of all other daily necessities for the residents of Wuhan and Hubei. Many food items like eggs, fish, beef and pork, were released from national reserves and arrangements were made for the increased production and distribution of fresh vegetables specifically for Wuhan, along with oversight to ensure prices remained stable or dropping rather than increasing.[47] Profiteering was virtually absent in China, with the notable exception of a few foreign firms. The MOC also ensured top priority for all vehicles carrying supplies to Wuhan,

---

43 "China central SOEs to offer 3.2b yuan to poor counties," The State Council, The People's Republic of China, *Top News,* updated March 7, 2020, http://english.www.gov.cn/news/topnews/202003/07/content_WS5e6338a8c6d0c201c2cbdbce.html.

44 Xinhua, "China SOEs pitch in to combat virus spread," *China Daily,* January 25, 2020, http://www.chinadaily.com.cn/a/202001/25/WS5e2b76faa3101282172732ab.html.

45 Xinhua, "China cranks up protective equipment supplies to fight new coronavirus," *Xinhua Net,* January 26, 2020, http://www.xinhuanet.com/english/2020-01/26/c_138733811.htm.

46 CGTN, "387 railway stations using temperature checks," *Global Times,* January 26, 2020, https://www.globaltimes.cn/content/1177867.shtml.

47 Xinhua, "China steps up mask, food supply for Wuhan," *China Daily,* January 25, 2020, https://global.chinadaily.com.cn/a/202001/25/WS5e2b8102a3101282172732c0.html.

and all supply firms, including even restaurants, were encouraged to provide home delivery to help maintain the quarantine with a minimum of inconvenience.

DISCOVERIES AND TREATMENTS

The pressure for urgent treatment was such that it was only on February 15 that the world's first autopsy on a COVID-19 patient was conducted, six weeks after the pathogen was first identified. It was then that the doctors discovered that the virus attacked not only the lungs, but also other organs such as the heart and kidneys as well as the circulatory system, thus altering the treatment methods but also inflicting even more pressure on the overworked medical staff. Still, it was then that Chinese physicians began the use of blood plasma from recovered patients as well as the nearly universal application of Traditional Chinese Medicine. It was these discoveries and treatments that almost instantly halved the mortality rate, especially from the more severe infections, and speeded up the recovery time. The Western media completely ignored this aspect, but it was widely proven that TCM was perhaps the primary factor in reducing the mortality rate by boosting the patients' immune systems.

By the end of March, the crisis in Wuhan was abating while the demand for medical supplies was increasing exponentially worldwide, with most relevant factories in China running 24 hours a day simultaneously trying to maintain quality and source raw materials internationally. There was a great deal of organization required behind the scenes to coordinate the manufacture as well as to expand domestic and international transport channels which were greatly suffering due to the collapse of the airline transport industry and the resultant lack of cargo space. The logistical hurdles were enormous in all categories, and a great part of China's commercial society leaped into the fray in a sincere effort to assist what was now a worldwide pandemic. Chinese auto manufacturers, idle due to the pandemic, retooled within a week and began manufacturing masks, hazmat suits and other supplies by the billions. The international demand was such that more than 12,000 companies in China began producing masks and ventilators, bringing the total to well over 50,000 such firms with about one-third of them being certified exporters.[48]

Thanks to their media who were too busy bashing China to understand the events unfolding, Westerners hadn't a clue about either the overwhelming demand for medical supplies nor the urgency of those demands. One company alone, Beijing Aeonmed, which makes ventilators, kept running 24\7 but was overwhelmed by tens of thousands of simultaneous overseas orders from nearly 50

---

48 "China keeps engine roaring to ensure global medical supplies amid pandemic," *Global Times,* March 29, 2020, https://www.globaltimes.cn/content/1184127.shtml.

countries.[49] And it wasn't alone. A large number of other manufacturers retooled in an attempt to respond to other nations then living through Wuhan's experience, in many cases, such as the U.S., with little or no central government support.

The situation was so dire that many countries, notably Italy, and many cities, notably New York, were so lacking in supplies they were openly stating their medical staff were every day being forced to decide who would live and who would die. It was in this context that Chinese firms, entirely on their own initiative, absorbed the expense of retooling, of arranging specially-chartered aircraft and trains to bring back their staff, of sourcing raw materials, then diving head-first into a new industry to help combat a worldwide pandemic the extent and mortality of which were still largely unknown. And it was in this context that the U.S. media spent all their time denigrating "China" for "sluggish and insufficient" effort, for the usual "lack of transparency," and blowing out of all proportion the few complaints of unsatisfactory quality. In this context where Chinese auto manufacturers and packagers of canned salmon are suddenly manufacturing surgical masks and hazmat suits, we can be genuinely astonished the quality was as good as it was.

We should bear in mind: these were private businesses, with nobody guaranteeing their profits. It is a huge risk for a company to retool for an entirely new industry and product because if they fail the entire loss is theirs to bear. They took the risk because they wanted to help, not because they could price-gouge. The potential losses were large and were real.

While China was still not out of the woods, the Chinese government was doing its best to donate supplies to needy countries all around the world, but local demand was still high and commercial export demand was rising exponentially, far more than China's combined potential supply. As an example, on one weekend alone, France ordered one billion masks which required 56 cargo flights to transport them, to say nothing of the manufacturing logistics. Part of the problem was that the majority of air cargo is carried in scheduled flights on passenger planes but, with the collapse of the airline industry, there were no passenger planes. In order to accommodate the dire international need, China Eastern Airlines stripped overnight all the seats from their passenger aircraft and loaded them with N95 masks for France—as they did for other nations. SF Express, one of China's prominent express firms, opened new routes including to New York, and delivered nearly 1,000 tons of medical supplies to more than 50 countries, with many other Chinese airlines and express firms doing about the same.[50]

There was yet more to the leadership, planning and organizing that was not apparent to anyone in the West. The Chinese government, while dealing with all

49 *Ibid.*
50 *Ibid.*

other domestic and international pressures from the pandemic, also remembered its students who were studying abroad and distributed over 11 million face masks and 500,000 health kits with disinfection supplies and health protection manuals, to Chinese students studying abroad.[51] These shipments bypassed the local governments, being delivered to the Chinese embassies and consulates for distribution directly to the students.

It wasn't only medical supplies but also medical staff transfers that were arranged by China's central government, to help the country deal with the epidemic. One of the government's first acts was to select about 500 of the top experts from the military's medical universities, those with prior experience with SARS and MERS, and with Ebola, and send them to Wuhan to help lead the battle. There were many other such teams, composed of experts in respiratory health, infectious diseases, hospital infection control and the establishing and managing of intensive care units, who were dispatched to the Wuhan hospitals with large numbers of virus-related pneumonia patients. Zhou Xianzhi, President of Air Force Medical University, said "We sent our best staff in various clinical departments. They have rich experience in battling contagious diseases. Some of them took part in major missions such as the battle against SARS and the fight against Ebola in Africa, as well as earthquake rescues." These were volunteers who canceled their plan to spend the Chinese Lunar New Year with their families, most saying they felt "extremely honored" to join this national mission.[52] As well, immediately upon the discovery of the effectiveness of TCM's ability to moderate serious infections, a team of 122 TCM specialists was sent to Wuhan from Shanghai with treatment plans already prepared for the combined application of Western and Chinese medicines.[53]

QUALITY CONCERNS

China's *Global Times* reported, "As China mounted a nationwide effort to produce desperately needed medical supplies, concerns over the quality of some Chinese-made equipment have been raised, and some foreign media outlets and politicians have even attempted to hype up recent incidents to smear China's manufacturing sector and its intention to help other countries."[54] The *Financial*

---

51 Xinhua, "China sends 500,000 health kits to its students studying abroad," *Xinhua Net,* April 2, 2020, http://www.xinhuanet.com/english/2020-04/02/c_138941573.htm.

52 Xinhua, "China sends 450 military medics to Wuhan in coronavirus fight," *Shine,* January 25, 2020, https://www.shine.cn/news/nation/2001250569/.

53 Cai Wenjun and Zhou Shengjie, "Teams of Shanghai TCM experts head to Wuhan," *Shine,* February 16, 2020, https://www.shine.cn/news/metro/2002152114/.

54 "Chinese medical supplies' 'quality concerns' overblown," *Global Times,* March 31, 2020, http://www.globaltimes.cn/content/1184245.shtml.

Times cited examples of the Netherlands, Spain and Turkey "rejecting" Chinese-made face masks and testing kits, others going so far as to claim Chinese masks could make people sick and even kill them.

There were a few instances of unsuitable products having been sold but, on examination of the eventual details, it appears the media reports were consciously hyped and much overblown, in every case blaming "China" for the products of one manufacturer and the actions a few incompetent or unscrupulous agents, most of whom were not Chinese. The overall quality environment was actually much too complicated to permit understanding within the scope of brief media sound bytes. While there were risks of quality issues in manufacturing, the use of improper procurement channels and fluctuating foreign regulations and standards were responsible for much of the trouble. A further issue was that in two or three prominent cases the purchasers had no experience in applying delicate medical tests or even in the storage and handling of such. To compound the problem even further, the virus proved to lend itself more readily to testing at later stages of progression.

China's *Global Times* did a creditable job of investigating the entire medical supply process, interviewing manufacturers and distributors, industry insiders and end users, and concluded that the vast majority of Chinese-made medical equipment was well up to standard, with most of the noise resulting primarily from the U.S. heavily politicizing China's role in the supply process and secondly from much deliberate misinformation on the part of the American media.

In one publicized case, Dutch authorities ordered a recall of 600,000 face masks[55] for lack of ability to filter out a full 95% of airborne particles. An executive at the Chinese manufacturer stated that the world experienced such a shortage of appropriate meltblown fabric that it had become increasingly difficult to make masks that exceed 70% (instead of 95%), since almost all of this fabric was being imported from Switzerland and Turkey. The fault, such as it was, was not due to low-quality manufacturing in China but to the degraded production ability of companies in Switzerland and Turkey who provided the raw materials. Nevertheless, "China" took the full blame on the chin. The mask quality issue became even more preposterous since the Netherlands and Belgium had already made clear that those China-made masks obtained by local agents were "commercial products made for non-medical use," in other words sanding or paint-spraying masks and such.[56]

---

55 *Ibid.*

56 Xinhua, "China-bashing syndrome makes coronavirus pandemic deadlier," *China Daily,* April 6, 2020, https://www.chinadailyhk.com/article/126796#China-bashing-syndrome-makes-coronavirus-pandemic-deadlier.

Having said that, it is true Chinese authorities discovered some companies engaged in the illegal production and sale of masks and other medical products and, though they did respond with an immediate and aggressive crack-down, some of that product did indeed reach foreign markets. The government conducted more than a dozen sweeps throughout the nation and heavily publicized the product confiscations and fines issued to deter such practices.

But their response to these issues was much more wide-ranging than this. China's national government established lists of companies qualified to manufacture various medical supplies for use against the coronavirus, and strongly recommended purchases be made from only those firms and only through officially-recommended channels. However, due to the urgency of the need and occasional panic, many agents, buyers, and foreign end users ignored the Chinese government instructions with predictable results in quality standards. As well, the EU generally was so eager for supplies they waived formal requirements and permitted the importation of products prior to those gaining regulatory approval.

"Though local medical authorities and Chinese embassies have explained the misunderstanding and misuse of the test kits, media coverage of life-saving Chinese products has turned a blind eye to these clarifications, revealing some countries' unfriendly motives. I think the quality issue reported by some media has been politicized. They can't prove the reported testing kits have quality issues, because the use and transport [of the kits] may influence their stability and sensitivity," an employee at test kit provider Beijing Beier Bioengineering told the *Global Times*. Medical workers unfamiliar with the products may have some difficulties, which could affect the accuracy of their results. The Beier employee added that Chinese medical staff also had issues when using the test kits in the early stages of the outbreak and any confusion was resolved after technical training.[57]

There were also instances of testing kits facing claims of insensitivity or inaccuracy. Spain withdrew about 8,000 such tests, and the Western media created much noise about claims from the Czech Republic of inaccurate or insensitive tests. However, in the Czech case, their officials simply had no understanding of proper methods of application. The manufacturer finally prepared instruction videos illustrating and explaining the precise methods of administering the tests, after which the results were perfectly acceptable. This occurred more than once, and even test kits manufactured by companies not yet on the approved list had the same successful result when proper methods were employed. It occurred surprisingly often in Western countries that the medical staff eventually admitted

---

57 Zhang Dan and Shen Weiduo, "China's test kit providers call on world to stop smearing Chinese assistance," *Global Times,* April 2, 2020, https://www.globaltimes.cn/content/1184530.shtml.

they had never administered such tests and had no clear idea of proper procedure, and in many cases simply did not follow the instructions.

A major part of the overall quality problem was that foreign companies and governments were too eager to fill their large and increasing demand for supplies and, rather than wait in a queue at a recognized factory, would hire their own private agents in attempts to short-circuit the process, agents who, to satisfy their anxious customers, would often resort to unapproved manufacturers in the hope their actions would not later be discovered. The result was that "China" took this blame on the chin as well, with the great assistance of the politicized Western media.

As one illustrative example of the media presentation of issues with medical supplies, a UK *Telegraph* article said, "Government seeks refund for millions of coronavirus antibody tests,"[58] stating they were "too unreliable to be used by the public." According to the *Telegraph*, the UK government ordered 3.5 million such tests "mainly from Chinese manufacturers," then noting that an additional 17.5 million had been purchased from firms in the U.S. and UK, with none being found sufficiently reliable. But by that time, China's 10% of the purchases had taken the media hit for the entire lot. But once the media smoke cleared and "China" had sufficiently been tarred and denigrated yet again, the UK government health officials admitted that the tests developed in China were created and designed primarily for use with patients "with a very large viral load," in other words those more severely infected, and not intended for patients suffering only mild symptoms from minor infections. The difficulty with the UK tests lay not with a quality problem from "China" but with UK physicians hoping for tests with a wider detection range. This was a bit like purchasing a "vehicle" then being disappointed it was unable to function as both sports car and dump truck, hardly the fault of the manufacturer. And finally, in the article's penultimate paragraph, the *Telegraph* remembered to report that the UK government was not actually demanding refunds but was negotiating with the manufacturers to increase the sensitivity of the tests. In the end, much ado about nothing.

Fox News joined the parade by yelling "CHINA CASHES IN OFF CORONAVIRUS, SELLING SPAIN $467 MILLION IN SUPPLIES, SOME OF THEM SUBSTANDARD." Spain purchased 950 ventilators, 5.5 million test kits, 11 million gloves and 500 million masks. The "substandard" part was 9,000 quick-test kits (out of 5.5 million) that lacked the sensitivity Spain wanted.[59]

---

58 Bill Gardner and Amy Jones, "Government seeks refund for millions of coronavirus antibody tests," *The Telegraph,* April 6, 2020, https://www.telegraph.co.uk/news/2020/04/06/government-seeks-refund-millions-coronavirus-antibody-tests/.

59 Barnini Chakraborty, "Netherlands becomes latest country to reject China-made coronavirus test kits, gear," *Fox News,* March 30, 2020, https://www.foxnews.com/world/

White House trade advisor Peter Navarro accused China of shipping "low-quality and even counterfeit" antibody testing kits to the U.S. and of "profiteering" from the outbreak.[60] The Chinese Foreign Ministry responded that Navarro's remarks were "groundless and extremely irresponsible," stating that China had exported tens of millions of COVID-19 tests, which had won wide acclaim from the international community, and the country had not received any feedback from the U.S. purchasers and users on quality problems.[61,62]

By the end of April of 2020, Chinese firms had indeed exported tens of millions of testing kits in addition to billions of masks and thousands of tons of other supplies to nearly 200 countries, all of which were widely praised by the international community. Barbara Woodward, British ambassador to China, expressed her deep appreciation and satisfaction with the products and speed of response, and many other nations were effuse in their gratitude for both commercial shipments and donations from China.[63] Chinese firms shipped enormous volumes of all nature of medical supplies to the U.S. with not a word of complaint from U.S. purchasers or users regarding the quality of test kits and other products. But also not a single word of praise or appreciation from the Americans. Instead, the recipient U.S. hospitals were silent while the U.S. government and the media were replete with non-stop smears for months.

In all the confusion, the U.S. media failed to notice that the U.S. itself led the world competition for defective medical products. As of the middle of February, 2020, AFP was reporting that even small countries like South Korea had performed hundreds of thousands of tests while the U.S. was below about 8,000, the reason being that all the tests produced by the CDC and American companies

---

netherlands-becomes-latest-country-to-reject-china-made-coronavirus-test-kits-gear.

60 Xinhua, "U.S. accusation against COVID-19 test kits from China 'groundless, irresponsible': spokesperson," *China.org.cn,* April 29, 2020, http://www.china.org.cn/china/Off_the_Wire/2020-04/29/content_75987996.htm.

61 "White House adviser Navarro lashes out at China over 'fake' test kits," *Reuters,* April 27, 2020, https://www.reuters.com/article/us-health-coronavirus-usa-china-idUSKCN2292S8.

62 Zhong Nan, "US official's claims on quality of China testing kits 'groundless,'" *China Daily,* April 29, 2020, https://www.chinadailyhk.com/article/129146.

63 China Daily, "Washington rebuked for smear over testing kits," *People's Daily News,* April 30, 2020, https://peoplesdaily.pdnews.cn/2020/04/30/world/washington-rebuked-for-smear-over-testing-kits-148227.html.

were flawed and useless.[64,65,66] The kits would produce opposite results on the same patient at the same time, or clearly miss serious infections while declaring infections in clean patients. The CDC eventually had to instruct all hospitals and clinics to discard the tests as unusable.[67] Again, in early to mid-April, the U.S. media were reporting the CDC was still unable to produce usable tests, this time because the test kits themselves were contaminated with the coronavirus for which they were to be testing. This was attributed to "a glaring scientific breakdown" at the CDC's central lab.[68,69]

To make matters worse, the CDC shipped those faulty tests not only across the country but sold them to 34 countries around the world, and no evidence emerged anywhere to suggest the CDC informed those other nations of the uselessness of their tests. The UK was not the only nation to discover this—at their own expense.[70] To say that the exported CDC tests were unusable would be quite an understatement. President John Magufuli of Tanzania complained that various fruits, a goat and a quail tested positive for coronavirus using the American tests.[71]

---

64 Denise Grady, "Coronavirus Test Kits Sent to States Are Flawed, C.D.C. Says," *The New York Times,* February 12, 2020, https://www.nytimes.com/2020/02/12/health/coronavirus-test-kits-cdc.html.

65 Danielle Zoellner, "Coronavirus: US government test kits are faulty and 'cannot be relied upon', New York reports," *Independent,* February 28, 2020, https://www.independent.co.uk/news/world/americas/coronavirus-tests-new-york-us-cases-kits-trump-cdc-results-a9365921.html.

66 AFP, "US health authority shipped faulty coronavirus test kits across country," *Yahoo! News,* February 12, 2020, https://news.yahoo.com/us-health-authority-shipped-faulty-coronavirus-test-kits-205948746.html.

67 "US Health Authority Shipped Faulty Coronavirus Test Kits Across Country: Official," *Channel News Asia,* February 13, 2020, https://www.globalresearch.ca/us-health-authority-shipped-faulty-coronavirus-test-kits-across-country-official/5703909.

68 Dan Mangan, "Coronavirus tests were delayed by contamination at CDC lab, report says," *CNBC,* updated April 20, 2020, https://www.cnbc.com/2020/04/18/coronavirus-tests-delayed-by-covid-19-contamination-at-cdc-lab.html.

69 David Willman, "Contamination at CDC lab delayed rollout of coronavirus tests," *The Washington Post,* April 18, 2020, https://www.washingtonpost.com/investigations/contamination-at-cdc-lab-delayed-rollout-of-coronavirus-tests/2020/04/18/fd7d3824-7139-11ea-aa80-c2470c6b2034_story.html.

70 "US health authority shipped faulty coronavirus test kits across country: Official," *CNA,* updated February 13, 2020, https://www.channelnewsasia.com/news/world/covid19-coronavirus-united-states-faulty-test-kits-12429566.

71 "COVID-19: Pawpaw and goat test positive for virus - President Magufuli," *MSN Briefly,* May 4, 2020, https://www.msn.com/en-za/news/africa/covid-19-pawpaw-and-goat-test-positive-for-virus-president-magufuli/ar-BB13AJWO.

It appears the U.S. 'national stockpile' was not an improvement on the CDC.[72] In early April, the media were reporting that many states received medical masks that were rotten, with an expiry date in 2010, and that 150 ventilators (at $30,000 each) sent to Los Angeles were broken, defective, and missing parts.[73,74,75] But, no problem. ABC News and other U.S. media including U.S. military channels ran dozens of articles titled, "Have a clean T-shirt? That's all you need to make this mask."[76]

And in late April, the UK *Telegraph* was reporting that the UK NHS staff "had been given flawed coronavirus tests" but, kindly, no mention that the U.S. CDC had supplied them.[77] And even the criticism was muted: the tests were described as "less reliable than first thought because of 'degraded' performance," and that they produced "discordant results," and "have been found to be flawed and should no longer be relied on."[78] Health Minister Helen Whately admitted "Some of the early tests were evaluated and the evaluation was that they weren't effective enough" saying that all patients would be called in for a second test, and

---

72 Toluse Olorunnipa, Josh Dawsey, Chelsea Janes, and Isaac Stanley-Becker, "Governors plead for medical equipment from Federal stockpile plagued by shortages and confusion," *The Washington Post,* March 31, 2020, https://www.washingtonpost.com/politics/governors-plead-for-medical-equipment-from-federal-stockpile-plagued-by-shortages-and-confusion/2020/03/31/18aadda0-728d-11ea-87da-77a8136c1a6d_story.html.

73 Associated Press, "Some states receive masks with dry rot, broken ventilators," *New York Post,* April 4, 2020, https://nypost.com/2020/04/04/states-receive-masks-with-dry-rot-broken-ventilators/.

74 Kim Chandler, "County received 5,000 rotted masks from national stockpile," *AP News,* April 2, 2020, https://apnews.com/2b1c7d508dbee187aba31b675f8c5685.

75 Danielle Garrand, "California received '170 broken ventilators' from federal government, governor says," *CBS News,* March 29, 2020, https://www.cbsnews.com/news/california-received-broken-ventilators-from-federal-government-governor-gavin-newsom-says/.

76 "Have a clean T-shirt to spare? That's all you need to make this face mask," *ABC News* video, 1:43, https://abcnews.go.com/GMA/Living/video/clean-shirt-spare-make-face-mask-69944363.

77 Laura Donnelly, "Revealed: NHS staff given flawed coronavirus tests," *The Telegraph,* April 21, 2020, https://www.telegraph.co.uk/news/2020/04/21/public-health-england-admits-coronavirus-tests-used-send-nhs/.

78 Greg Heffer, "NHS staff offered new COVID-19 tests after initial checks found to be flawed," MSN, April 22, 2020, https://www.msn.com/en-gb/news/coronavirus/nhs-staff-offered-new-covid-19-tests-after-initial-checks-found-to-be-flawed/ar-BB131rbF.

that this was a "normal process" when testing for a new illness.[79] No slander, no vitriol, no condemnation. Instead, the Brits and their media were quick to note that all tests have a margin of error accuracy which depends on the skill with which they are administered, among other factors. If only they had been so kind and understanding towards China.

Shanghai Dasheng is one of the world's largest manufacturers (and the world gold standard) of N95 face masks and one of the few certified to make U.S. NIOSH-approved N95s. The company deals directly with medical purchasers only, and states on its website: "We do not have any distributors, dealers or branch factories. Beware of counterfeits." But some masks (that were clearly fake since they were models the company did not export) bearing this company's name appeared in the U.S., apparently purchased through unknown third parties.[80] Associated Press added: "AP could not independently verify if [Dasheng] are making their own counterfeits." Charming.

DEATH RATES

At the end of the epidemic, China reported 4,645 coronavirus deaths while the U.S. total of 90,000 fatalities was still climbing rapidly. The death rates per 100,000 of population were 26.0 for the U.S. and 0.33 for China.

There are many reasons for China's relatively low infection and death rates. First, if two countries have the same death toll, the death per 100,000 people for the country with a larger population will be lower; China's population is nearly four times that of the U.S. Secondly, due to the immediate lockdown of Wuhan and Hubei, almost all of China's fatalities were restricted to that one area: of China's 4,645 deaths, 4512 (97%) were in Hubei with the entire remainder of the country having little more than 100 deaths. The statistical result was that Wuhan's rate was 35.2, Hubei's 7.6, and China's 0.33, comparable to 26 for the U.S. Further, all provinces and major cities executed their own version of lockdown and quarantine, literally preventing the virus from entering even if it should escape Hubei. China's measures broke the transmission chain and contained the contagion within Hubei Province. The tough measures in Wuhan bought the rest of China time to prepare and execute their own restrictions, and China bought the rest of the world at least two and probably three months in which to prepare

---

79 Mikey Smith, "Coronavirus: NHS staff called back for re-testing after tests found to be flawed," *Mirror,* April 22, 2020, https://www.mirror.co.uk/news/politics/breaking-coronavirus-nhs-staff-called-21905571.

80 Juliet Linderman and Martha Mendoza, "Counterfeit masks reaching frontline health workers in US," *AP News,* May 13, 2020, https://apnews.com/850d9e6834fc71967af6d3dda65ad874.

for the epidemic. Looking at the statistics below, you can see which countries followed China's example and which did not.

Still, on the above scale for the U.S., New York was at 140.0, New Jersey at 107.0, Connecticut at 85 and Massachusetts at 75, while some states were near zero.[81] Comparably within China, and due to the aggressive quarantines, Shanghai was at 0.02 and Beijing similar. Turning to Europe (on the same scale of death rate per 100,000), Belgium was hit very hard with 76, with Spain, Italy, the UK, France, Sweden and the Netherlands ranging down from around 60.0 to about 35.0.[82]

North America and Europe were hit very hard while Asia was not. At the time of writing, the Philippines had the highest death rate in Asia, at 0.83 on the same scale as above. Japan was at 0.61, South Korea at 0.52, Australia and Malaysia at 0.40, Singapore at 0.38, China at 0.33, Hong Kong at 0.06, Taiwan at 0.03, India at 0.23, Thailand at 0.08 and Vietnam at 0.00.

DONATIONS

When COVID-19 first erupted in China, several countries immediately came to China's aid with scarce and badly-needed medical supplies. South Korea was one, and in return, as the situation worsened in South Korea, the Chinese government sent large amounts of medical supplies and more than 20 local governments in China donated masks, protective clothing, goggles, test kits, thermometers and other materials. The situation was similar with Pakistan, who sent aircraft loaded with medical supplies, the Chinese government later returning the favor with large volumes of supplies and assistance in building a quarantine hospital.[83] Many provinces and cities in China independently donated masks to Islamabad and Karachi.

China was sending supplies and assistance to other countries long before it fully recovered from its own difficulties. President Xi Jinping stressed on multiple occasions that public health security was a common challenge faced by humanity, and all countries should join hands to tackle it. China saw itself as perhaps the only country in the world able to help smaller nations in various states of medical

---

81 John Elflein, "Death rates from coronavirus (COVID-19) in the United States as of May 29, 2020, by state (per 100,000 people)," *Statista,* accessed May 29, 2020, https://www.statista.com/statistics/1109011/coronavirus-covid19-death-rates-us-by-state/.

82 Chen Jie and Shen Xinyi, "Latest coronavirus pictographs in Shanghai, China and around the world," *Shine,* accessed May 30, 2020, https://www.shine.cn/news/world/2003124144/.

83 "China announces to help 82 countries fight COVID-19," *CGTN,* updated March 21, 2020, https://news.cgtn.com/news/2020-03-20/China-announces-to-help-82-countries-fight-COVID-19-P1hcQcQKe4/index.html.

emergency. European Commission President Ursula von der Leyen expressed her gratitude in a videotaped speech broadcast throughout Europe.[84]

China also shared hundreds of documents on the prevention and control of COVID-19 and its diagnosis and treatment, with groups in more than 100 countries, followed by multiple technical exchanges that included personal discussions and teleconferencing.[85] In a short space of time, China released seven different editions of a guideline on diagnosis and treatment of the disease and six editions of a prevention and control plan for the disease, both of which have been translated into dozens of languages.

China's telecom giant Huawei donated countless millions of masks and other items to most countries where it has staff and does business. When the U.S. cancelled all medical supply exports to Canada in April, the country's supply shortage became desperate so Huawei quietly shipped millions of masks, plus goggles, gloves, and other protective equipment to Canada to help front-line medical workers to cope.[86] But Canada refused to publicly acknowledge the gifts. Canadian Prime Minister Justin Trudeau merely told the media that Canada would be receiving a shipment of millions of masks from "unnamed countries and companies," and the British Columbia government which was the prime beneficiary of the supplies was so mean-spirited as to tell the Canadian media, "The province has many supply sources . . . We don't share details about our suppliers." Others in Canada went so far as to accuse Huawei of "political generosity," and Trudeau even made a point of saying that donations of medical supplies from foreign companies "will not change how the government views those companies going forward."

China's Fosun Group donated a large batch of medical supplies to Portugal, including 1 million face masks and 200,000 test kits, as did many other Chinese companies. The Fosun Foundation in Shanghai donated large batches of face masks to hospitals in Italy, and coordinated with other companies and foundations in more than 10 shipments of medical supplies to countries that included Italy, Japan, Britain and France.[87] The Chinese automaker Geely donated large amounts of medical supplies to 14 countries including Sweden, Germany, Italy, Spain,

---

84 "China selflessly extends helping hand to countries around world in global battle against COVID-19," *People's Online Daily,* March 25, 2020, http://en.people.cn/n3/2020/0325/c90000-9672307.html.

85 *Ibid.*

86 Rena Li, "Huawei quietly pitches in to help Canada," *China Daily,* April 9, 2020, http://www.chinadaily.com.cn/a/202004/09/WS5e8e772ba310e232631a4e08.html.

87 "Singers from 12 countries perform song to fight COVID-19," *China Daily,* May 8, 2020, http://global.chinadaily.com.cn/a/202005/08/WS5eb4d906a310a8b24115437d.html.

Belarus and Britain. Chinese privately-owned firms and SOEs built and supplied complete COVID-19 testing labs and constructed or renovated hospitals in many countries. China's BGI Group built two testing labs in Serbia in 12 days and donated all the core equipment and instruments.[88] China State Construction Engineering offered free renovation service for a hospital in Ethiopia, transforming regular wards into virus facilities.[89,90]

Many Chinese foundations donated medical supplies to support smaller countries. The Jack Ma Foundation and the Alibaba Foundation donated 7.5 million face masks, 485,000 test kits and 100,000 sets of protective clothing, as well as ventilators and thermometers to 23 countries that included Azerbaijan, Bhutan, India, Kazakhstan, Kyrgyzstan, Uzbekistan and Vietnam.[91] The Jack Ma Foundation also donated a large amount of medical supplies to 54 African countries.[92] China's northwest Gansu Province, probably China's poorest province, donated two consignments including tens of thousands of face masks and protective suits to Zimbabwe, added to large donations of medical supplies from other Chinese foundations.[93] Various entities in China, including corporations, social agencies and the Chinese government, donated many air shipments of supplies to Iran, including test kits and respirators, these being especially important since U.S. economic sanctions prevented Iran from possessing the foreign currency to purchase medical supplies abroad.[94] China also sent several teams of medical experts to Iran, to help assess the situation and provide guidance and assistance.

Even small Chinese associations were active in their assistance. Chinese Community Groups in the UK raised money and collected medical supplies from more than 100 local Chinese communities and Chinese people in the UK, donating

88 "China-built COVID-19 testing lab completed in Serbia," *People's Daily Online*, April 22, 2020, https://www.globalsecurity.org/security/library/news/2020/04/sec-200422-pdo07.htm.

89 Li YingYan, "Chinese enterprises lend a big hand to Africa to combat COVID-19," *People's Daily*, April 28, 2020, http://en.people.cn/n3/2020/0428/c90000-9684957.html.

90 "Chinese enterprises lend a big hand to Africa to combat COVID-19," *People's Daily*, April 28, 2020, https://newsghana.com.gh/chinese-enterprises-lend-a-big-hand-to-africa-to-combat-covid-19/.

91 Xinhua, "Chinese foundations donate to countries in fight against COVID-19," *Shine*, March 29, 2020, https://www.shine.cn/news/world/2003295304/.

92 "China selflessly extends helping hand to countries around world in global battle against COVID-19," *op cit.*

93 Xinhua, "China's Gansu province donates medical supplies to Zimbabwe to combat COVID-19," *People's Daily*, May 7, 2020, http://en.people.cn/n3/2020/0507/c90000-9687490.html.

94 China Daily, "Medical supplies from China arrive to help Iran," *People's Daily*, March 21, 2020, http://en.people.cn/n3/2020/0321/c90000-9670897.html.

tens of thousands of medical gowns, surgical masks, and other items. The China Chamber of Commerce in the UK and the Bank of China donated 20 ventilators and nearly 2 million pieces of PPE to local English hospitals.[95,96]

By early April, China had already sent more than 300 charter flights carrying medical professionals and emergency supplies to support global anti-epidemic efforts, the flights carrying more than 110 medical specialists, and nearly 5,000 tons of medical supplies to about 50 countries, as well as a special flight to Ghana carrying nearly 40 tons of medical supplies for Africa.[97] These supplies include ventilators, N95 face masks, protective clothing, gloves and other medical devices and protective equipment.

In many cases, smaller nations had no idea of the procurement process for medical supplies, and the Chinese national government lent assistance to assure proper purchase and timely delivery.

However, while claiming it had offered $274 million to assist 64 different countries and UNHCR in combatting the pandemic, the U.S. ran into problems with its medical donations. When the State Department helped send 17.8 tons of personal protective equipment, or PPE, and other medical supplies from U.S. charities, including Samaritan's Purse and the Mormon Church, to Wuhan in early February, Pompeo was pummeled by the media and Democrats for sending China medical supplies that were desperately needed at home.[98] By the end of March, the U.S. was forced to begin ordering medical supplies from China, which then airlifted a massive amount of vital medical supplies from Shanghai to the U.S., including 12 million gloves, 130,000 N-95 masks, 1.7 million surgical masks, 50,000 gowns, 130,000 hand sanitizer units and 36,000 thermometers.[99] The assistance increased rapidly. In one week of April alone, there were 75 cargo

---

95 Sun Wei, "British Chinese communities donate 30,000 PPE gowns to NHS," *Global Times,* April 22, 2020, http://www.globaltimes.cn/content/1186348.shtml.

96 Jian Sun, "PPE Donation from British Chinese Community Group," *Times Publications Group,* April 22, 2020, https://times-publications.com/2020/04/22/2333/uk-trade-and-business/.

97 Xinhua, "China sends 302 charter flights for int'l anti-epidemic work," *China. cn.org,* April 7, 2020, http://www.china.org.cn/china/Off_the_Wire/2020-04/07/content_75903130.htm.

98 Global Times, "Capacity of state in China to deal with epidemic far more developed than Western govt: Martin Jacques," *op cit.*

99 "First aircraft carrying medical supplies from China arrives in U.S.," *CGTN,* March 30, 2020, https://news.cgtn.com/news/2020-03-30/First-aircraft-carrying-medical-supplies-from-China-arrives-in-U-S--Ph2wcnA0Ok/index.html.

flights from Shanghai, Beijing and Shenzhen to New York and Los Angeles, each carrying around 80 tons of supplies.[100]

China also provided treatment assistance to the U.S. Zhong Nanshan, China's top respiratory scientist, held multiple video-link teaching sessions with intensive care specialists from Harvard's Medical School, explaining the clinical manifestations and difficulties involved in treating severe and critical novel coronavirus patients. A professor at the Johns Hopkins University School of Medicine said Chinese experts "spared no effort to share their experience."[101] As well, the nation's leading Traditional Chinese Medicine (TCM) experts shared with U.S. counterparts their diagnosis and treatment experience that had proved effective in Wuhan.[102]

A great many Chinese companies, foundations, provinces, and social groups made private donations directly to U.S. hospitals or states by various.[103] The Wanxiang Group, a Chinese multinational manufacturer in Hangzhou, donated 1.1 million face masks and 50,000 protective masks to 12 U.S. states.[104] China's Fujian Province, which was Oregon's sister state, donated 50,000 medical face masks for distribution to frontline workers, in addition to 12,000 masks provided personally by Ambassador Wang Donghua, Consul General of the People's Republic of China in San Francisco, as a gift to the people of Oregon.[105]

However, the treatment of China in the U.S. media overall remained nothing short of reprehensible, the press and airwaves filled for months with a ceaseless flood of denigrating rubbish with the result that Pew polls showed that more than two-thirds of Americans held a negative or strongly negative view of China, which was unquestionably the intent of the media assault. As Martin Jacques said in a live interview in Beijing cited above, the American behavior was "absolutely

---

100 Tu Lei, "Chinese airlines keep flying to US with medical supplies," *Global Times*, April 26, 2020, https://www.globaltimes.cn/content/1186786.shtml.

101 "China selflessly extends helping hand to countries around world in global battle against COVID-19," *People's Daily Online, op cit.*

102 Wu Yong and Huang Zhiling, "TCM experience shared with US counterparts to fight virus," *China Daily*, March 20, 2020, http://www.chinadaily.com.cn/a/202003/20/WS5e740a2ca31012821728094e.html.

103 Alexandra Stevenson, Nicholas Kulish, and David Gelles, "Frantic for Coronavirus Gear, Americans in Need Turn to China's Elite," *The New York Times*, April 24, 2020, https://www.nytimes.com/2020/04/24/business/us-china-coronavirus-donations.html.

104 Xinhua, "Chinese company donates 1.1 mln face masks to 12 US states," *China. org.cn*, May 6, 2020, http://www.china.org.cn/world/2020-05/06/content_76010588.htm.

105 Sam West, "China's Fujian province donates 50,000 face masks to sister state Oregon," *People's Daily Online*, April 29, 2020, http://en.people.cn/n3/2020/0429/c90000-9685576.html.

disgraceful," He went on to say, "Too many Western politicians and the Western media responded to what was a grave medical health crisis in China in a way that was completely lacking in compassion and simply used as a stick to beat China. And in doing so also explicitly or implicitly, they encouraged a certain kind of racism against the Chinese, not just the Chinese in China, but Chinese everywhere."[106]

Some in the West, led by the U.S., heavily politicized China's assistance to other nations, claiming China's acts were done with murky motives and sinister geopolitical intent. The efforts of the Chinese government to help others were categorized as attempts to vie for global influence by vacuuming up America's allies with bribes. And, since the global pandemic was "all China's fault," those donations were merely gestures of atonement camouflaged as charity.[107]

The Chinese people generally were not very sympathetic to the U.S., many comparing America's confused and corrupted efforts with China's leadership. One post that received hundreds of millions of views said, "It took China two months to defeat the coronavirus, while it took the coronavirus two months to defeat the U.S."[108] Similar topics equally drew 250 or 300 million views. One Weibo post received 150 million views almost immediately when suggesting President Trump responded only after 1 million citizens became infected.

Today's urban Chinese are much less naive about international affairs, and were quite aware of the Zionist-American hate propaganda that was filling Western airwaves and sheets of print, and of the resulting racism and hatred being generated toward China and the Chinese people, many of them having been victims of abuse in the U.S. They were also aware of the vast efforts made by their own nation to not only protect the lives of Chinese citizens but of the truly enormous contributions their government, corporations and societies had made to helping other nations while the U.S. denied vital supplies to other countries.[109]

---

106 Global Times, "Capacity of state in China to deal with epidemic far more developed than Western govt: Martin Jacques," *op cit.*

107 Conor Finnegan, "Despite calls for global cooperation, US and China fight over leading coronavirus response," *ABC News,* March 31, 2020, https://abcnews.go.com/Politics/calls-global-cooperation-us-china-fight-leading-coronavirus/story?id=69898820.

108 Yan Yunming, "Chinese netizens concerned as 'coronavirus defeats US' with over 1m cases," *Global Times,* April 29, 2020, https://www.globaltimes.cn/content/1187121.shtml.

109 The US government (primarily FEMA and/or the CIA, in conjunction with Israel's Mossad) were widely accused by France, Germany, and other nations of repeatedly hijacking—on airport tarmacs—shipments of medical supplies destined for other countries. These actions were simultaneous with FEMA's seizures of medical supplies from hospitals and importers all across the US, and there appeared to be substantial evidence much of these supplies were sent to Israel—while US hospitals were bleeding.*

The enormity of anti-China hate literature during the past decade is producing sentiments like, "Send the supplies to Iran, Venezuela and Cuba, and let the Americans learn a lesson." I had a long conversation with a senior Chinese executive who told me of operating his factory 24/7 and pushing his staff to work 12-hour days to produce vital medical supplies for the U.S. while partially sacrificing his commitments to China. After being exposed to the outrageous denigration of China in the U.S. media, he said he would never again take any action to assist Americans. His final comment to me: "After this, I wouldn't cross the road to piss on the U.S. if it were on fire."

---

*There isn't space to follow the story here, but you can follow this set of links below to research the subject.

- https://www.rt.com/news/484743-cuba-covid19-us-blockade/
- https://www.nytimes.com/2020/04/17/opinion/cuba-coronavirus-trump.html
- https://www.ctvnews.ca/health/coronavirus/cuba-u-s-embargo-blocks-coronavirus-aid-shipment-from-asia-1.4881479
- https://www.theguardian.com/world/2020/apr/02/global-battle-coronavirus-equipment-masks-tests
- https://germany.timesofnews.com/breaking-news/us-accused-of-seizing-face-mask-shipments-bound-for-europe-canada
- https://dnyuz.com/2020/04/03/us-accused-of-seizing-face-mask-shipments-bound-for-europe-canada/
- https://abcnews.go.com/Politics/us-works-assure-allies-deny-allegations-seizing-supplies/story?id=70019576
- https://edition.cnn.com/2020/04/04/europe/coronavirus-masks-war-intl/index.html
- https://www.rtl.fr/actu/debats-societe/masques-detournes-les-americains-sortent-le-cash-il-faut-se-battre-dit-jean-rottner-sur-rtl-7800346680
- https://www.lefigaro.fr/international/coronavirus-l-amerique-relance-la-guerre-des-masques-20200402
- https://www.huffingtonpost.fr/entry/coronavirus-des-masques-commandes-par-la-france-detournes-par-des-americains-des-masques-commandes-par-la-france-detournes-par-des-americains_fr_5e84eb13c5b6f55ebf47271a
- https://www.huffingtonpost.in/entry/coronavirus-medical-supplies-countries_in_5e873034c5b63e06281ccebd
- https://abcnews.go.com/Politics/us-works-assure-allies-deny-allegations-seizing-supplies/story?id=70019576
- https://edition.cnn.com/2020/04/04/europe/coronavirus-masks-war-intl/index.html
- https://www.globaltimes.cn/content/1185063.shtml

- https://www.globaltimes.cn/content/1186406.shtml
- https://www.reuters.com/article/us-huawei-tech-fedex-exclusive-idUSKCN1SX1RZ
- https://www.journaldemontreal.com/2020/04/03/des-masques-pour-le-quebec-detournes
- https://nationalpost.com/news/what-happened-when-five-million-medical-masks-for-canadas-covid-19-fight-were-hijacked-at-an-airport-in-china?video_autoplay=true
- https://dnyuz.com/2020/04/03/us-accused-of-seizing-face-mask-shipments-bound-for-europe-canada/
- https://abcnews.go.com/Politics/us-works-assure-allies-deny-allegations-seizing-supplies/story?id=70019576
- https://edition.cnn.com/2020/04/04/europe/coronavirus-masks-war-intl/index.html
- https://www.telegraph.co.uk/news/2020/04/19/flight-carrying-vital-ppe-supplies-nhs-delayed-turkey/
- https://www.telegraph.co.uk/politics/2020/04/18/ministers-plead-overseas-counterparts-allow-shipments-ppe-shortage/
- https://www.telegraph.co.uk/news/2020/05/06/exclusive-gowns-delayed-ppe-shipment-turkey-impounded-failing/
- https://www.al-monitor.com/pulse/originals/2020/04/turkey-aid-covid19-coronavirus-erdogan-satterfield-sweden.html
- https://apnews.com/b940aca2ab2d0c31af2826da9c30d222
- https://www.opednews.com/articles/Are-the-Face-Masks-Stolen-by-Meryl-Ann-Butler-Corona-Virus-Coronavirus-Covid-19-200410-528.html
- https://www.msn.com/en-us/news/us/not-an-ideal-solution-maryland-national-guard-members-advised-to-make-their-own-cloth-masks/ar-BB12eKEL
- https://www.armytimes.com/news/your-army/2020/04/24/army-researchers-say-this-is-the-best-material-for-a-homemade-face-mask-theyve-found-so-far/
- https://twitter.com/TsahiDabush/status/1247601103006502914
- https://urmedium.com/c/presstv/12226
- While American health workers beg for PPE, Trump just shipped a million masks to the Israeli army: https://t.co/2sVFLMteo9 — Ali Abunimah (@AliAbunimah) April 8, 2020
- https://www.jpost.com/Israel-News/US-Department-of-Defense-give-1-million-masks-to-IDF-for-coronavirus-use-623976
- https://www.globalsecurity.org/security/library/news/2020/04/sec-200408-presstv01.htm
- https://www.jpost.com/Israel-News/Mossad-bought-10-million-coronavirus-masks-last-week-622890

- https://abcnews.go.com/Politics/fema-relied-inexperienced-volunteers-find-coronavirus-protective-equipment/story?id=70519484
- https://www.washingtonpost.com/politics/kushner-coronavirus-effort-said-to-be-hampered-by-inexperienced-volunteers/2020/05/05/6166ef0c-8e1c-11ea-9e23-6914ee410a5f_story.html
- https://abcnews.go.com/Politics/fema-relied-inexperienced-volunteers-find-coronavirus-protective-equipment/story?id=70519484
- https://abcnews.go.com/Health/us-short-ppe/story?id=70093430
- https://abcnews.go.com/Politics/kushner-backed-program-charters-flights-medical-supplies-behalf/story?id=70291872
- https://abcnews.go.com/Politics/white-house-wind-coronavirus-task-force-trump-shifts/story?id=70518706
- https://apnews.com/8cd84c260cb6d951ac57a6248542a44f

CHAPTER THREE

难忘半月----从春节到元宵节
舰桥博士

LOCKDOWN:
THE UNFORGETTABLE 15 DAYS FROM THE SPRING FESTIVAL TO LANTERN FESTIVAL 2020

Anonymous

疾风知劲草，烈火炼真金。

Adversity reveals genius, and genuine gold stands raging fire.
—Chinese proverb

我们唯一害怕的就是害怕本身。
—1933年3月4日，富兰克林·罗斯福

The only thing we have to fear is fear itself.
—Franklin Roosevelt, March 4,1933

　　春节是中国民间最隆重盛大的传统节日，是集祈福禳灾、欢庆娱乐和饮食为一体的民俗大节。除夕的家庭团圆，形成了中国一个月内35亿人次的人口流动。中国为此发明了一个特有名词叫"春运"。而新春的贺岁活动更是内容丰富，热闹喜庆，到处充满着浓浓的年味。这些庆祝活动从春节一直延续到中国农历正月十五的元宵节。

　　The Spring Festival is the most solemn and grand traditional festival among Chinese people. It is a folk festival combining blessing and praying, entertainment and the enjoyment of food. The family reunion on New Year's eve leads to the flow of 3.5 billion people in one month. China has invented a special term for this called "chunyun." And the New Year's activities are rich in content, with lively festivals, full of the flavor of the year. These celebrations extend from the beginning of the Spring Festival to the Lantern Festival on the 15th day of the first month of the Chinese lunar calendar.

中国春节通常都在每年的公历二月份。但是今年的春节来得特别早，1月24日就是春节的除夕之夜，相当于西方的圣诞节平安夜。这一天，我所居住的这座中国南方滨海城市，街上到处张灯结彩、花团锦簇、车水马龙、熙熙攘攘，喜庆祥和之气伴着和煦的春风弥漫在城市的每一个角落。此情此景不禁让人想起宋代宰相诗人王安石的名诗："爆竹声中一岁除，春风送暖入屠苏。千门万户瞳瞳日，总把新桃换旧符。"

The Chinese New Year is usually in February of the Gregorian calendar. But the Spring Festival came early this year. January 24 was the eve of the Spring Festival, the western equivalent of Christmas Eve. On this day, in the coastal city in southern China where I live, the streets are decorated with lights, a multitude of flowers, and the traffic is heavy and bustling. This scene cannot help but remind people of the Song dynasty prime minister poet Wang Anshi's famous poem:

With crackers' cracking noise the old year passed away;
The vernal breeze brings us warm wine and warm spring day.
The rising sun sheds light on doors of each household,
New peachwood charm is put up to replace the old.
(or: "Firecrackers bloom a New Year, with breeze and wine we cheer.
The sun warms everyone, the new replaces the old everywhere.")

可是到了吃年夜饭时，突然听到了一则令人不安的消息。湖北省武汉市新近发现的新型冠状病毒大有漫延之势，为此武汉市已经宣布"封城"！政府号召大家采取各种必要的防疫措施，如戴口罩、常洗手、取消聚会，减少外出，甚至居家隔离等等。

But when it came time to eat dinner, I suddenly heard a piece of disturbing news. Wuhan, Hubei province, has declared a "city closure" after a newly discovered coronavirus spread. The government called on people to take all necessary precautions, such as wearing masks, washing their hands often, canceling parties, going out less, and even segregating themselves at home.

最热闹、最快乐的节日一夜之间变成最寂寞、最焦虑的日子。大年初一开始，街上除了快递小哥，几乎看不到人影。为了自己、也为了他人的安全，大部分人都足不出户，实行自我隔离。笔者也不例外。每天在室内，只能通过电视、广播、网络和微信获取与疫情有关的各种信息，以了解疫情发展、国家应对、百姓反应、友邦态度，等等等等。多亏信息时代，虽然坐井观天，却能窥见人间百态，风雨千般。中国有两句古语，一是"疾风知劲草"，一是"患难见真情"。这样的大难临头，也许更有利于我们体会人间冷暖、辨清宦吏忠奸，鉴别朋友真假，反省自身对错。因此，这半个月的隔离观察与思考，让人感触良多。

The most lively and the most happy holiday changed into the most lonely and the most anxious day, overnight. Since New Year's day, few people could be seen in the street except some mailmen. For the safety of oneself and the safety of others, most people stayed indoors and practiced self-segregation. The author was no exception. Every day in the room, I tried my best to collect all kinds of information related to the epidemic through TV, radio, Internet and WeChat to learn about the development of the epidemic, the national response, people's responses, their friendly attitudes, and so on. Thanks to the information age, though isolated, I can still follow the changing world. There are two old sayings in China. One is that a strong wind tells a strong grass. The other is that a friend in need is a friend indeed. Such a disaster, perhaps, is more conducive to our experience of the world's warmth and cold, enabling us to distinguish between officials: loyal or in bed with others; to identify friends: true or false; and to reflect on ourselves: right and wrong. Therefore, this half a month of isolation, observation and thinking, let me experience a lot.

抗击疫情，撼天震地
THE GREAT EFFORTS

这次武汉疫情的发展异常迅猛。从确诊病例数目的增加速度可见一斑：1月24日830人，25日增至1287人，26日1975人，27日2744人，28日4515人，29日5975人，30日7711人，31日9692人，2月1日11823人，2月2日14488人，2月3日17254人，2月4日20520人，2月5日24324人，2月6日31161人，2月7日34601人，2月8日37198人，2月9日40171人，而且病死率不低，平均每天几十人。

This outbreak in Wuhan is developing very rapidly. This can be seen in the rate at which the number of confirmed cases is increasing: On January 24th, there were 830 cases. On the 25th, 1287. On the 26th, 1975. On 27th, 2744. On the 28th, 4515. On the 29th, 5975. On the 30th, 7711. On the 31st, 9692. On February 1, 11823. On February 2, 14488. On the 3rd, 17254. On the 4th, 20520. On the 5th, 24324. On the 6th, 31161. On the 7th, 34601. On the 8th, 37198. On the 9th, 40171. And the case fatality rate is not low: dozens every day on average.

疫情爆发之后，中国党和国家领导人反应迅速，决策果敢，措施有力。中央政治局常委就同一个问题在短短的10天内两次召开会议，这在中国共产党党史上没有先例。更重要的是，会议特别强调"始终把人民群众生命安全和身体健康放在第一位，把疫情防控工作作为当前最重要的工作来抓"。会议对当前的疫情防控工作进行了全面的部署。1月25日第一次政治局会议后，总书记亲自指挥，总理亲临武汉一线指导。2月3日政治局常委会议专门听取了疫情防控工作的汇报后，进行了"再研究、再部署、再动员"。

After the outbreak, Chinese party and state leaders responded quickly, made resolute decisions and took forceful measures. There is no precedent in communist party history for members of the Politburo standing committee to meet twice in just 10 days on the same issue. More importantly, the meetings stressed that "we will always give top priority to the safety and health of the people and make the prevention and control of the epidemic the most important task at hand." The meetings made comprehensive arrangements for the prevention and control of the current epidemic. After the first meeting of the political bureau on January 25, the general secretary took command and the premier came to Wuhan to give guidance. On February 3, the standing committee of the political bureau heard a special report on the prevention and control of the epidemic, and conducted "re-study, re-deployment and re-mobilization."

在党中央的号召下，全国各省、自治区、直辖市、人民解放军实施总动员，打响了一场举国抗击疫情的可歌可泣、撼天动地的人民战争。全国各地向武汉迅速增援医护人员，紧急运送医疗物资，大量调集生活资料。全国平均每天有800多名医护人员增援武汉。每天向武汉输送各种物资数百万吨。解放军更是直接接管了一些重要的医疗机构。特别值得一提的是，在短短的半个月时间里，在武汉神速建成了两座现代化流行病医院：雷神山医院和火神山医院，大大改善了抗疫条件。雷神山、火神山两座医院的迅速设计谋划、迅速动员建设的过程，展现出中国建设队伍在重大战役中高超的指挥调度和统筹协调能力，生动体现了中国现行制度的优越性。全国交通运输系统实施战时运输模式，既要坚决阻断疫情传播，又要保障抗疫人员、物资、器材、设备的快速流通，保障疫区生活物资的正常供应。同时作出了乘客无偿退票的规定，尽可能减少疫期的人员流动。全国基层社区严格实行网格化管理，积极采取防疫检查与隔离的严格措施。全国十几个省市对口支援湖北省十几个地区，以解决当地医疗资源紧缺的燃眉之急。全国春节假期延长到2月2日，学校、幼儿园推迟到2月底开学。总之，中国几乎采取了一切应该采取和能够采取的措施抗击疫情，保护人民群众的生命安全和身体健康。中国的医学科研机构日夜奋战，迅速分离出病毒毒株，测试出基因序列，争分夺秒研制有效药物和疫苗，并及时实行病毒信息的国际共享。

At the call of the CPC central committee, all the provinces, autonomous regions, municipalities directly under the central government and the People's Liberation Army (PLA) launched a general mobilization campaign to fight the epidemic. From all over the country medical personnel, emergency delivery of medical supplies, means of livelihood reinforced Wuhan quickly. On average, more than 800 medical workers are sent to Wuhan every day from across the country. Millions of tons of supplies are sent to Wuhan every day. The PLA directly took over some important medical institutions. It is worth mentioning that in just half a month, two modern epidemic hospitals were built in Wuhan at a great speed: Raytheon Mountain Hospital and Vulcan Mountain Hospital, which greatly improved the anti-epidemic conditions. The rapid design and planning of these two hospitals, as well as the rapid mobilization and construction process, demonstrated the excellent command, dispatch and overall coordination capabilities of the Chinese construction team in major battles, and vividly demonstrated the superiority of China's current system. The implementation of the wartime transport model in the national transport system has not only resolutely prevented the spread of the epidemic, but also ensured the rapid circulation of anti-epidemic personnel, materials, facilities and equipment, and ensured the normal supply of the necessities of life in the affected areas. At the same time it has provided passengers with free refunds to reduce population movement due to the epidemic. The communities throughout the country strictly implement grid management, and take active measures to prevent and quarantine epidemics. More than a dozen provinces and cities across the country have provided assistance to more than a dozen regions in Hubei province to meet the urgent need for medical resources.

The national Spring Festival holiday was extended to February 2, and schools and kindergartens were postponed to the end of February. In short, China has taken almost all measures that should and can be taken to combat the epidemic and protect people's lives and health. Chinese medical research institutes have been working around the clock to isolate viral strains, test genetic sequences, racing against time to develop effective drugs and vaccines, and share virus information internationally.

中国对疫情的反应和投入，在人类抗击流行病史上，堪称速度空前，强度空前，规模空前。中国快速、高效、大量地调动国家资源以应对紧急事件的能力举世瞩目。加上中国抗疫行动的透明性与国际担当，所有这些都赢得了国际卫生组织和众多外国领导人的高度赞扬和崇敬。国际舆论称赞中国为人类抗击流行病树立了典范和标杆。

China's responses and input to overcome the outbreak have been unprecedented in speed, intensity and scale. China's ability to mobilize national resources quickly, efficiently and massively to respond to emergencies is remarkable. Together with the transparency and international responsibility of China's response to the outbreak, all these have won high praise and admiration from the WHO and many foreign leaders.

International public opinion has praised China for setting an example and a benchmark for humankind's fight against epidemic diseases.

赤子情怀，感天动地
THE NOBLE SPIRIT

中华民族的优秀子孙自古以来就有"先天下之忧而忧，后天下之乐而乐"的情怀，始终不忘"天下兴亡，匹夫有责"的使命担当。在这次与病毒的搏斗中，全体中国人民团结一心，众志成城。在民族的危急关头，表现出感天动地的赤子情怀，催人泪下。大年初一，全国各地的许多医护人员，得知疫情后立即决定中止家庭团聚，纷纷请愿要求驰援武汉的抗疫斗争。作为医护人员，他们不会不明白驰援疫区意味着什么，但"明知征途有艰险，越是艰险越向前"。有的甚至在写着"不计报酬、不管生死"的请愿书上，按下血红的手印。84岁高龄的钟南山院士，长时间深入抗疫一线。武汉一传染病医院院长，拖着得了绝症的病体，一瘸一拐地日夜奋战。他说，正因为自己时间不多了，更要格外珍惜时间，加倍抓紧工作。一位女护士在抗击疫情的斗争中感染了病毒被送入病房医治，治愈当天就提出立刻重返岗位的申请。一位传染科主任医生，得知一个科主任、自己的好友在岗位上不幸染毒病危，将不久人世，不禁潸然泪下。但他很快擦干眼泪，投入工作。他说：战友倒下了，但战斗还在继续，我不能有片刻的迟疑和耽搁。许多民营公司、社会团体、国内民众、海外华人纷纷慷慨解囊，捐款捐物。阿里巴巴捐款达10亿之巨。韩红的爱心慈善基金会募捐资金近3亿。一个南航墨尔本返航广州的航班，舱内空无一客，全是澳洲华人为了及时把物资运送回国内，号召大家购票后把无偿捐助的救援物资放在自己的座位上。

Since ancient times, the outstanding descendants of the Chinese nation have always had sentiments of "worry about the world first, and joy for the world later," and they never forget the concept of mission: "In the rise and fall of the world, every man has a responsibility." In this fight against the virus, all Chinese people unite as one. At this critical moment of the nation, they showed their noblest spirit.

On the first day of the New Year, many medical workers all over the country decided to suspend family reunions immediately after learning of the epidemic and petitioned for help in the fight against the disease in Wuhan. As medical staff, they understood well what it means to enter the epidemic area, but they also "know the journey is difficult, the more difficult the more forward." Some even pressed red handprints on petitions that read "regardless of pay, regardless of own life." Professor Zhong Nanshan, an 84-year-old academician, spent a long time in the frontline of anti-epidemic efforts. The head of a hospital for infectious diseases in Wuhan has been limping day and night, dragging his terminally ill body. He said, "because my time is not much, I have to cherish the time more, to work harder." A female nurse who was admitted to the ward after contracting the virus during the battle against the epidemic applied to return to work immediately the same day she was cured. A director of infectious diseases, learning that his friends in the post unfortunately were infected with poison and dying, cannot help but shed tears. But he soon dried his tears and went to work. He said, "My comrades are down, but the battle goes on." Many private companies, social organizations, domestic people, and overseas Chinese have donated generously. Alibaba donated a billion dollars. Han Hong's charity foundation raised nearly 300 million yuan. On a China Southern flight from Melbourne to Guangzhou, there were no passengers in the cabin. All of these Chinese Australians, after buying tickets, had called on everyone to put relief supplies donated for free on their seats in order to deliver the supplies back to China in time.

面对人类的共同敌人，绝大多数国家和民众，无论西方还是东方，无论是发达还是发展中，无论是富有还是贫穷，都表现出了高尚的人道精神和国际情怀。特别是巴基斯坦等欠发达国家，决意要与中国休戚与共，尽其所能援助中国的抗疫斗争。2 月5日，柬埔寨首相洪森特意访问中国，亲临现场声援中国的抗疫斗争。许多国际友人和普通民众同样积极捐款捐物，人道主义精神令人感动。除了中国以外，法国、澳大利亚、美国等众多顶尖医学科研机构展开了一场声势浩大的赶制疫苗的全球攻坚战。2月8号国际卫生组织决定于2月12日在日内瓦举行控制新型冠状病毒肺炎疫情的国际论坛。而当某国的政要声称中国的疫情有利于工作机会流向他的国家时，立即遭到包括他本国在内的国际舆论的广泛批评，斥责这种言论无知无情，近乎幸灾乐祸。

In the face of the common enemies of mankind, the vast majority of countries and people, whether in the east or the west, whether in the developed or developing countries, whether rich or poor, have shown their noble humanitarian spirit and international sentiments. In particular, Pakistan and other less developed countries are determined to share weal and woe with China and do their best to assist China in its fight against the epidemic. On February 5, Cambodian Prime Minister Hun Sen paid a special visit to China to support the country's fight against the epidemic. Many international friends and ordinary people are also active in donating money and goods. The humanitarian spirit is touching. In addition to China, France, Australia, the United States and many other top medical research institutions launched a massive global battle to rush to make vaccines. On February 8th the WHO decided to hold an international forum in Geneva on February 12th to control COVID 19. When a foreign politician claimed that the outbreak in China was conducive to the flow of jobs to his country, he was immediately widely criticized by international opinion, including his own, for being ignorant, heartless and bordering on schadenfreude.

认真反省，别有天地
THE DEEP LESSONS

2003年非典爆发，中国曾经陷入极大的被动，付出了沉重的代价。这一次新型冠状病毒爆发，中国陷入更大的被动，付出更大的代价。这是不是在同一个地方跌了两跤？而且这次比上一次跌得更重，摔得更惨。但是，有党和国家的高度重视，有全体国民的众志成城，艰苦卓绝，有国际力量的大力支持，大家对打赢这场对病毒的全面抗战抱有必胜的信心。中国一定赢，中国必须赢！但即便赢了，中国这一次可不能再好了伤疤忘了疼。而应该深刻总结、认真吸取教训。关于这个严肃而沉重的话题，笔者人微言轻，说与不说没有太大区别。但是同样受"天下兴亡，匹夫有责"信条的驱使，冒昧谈四点管见。

When SARS broke out in 2003, China fell into great passivity and paid a heavy price. At the outset of this outbreak of the new coronavirus, China was more passive and, as a result, has paid a higher price. Did it fall twice in the same place? And this outbreak was much worse than the last one. However, with the great importance attached to it by the party and the state, with the unity of all the people, their arduous work and the strong support of international forces, the Chinese people have the confidence to win the war against the virus. China will win! China must win! But even if they win, China can't mend its wounds this time. Instead, they should summarize and draw lessons from them. On this serious and heavy topic, the author is too insignificant to draw public attention. For him to say or not say makes little difference. However, also driven by the maxim "In the rise and fall of the world, the common man has a responsibility" the author ventures to elaborate four views.

第1，建立健全高效的防疫体系是保障平安的根本途径。防疫工作的重心是"防"而不是"抗"。对于任何传染病，都应该以防为主。防比抗容易，防比抗代价要低很多。因此应该在它流行之前，一方面要采取措施严防其传播。一方面深入研究它，测出病源体基因序列，研制出有效药物和疫苗。这样病毒就不大可能传播，即便传播了也不至于造成太大的危害。中国早在2018年就在武汉发现了新型冠状病毒，也初步了解其潜在危险，中央电视台还作了广播。中国国家疾病控制中心2019年12月就已经知道武汉新型冠状病毒已经传染到人，甚至预测了疫情即将爆发。张继先医生12月29日通过组织报告了疫情，李文亮等八位医生12月30日在网友圈提醒大家警惕疫情。但为什么国家从中央到地方没有采取必要的防范措施，为什么相关部门和研究机构不组织力量进行研究，制造药物和疫苗？非要等到暴发了再来"抗击"？这里的原因也许不止一个，但至少包括了中国目前防疫体系不健全特别是防疫法规和防疫组织不健全这一重要因素。如果防疫法规不完善、防疫队伍不健全，工作职责不分明，工作落实不到位，这样的防疫体系就不具备快速反应、有效运作的功能，充其量只有在高层领导的"高度重视"和强力推动下才能发挥作用。而实践证明这样发挥的作用往往是滞后的。因此，必须从立法上、组织上采取有力措施，让防疫工作有法可依，有章可循，违法必罚，违章必究。让防疫队伍实现组织完善，职责分明，保障有力，运作高效。

First, establishing and improving an efficient epidemic prevention system is the fundamental way to ensure safety.

The focus of epidemic prevention is "prevention" rather than containment. For any infectious disease, we should give priority to prevention. Prevention is easier and much cheaper than containment. Therefore, measures should be taken to prevent epidemic spread in advance. On the one hand, the Chinese people should conduct an in-depth study of it, detect the source of its gene sequence, and develop effective drugs and vaccines. This makes it less likely that the virus will spread, and if it does, it won't do much harm. China discovered the new coronavirus in Wuhan in 2018, and got a preliminary understanding of its potential dangers. CCTV also broadcast about it in the same year. China's national center for disease control knew in December 2019 that the Wuhan coronavirus had spread to humans, even predicting an imminent outbreak. Doctor Zhang Jixian reported the epidemic situation through the organization on December 29, and Doctor Li Wenliang and seven other doctors brought everyone's attention to the epidemic situation in the net circle on December 30. But why didn't the country—from the central government to the local government—take the necessary preventive measures, and why didn't the relevant departments and research institutions organize efforts to conduct research and manufacture drugs and vaccines? Why wait until the outbreak to "fight"? There may be more than one reason for this, but at least one important factor is that China's epidemic prevention system is not sound, especially its epidemic prevention laws and regulations and its epidemic prevention organizations are not sound. If the epidemic prevention laws and regulations are not perfect, the epidemic prevention team is not sound, the work responsibilities are not clear, the implementation of the work is not in place, such an epidemic prevention system will not function as a rapid response, effective operation. At best in such a situation, only the senior leadership's "heightened attention" and strong promotion can play a role. Such a role has been proved in practice to often be lagging. Therefore, we must take effective measures in legislation and organization to ensure that epidemic prevention work has laws to follow and rules to follow. Let the epidemic prevention team achieve organizational perfection, with clear responsibilities, strong support, and efficient operation.

第2，改善卫生环境、提高国民文明素质是防疫、抗疫的重要基础。历史经验证明，疫情的暴发往往与社会的卫生环境和群众的不文明生活习惯紧密相关。特别是食用野生动物的恶习与传染病的传播有很大关系。而疫情发生后发展的快慢，同样与社会的医疗卫生条件和民众的素质息息相关。感染人群如果不能得到及时有效的治疗、隔离，疫情就会在疫区迅速漫延。疫区人群如果不以大局为重，大量流向非疫区，外部地区将很快遭殃，其后果不堪设想。这次武汉疫情在当地传播如此之快，与没有及时隔离、有效治疗紧密相关。病毒之所以迅速漫延到全国各地甚至国外，不能不说与疫情发生后，恐慌之数以百万计的人口离开武汉有关。历史表明，疫情发生时，不同的国民素质会有截然不同的反应，会对疫情的后续发展产生截然不同的影响。当年欧洲发生黑死病疫情时，同样有大量的疫区人员流向非疫区，造成将近一半人口的死亡。但在英国也有一个疫区与非疫区交界的村庄，全体村民虽然已被传染却宁可就地病死也不逃向非疫区，从而以自己的牺牲保护了相邻的村民。他们的信条是：宁可死亡也要把善良传给后代。要在短时间内大幅改善全社会的医疗卫生条件，对任何国家都不是一件容易的事情，但中国目前已经较有财力物力，更有迅速调动国家资源集中使用的体制优势。只要国家尽快完善相关法律法规，加大财政投入，民间社团和企业积极响应，广大民众主动配合，就一定能够做到。而提高国民文明素质决非易事，中国更是任重道远，但只要从健全法律法规与加强教育两方面入手，坚持不懈，就一定能够较快实现。

Second, Improving the sanitary environment and the civilizational level of the people are important bases for epidemic prevention and anti-epidemic organization.

Historical experience has proved that the outbreak of an epidemic is often closely related to the social health environment and the uncivilized living habits of the masses. The vice of consuming wild animals in particular has much to do with the spread of infectious diseases. The speed of development after the outbreak is also closely related to the medical and health conditions of the society and the civilizational level of the people. If the infected population cannot get timely and effective treatment, and be isolated, the epidemic will spread rapidly in the affected areas. If the affected areas do not focus on the overall situation, a large number of people will flow to non-affected areas, and the external areas will soon suffer. The consequences are unimaginable. The Wuhan outbreak is spreading so quickly locally, which is closely related to the lack of timely isolation and effective treatment. The rapid spread of the virus throughout the country and even abroad has to do with the panic of millions of people leaving Wuhan after the outbreak. History shows that when an epidemic occurs, different national qualities will have different responses and this will have different impacts on the subsequent development of the epidemic. During the black death epidemic in Europe, a large number of people from affected areas also moved to non-affected areas, killing nearly half of the population. However, in Britain, there was also a village at the border between the epidemic area and the non-epidemic area. Although all the villagers had been infected, they would rather die on the spot than flee to the non-epidemic area, thus protecting the neighboring villagers with their own sacrifice. Their creed was: To preach good, choose death. It is not easy for any country to improve the medical and health conditions of the whole society in a short period of time, but China already has more financial and material resources and more institutional advantages to mobilize the national resources quickly and intensively. As long as the state improves relevant laws and regulations as soon as possible, increases financial input, civil societies and enterprises actively respond, and the general public take the initiative to cooperate, we will be able to do so. China has a long way to go. However, as long as we continue to improve laws and regulations and strengthen education, we will be able to achieve this goal fairly quickly.

第3，科学的用人制度是防疫抗疫的组织保障。事实已经反复证明，如果一种用人制度，使得被用干部只在乎上级领导而不在乎下级和群众，那他们就会惧上不惧下，进而欺上而压下。为了显示所谓的政绩，让上级满意，有些干部就会报喜不报忧。发生疫情显然多少会影响相关官员的政绩，他们因而就可能产生拖报甚至瞒报疫情的动机。但是，疫情的侦测与报告恰恰必须分秒必争。疫情报告如同火情报告、战情报告，生死攸关，十万火急。任何的拖延和隐瞒都是对国家安全和人民生命财产的严重危胁，都是滔天之罪。当年非典之所以酿成大祸，跟疫情报告不及时有关，如今新型冠状病毒肆虐，同样也有相同的原因。这次疫区的一些官员，面对突发疫情不但没有尽快向市民发出警报，火速采取防控措施，而是千方百计地隐瞒、拖报。只想维护自己的"政绩"，不在乎百姓的死活。会出现这样的官员，应该从用人机制上找原因。拿出腕骨的勇气，改革用人机制，从根本处解决问题。

Third, the scientific system of engaging the people is the organizational guarantee of epidemic prevention and epidemic resistance. It has been proved time and again that if a system of employing cadres makes them care only for the superior and not for the subordinate and the masses, they will be afraid of the superior instead of the subordinate, flatter the superior while suppressing the inferior. In order to show their so-called achievements and satisfy the superiors, some cadres will report the good news but not the bad news. An outbreak obviously affects the performance of officials in some way, so they may have an incentive to delay or even conceal reporting an outbreak. But the detection and reporting of outbreaks must be done, racing against the clock. Outbreak reports are like fire reports, war reports. It's a matter of life and death. Any delay or concealment is a grave threat to national security and people's lives and property, and is a heinous crime. The same reason why SARS had such a disastrous impact was related to the untimely reporting of the epidemic. Now the epidemic of this new coronavirus is related to the same reasons. In the face of the outbreak some officials in the affected areas not only did not alert the public as soon as possible, or take measures to prevent and control, but rather they did everything possible to conceal and delay the report. They just wanted to protect their own "achievements," did not care about the lives of the people. To explain why such officials appear we should look for reasons in the employment mechanism. We have to take great pains to reform the personnel mechanism so as to solve the problem from the root.

Fourth, investigating who is guilty of negligence and punishing wrongdoers are necessary measures to put an end to future trouble. Outbreaks are natural disasters. But the extent of natural disasters often depends on human mistakes. This outbreak is doing just that. One of the serious problems is the delay in reporting and concealment of outbreaks by relevant agencies and departments. It is this delay and cover-up that has contributed to the local and international spread of the disease. Different positions, different departments have different responsibilities. Here is a brief analysis of the three departments and agencies.

1. 中国疾控中心。2020年1月22日，中国疾控中心主任向世界著名医学刊物英国的《新英格兰通讯》投送了新型冠状病毒的研究论文。这篇论文预计："通过分析12月10日至1月4日期间发病病例的数据，来估算疫情的增长速度，因为我们预计在12月13日武汉疫情正式宣布之后，发现的感染比例将很快增加"。由此可见，他和他所领导的中心知道这种病毒具有高传染性。既然如此，他为什么在面对国内大众时却说：大家放心过年，冠状病毒不会人传人。疫情可防、可控、可治，不要相信谣言。一经发现造谣者，立马严惩不贷。就在他忙于撰写论文、叫大家放心过年的半个月时间内，武汉数百万人口流向全国各地。他到底良知何在？职业道德何在？在他撰写论文之前，即1月5日之前，中国疾控中心向有关上级部门报告疫情了没有？提出对策建议了没有？如果没有就是严重的失职！这类似于总参作战部收到敌军马上要对本国发动核打击的确切情报，作战部长却只是组织一班人马把它写成一篇爆炸性新闻拿到报社投稿！千古奇闻，万年遗臭！

Chinese Center for Disease Control. On January 22, 2020, the director of the Chinese Center for Disease Control presented a research paper on the new coronavirus to the world-famous medical journal, *New England Journal of Medicine*. The paper predicts: "the growth rate of the outbreak was estimated by analyzing the data of cases that occurred during the period of December 10 solstice and January 4, as we expect the rate of infection to increase rapidly after the official announcement of the outbreak in Wuhan on December 13." So he and his center staff already knew the virus was highly contagious. That being the case, why did he say to the public at home: people can rest assured that the coronavirus will not spread from person to person. The epidemic can be prevented, controlled and treatable. Don't believe rumors. Once the rumor mongers are found, they will be severely punished immediately. During the half month that he was busy writing a paper and let everyone rest assured for the New Year, millions of people in Wuhan flew to other parts of the country. Where is his conscience? Where is his work ethic? Before he wrote his paper, that is, before January 5, did the Chinese Center for Disease Control report the outbreak to the relevant superior departments? Had it suggested any countermeasures? It would be a grave dereliction of duty if it didn't! This is similar to a situation where the general staff of a war department received exact intelligence that the enemy is about to launch a nuclear attack on the country, but the minister of operations just organized a team to write the sensational news in a newspaper! The behavior is so strange that it will go down in history as a symbol of infamy.

2.武汉疾控中心。作为武汉地区疾病监控前哨阵地的武汉疾控中心，对于本次武汉流行病大爆发具有不可推卸的责任。在整个疫情酝酿和爆发的过程中它发挥了多大作用，是正面还是负面作用，相信中央调查组一定会调查清楚。在这里不妨提供一些相互关联的事实。2019年12月8日武汉出现第一例新型冠状病毒性肺炎，12月26~29日湖北省中西医结合医院张继先医生陆续接待7个与该病有同样病症的患者，并及时报告领导，12月30日李文亮、刘文等8个医生在微信圈提醒大家要警惕新型肺炎，1月10~11日累计7名医务人员发现被传染，1月15日中国疾控中心内部发文，启动一级应急响应，1月16日发布通报：不排除有限的人传人。就在这传染性疾病开始流行的危急关头，武汉宣布封城的4天前，即1月19日，武汉疾控中心主任竟然发表电视讲话，断言此次新型肺炎传染性不强。一个疾控中心在疫情来袭时不是唤起民众警惕，向政府献计献策积极防控，而是继续麻痹大众。这也好有一比：敌军的核弹正向本国领土飞来，作战部长对国民发表电视讲话：不要紧，敌人核弹的当量不大！

千古罪人啊！如果不是第二天钟南山院士明确宣布该病毒会人传人，中央进而决定采取封城的果断措施，中国将万劫不复！

The Center for Disease Control in Wuhan. As an outpost of disease monitoring in Wuhan, The Center for Disease Control in Wuhan has an inescapable responsibility for the outbreak of epidemic disease in Wuhan. The public believes the central investigation team from Beijing will find out the extent of the role it played in the whole process of the outbreak, whether it was positive or negative. Here, some interrelated facts may be provided. On December 8, 2019 in Wuhan, the first case of a new type of coronary viral pneumonia appeared in the combined traditional Chinese and western medicine hospital in Hubei province. On December 26-29 Dr. Zhang Jixian dealt with 7 cases having the same symptoms of coronary viral pneumonia, and promptly reported this to the leadership. On December 30 Wen-liang Li, Liu Wen and another 6 doctors in WeChat alerted everybody to beware the outbreak of a pneumonia. January 10-11, a total of seven medical staff were found to be infected. On January 15, the Chinese Center for Disease Control issued an internal alert as an emergency response. On January 16 the Center issued a report saying: do not rule out limited human-to-human transmission. At this critical juncture of the outbreak, four days before Wuhan announced the closure of the city, that is, on January 19, the director of the Center for Disease Control in Wuhan gave a television address, declaring that the new pneumonia infectiousness was not strong. Instead of raising awareness and offering advice to the government, the CDC continued to paralyze the public. Compare this to a situation where, when the enemy's nuclear bombs are en route to their territory, the minister of war counsels by means of a national television speech: never mind, the yield of the enemy's nuclear bombs is not big!

If it had not been for Professor Zhong Nanshan's clear announcement the next day that the virus would spread from person to person, the central government would have failed to take the decisive step of sealing the city, China would have been doomed!

3.省市政府部门。疫情发生后，湖北省政府、武汉市政府有没有及时向中央报告？我们不得而知。但我们看到的是，中央决定武汉封城之前，这两级政府并没有全力以赴，采取一切必要的措施抗击疫情。相反，封城之前武汉灯红酒绿，莺歌燕舞，大型集会此起彼伏，机场、车站、码头人流涌动。半个月之内，数百万人流出武汉。更有甚者，当地政府部门对于发生疫情的消息进行封锁。对在媒体上发布疫情消息的人士进行打压。武汉市公安局把在网上发布疫情消息的李文亮（已经于2020年2月7日死于新型冠状病毒，享年34岁。）等八位医生当作"造谣"者传唤至派出所加以训诫，施以惩处。另外，如果没有领导的意图，1月19日武汉疾控中心主任岂敢发表麻痹公众的电视讲话？

Provincial and municipal government departments. Did the Hubei provincial government and Wuhan municipal government report the outbreak to the central government in time?

We don't know. But what we see is that before the central government decided to seal off Wuhan, the two levels of government did not fully take all necessary measures to combat the epidemic. On the contrary, before the closure of the city, Wuhan had been indulging in a false peace and prosperity. Large gatherings took place, one after another. The airports, stations and wharf were crowded with people. Within half a month, millions of people left Wuhan. What's more, local government departments blocked news of the outbreak, cracking down on those who leaked any information about the outbreak to the media. The public security bureau in Wuhan summoned Li Wenliang (who died of the new coronavirus on February 7, 2020, at the age of 34) and other eight doctors who warned local citizens of a possible outbreak of coronavirus to the police station to reprimand, and impose punishment on them as "rumormongers." In addition, if not incited by some authority, how could the director of the Wuhan Center for Disease Control and Prevention dare to make such a public television address on January 19, to paralyse the local people?

再者，国民感到十分困惑的是，中国外交部新闻发言人说，中国早在1月3日起共30次向国外通报了疫情和防控措施。而国内绝大多数民众正式得到疫情通报却迟到大年三十，也就是1月24日。发生在中国的疫情要先向外国人报告，而且报告那么勤，中国人却要晚3周才有知情权，这是为什么？

What's more, to the great confusion of the Chinese people, the spokesman of the Chinese foreign ministry said that China had notified the foreign countries of the outbreak and control measures 30 times since January 3. The vast majority of people in the country were only officially notified of the outbreak on January 24, the eve of the Chinese lunar New Year. The outbreak in China should be reported to foreigners first, and so often, but the Chinese people, who had the right to know, were only advised about it three weeks later. Why?

这一次，深受其害的国民真是忍无可忍了！纷纷在各种非官方媒体愤怒发声，强烈要求依法对防疫中的失职者、渎职者特别是企图掩盖疫情的罪犯彻底清查，严惩不贷。2月7日，经中央批准，国家监察委员会决定派出调查组赴湖北省武汉市，就群众反映的涉及李文亮医生的有关问题作全面调查。网民对此反应热烈，并且希望国家监察委员会也将派出调查组赴中国疾病控制中心认真调查。他们说，还原真相，就能稳定人心；呵护正义，就能凝心聚力；捍卫法治尊严，更能凝聚起团结一心的强大力量。还白衣勇士们一个清白，给祸国殃民者应有下场，向全国人民作出交待。否则，不仅天理不容，而且这种人间惨剧还将重演。

This time, the suffering of the people is really unbearable! They have voiced their anger in various non-official media, calling for a thorough investigation and punishment in accordance with the law for those who fail to perform their duties, especially those who attempt to cover up the epidemic. On February 7, with the approval of the central government, the national supervisory commission decided to send an investigation team to Wuhan, Hubei province, to conduct a comprehensive investigation into the public's concerns about Li Wenliang. The citizens responded enthusiastically and hoped that the national supervisory commission would send an investigation team to the Chinese Center for Disease Control. They said: if you restore the truth, you can stabilize people. If you care for justice, we will be able to concentrate our efforts. If you safeguard the dignity of the rule of law, we will be able to rally a strong force of unity.. Those who brought misfortune to the country and the people deserve to be punished. To make their confession to the people of the country. Otherwise, heaven forbid, this human tragedy will be repeated.

如果以上四条教训能够吸取，有理由相信中国的防疫工作必将展现一片新的天地。

If the above four lessons can be learned, there are reasons to believe that China's epidemic prevention work will open up a new horizon.

CHAPTER FOUR

LIVING THROUGH THE LOCKDOWN:
AN AFRICAN WOMAN'S COVID-19 DIARY

Anonymous

I AM BLACK

Being Black during the COVID-19 outbreak in China will forever resonate with me partly as a racial situation as well as an epidemic. I am one person who tries as much as possible to overlook racial issues and I try not to be sensitive or count it as one of those things. But I knew from day one that the effects of this epidemic could be devastating for people of African origin. This chapter is a story-telling experience of my time during the lockdown.

Warning: If you get sensitive about racial issues, please do not read further.

It has been 77 days since the word "coronavirus" has entered daily vocabulary. At this point, one cannot tell how many times I have used it. I heard it first on the subway as I was heading to town. I immediately took a quick stop in the middle of that trip at the next station. I knew I could probably find a FamilyMart[1] store and buy a pack of masks. I was fortunate enough, so I purchased the only one available for ¥10, and it contained 10 pieces. The only thoughts in my head were *"I am Black I can't fall sick,"* and I kept repeating that till I joined another train. That was Day 1.

DAY 1

I made it back to where I was going, looking weird with my mask on. I was taking no chances! So I made a quick mental calculation... *"If I got on a train... What if someone coughs?"* So I decided on taking a cab back.

My driver started coughing! He is probably a smoker because the vehicle had the unpleasant smell of cigarettes and herbal tea. I told him to stop, but then again, I had no right. He probably hasn't read the crazy things I had been reading on

---

1 FamilyMart is Japan's largest convenience store chain, also very common in almost all Chinese major cities.

WeChat[2] a few hours ago about a virus spreading in Wuhan. So even though I told him not to spit out of the window, I also shifted to the other side of the window, wore my sunshades and looked officially crazy.

I am Black, I can't fall sick!! Now the battle has begun.

On my ride home, I pondered so much on this strange sickness. Where was it from, and where is Wuhan? Do Black people have it? They said it was from an animal market, is it like the swine flu or SARS!? I did not care much about other people at that point, because I worried about the origin of the virus. If it was a family of the Ebola Virus strain, then Africans are in big trouble. In that 40-minute ride, I worried so much about the effect of the virus racially in China. I did not know that while I was writing this on day 79, it would have spread right over the Great Wall, settling in Italy then swiftly moving to the West.

"I am Black, I cannot afford to catch any Virus." By now, you must be tired of my repetitive phrase. Let me break it down.

Five months before the outbreak of the Coronavirus, I had an accident and was taken to the ER. For about 20 minutes, no one attended to me. I guess I was foreign, and they don't understand English. I was just placed on the stretcher, my blood pressure was checked, and that was it! I was only saved when my colleague's wife, who was Chinese, came to my rescue. I was placed in a separate room alone because I requested it, as I will not want to raise my skirt in a ward where there are men and women. The communication was unbearable even with the translator device provided by my office. My wound was not cleaned until the next day. I was allergic to a prescription in my drip, my hands began to swell, but nothing was done for hours. And by the time it was, the nurse yanked the needle off, and my blood splattered on the floor while she added that she was not going to give me any more medicine. It was not cleaned until the next janitor's shift. I was just relieved she does not have to poke me anymore with that needle as my veins were not easy to locate as I had so much melanin. After seeing some nice doctors and running a lot of tests I left the hospital before I was discharged. It was uncomfortable for me.

I was not going to have that experience anymore. So, if that virus was floating anywhere, I do not want it near me. It was hard being a Black English-speaking foreigner in a Chinese hospital.

DAY 8

Everyone is now aware of the virus. I was scared, so I stayed indoors. Most of my colleagues had left our apartment complex and gone somewhere else for vacation. The Coronavirus was spreading in Wuhan, the numbers were going up

---

2 The most common or widely used Chinese Messaging app.

daily. It was time to officially stock up on groceries. I dashed out, walking on needles. *I wore gloves, two masks, grabbed my bottle of sanitizer and rode my e-bike to the closest mall.* The supermarket was filled up. I thought everyone was supposed to stay indoors. But then if they were like me, they needed to stock up on supplies. So I grabbed instant noodles first because it was going out fast. Yes, *Indomie*[3] first!!!

Vegetables were gone, lemons were expensive, we were all moving fast! *Garlic, Ginger, fruits, sanitary pads, handwash, hmm meat (they were well preserved), bread, cola.* The queue was so long, but we were all going to stock up even if it was the longest in the world Then I noticed it—no one was staring at me. That was strange. It was a good thing, but it felt weird at the same time. My visit to public places like malls does not go without someone pointing at me, looking at me like I was out of place. Children and adults will whisper *"hei ren, hei ren,"* 黑人，黑人.[4] I know I am Black, but the incessant rhythmic tone of it drove me crazy when I first arrived here. But now it stopped. This was a part of me, but now the virus was king over it, as everyone minded their own business. This mask and the need to stay alive for the first time knows no skin colour. The virus came with a crown, Corona is King. While I breathed a sigh of relief, in the world out there, some other people were fighting not to be the face of the virus. The media was filled with campaigns against discrimination against Asians. I went to my Facebook and wrote a long post on why the virus is the enemy, not humans. *"We are humans, not virus."* I added that as an African, I too am not a *virus,* just because Ebola was in Africa some years back.

Day 18

As the days went by I began to wonder if it would eventually be a good thing that Africans were not being infected by the disease. There was only one student who had been on the news, and he was discharged a few days later. I foolishly thought that maybe we were immune to this virus. I wondered if people thought *"Oh, maybe Africans can't contact the Virus."* That did not make me in any way careless, but I was in a way relieved for Africans because I feared soon people will find a way to say it was from Africa. I still occasionally got the Ebola stop and search at airports last year even though I had been coming from Europe and had only stopped over in Belgium. Yes, it is better to keep the country safe, but when the other Black family on my flight was not stopped because they had British passports, then I wondered if it is an offence to be African.

---

3 Indomie is a brand of instant noodles produced by an Indonesian company. It is widely distributed in so many countries especially Nigeria and luckily in China

4 *Hei ren* = Black person.

I had been reading weblinks of Africans volunteering at the railway stations, I saw pictures of our brothers holding thermometers and performing health checks. I was proud of them. We do our best, we love everyone, we go out of our way to help. I wondered if this is all going to last. We all sang, cried and shouted *"*中国加油，武汉加油，*Zhongguo Jiayou, Wuhan Jiayou!"* (*China keep fighting, Wuhan Keep fighting!*) This virus is our fight, it does not matter who is affected, white or black, we keep fighting!

I still wondered how all this is going to pan out, will we go back to being sneered at on the train? But first, we fight a common enemy. *Coronavirus!*

Day 29

Back home in Nigeria, the comments on social media were brutal! It felt like the world was against us. Nigerians in Wuhan wanted to be evacuated as some other countries had evacuated their citizens. We were all emotional. People's social media accounts were blocked because they were tagging authorities for help. I would never forget how we were laughed at in a video on national TV. It was a mess!! Then came Nigerians on social media. We were mocked and rejected like it was a crime if people moved abroad. There was no empathy!!! I finally broke. *I cried!*

I was only contented by the fact that people were being discharged in Wuhan and some other cities now. China was winning against the virus. Yes! I started putting much hope in the country that feeds me, not the one I am from. The Wuhan Nigerians got some relief materials as seen in some online news outlets. Soon enough people calmed down or lost hope. I did not pretend to know how they felt because I was far away from the epicentre.

By the end of February, my friends and family would check on me, via Whatsapp, but I remember at one point, I could not take it anymore. I wanted to break. They asked short random questions, but it was not warm enough to envelop the deep hole in me. At a point, I had been indoors for 18 days. I tried to go out of the gate, but the management said No. I thought about jumping, but I was on the 7th floor, and I am not in any way suicidal. I would have loved to jump to my *freedom,* not my death. I just wanted to see people. No one outside my sphere of influence or even my circle of friends outside understood how I felt. I did not want to die, but I wanted to fly. I was saved by work. Online school or teaching in my case, saved my life!

Day 50

The joy of seeing their faces and being able to solve their academic challenges or even making them smile by cracking a dry joke, making crazy faces and sending teacher emojis, made me look forward to my mornings. They would show up in the little spaced-out boxes on Zoom platform trying to be of good cheer. I wondered every time what imperfections lie beyond the positive glares of these teenagers in front of me. They came early to class, especially when they do not have internet connection problems. I could see it in their eyes that it was hard adapting to this life, but we were all helpless, and I try to make do with the shift in our usual teaching curriculum which worked most days. My students have changed, they turned in homework effectively and on time and most importantly, they were communicating. They would ask questions using the Microsoft Teams chatting platform, and this made me happy because they are not used to asking open questions. We are still trying to challenge every new development, even though we have been at this for 7 weeks. In the 10th week of this semester we will be resuming physical school.

DAY 76

Yesterday I went out of my apartment gate after 9 days. I felt like an adolescent girl who was released the first time in her life to go see boys. I rode my bike around for a while. Stopped to get some groceries and also checked out a new bookshop beside the mall. I felt free. But my heart aches for the nations out there where the death toll is surging. My Italian friend called me out of the blue, two or three weeks back. I could feel the weight of the situation in his voice. He said they had lost over 700 people that day. It was so sad because Italy is one of my favorite countries on earth. Therefore, thinking a part of it was crumbling away made me so sad. My country has had a limited number of cases. The government is trying to handle it, but there is limited medical equipment and supplies. There were donations from Jack Ma, as seen on the news and social media, and there is a long list of Billionaire Nigerians who have donated money, but there is still a lack. The Medical Association once sent out a letter listing their expectations. I cannot but ask myself, *"where are the large donations really going? What happened to Jack Ma's provisions?"*

DAY 78

The hate is back. I woke up to series of videos flying around on WeChat showing stranded Nigerians in Guangzhou, a city with the most Black people in China. I saw some clips about Nigerians who were on business trips and had quarantined for 14 days, but now they are displaced on the streets. There was information being passed around that some foreigners were refused accommodation in hotels. There were other short videos of some Chinese stores avoiding Black foreigners.

I try not to personalize negative experiences against Africans or Black people in China until I am sure of the stories. Even at that, I try to be as open-minded, and also to be very finicky with my comments, especially on social media, most notably because of misinformation. I would do nothing that will tarnish my name or make my somewhat new existence uncomfortable. Therefore, I did not want to get myself in this fresh tension between the African Community and the Guangzhou authorities. And for a fact, I live far away from there. However, I could not help but think that, yet again, this Coronavirus is slowly beginning to pose Africans as the "threat or the disease." Reports came in that Africans, especially Nigerians, were separated from others and asked to get the Nucleic Acid tests. An account said his Mexican friend or housemate had requested to take the test and they were told it's just for Africans. This made my blood boil, but there was nothing I could do. It's the job of the Embassy to help its citizens. I am sure you think I should call them out; I should uphold and defend the Black race. I won't, now it is time for my government to stand up. It's time for mother Africa to help her children. Will you abandon us again? I went to bed on this day crippled by my thoughts.

Day 80

This is the eightieth day since I heard about this virus. It's shaking the world. And our lives will never be the same. In the past few days, some Nigerians in Guangzhou were reported to have been separately tested by health workers showing up in their houses and specifically asking to conduct a Nucleic Acid test on just Africans. Some days before a Nigerian had made the news for allegedly beating a nurse trying to treat him. I knew this action was brewing big trouble for the Nigerian community in that city or all over the country. Ignorant netizens will tear Black people apart with their words online. As it is now, the virus is allegedly spread by foreigners. Some foreigners were refused entrance to restaurants, malls, and I read a chat history where a foreigner was tagged "DANGER." These are crazy times. Even though at the height of the spread we all wanted to survive and no one cared about skin colour, as the world around me slowly returns back to normal, fingers are being pointed again

Day 82

I had been debating back and forth with a friend today. He had confronted me about the maltreatment of Nigerians or Africans in Guangzhou and insensitively emphasizing on a clap back question on whether I would or wouldn't have questioned the Nucleic Acid Test if it had been on my doorstep and I was singled out as an African and asked to take the test. This is a profound question. He is testing me. He wanted to know where my loyalty lies. So, I laid it all out. If I was asked to do a nucleic acid test even though I had not been out of my city this year, the request would have passed through my workplace. I will ask questions about why I was the "only" one taking it. If the answers are not forthcoming or not transparent enough. I will ask about the procedure, especially if it is invasive. Then I will let my colleagues or supervisor know that I was asked to be tested. If they are not available, then I will record the whole situation with their approval. I will not fight because I am in my right senses, and even though the case is racial, the world is in a medical emergency. Even though a broadcast a few days earlier of two French doctors talking about using Africans as lab rats supposedly had sparked tensions all over the world. I will still take the test because my health matters and it may cost me my job. Yes, call me a coward, but *"no one knows where the shoe pinches, but he who wears it."*

Day 90

Living as an African in China during this epidemic makes you sensitive. Even when the strict regulations put in place now are for all foreigners, it feels as if it is an attack directed at you. We had struggled before COVID-19, but now it is a mix of both. And if you dare complain, you get the measured response of, *"Go back to your country."* America wants us to go back to our continent, China says go back to your country. This brings me back to the first day on that train; *"I do not want this virus near me, I am Black, I do not want to be sick, because fingers will be pointed."*

I can still listen to my voice echoing right behind me. I will always hear it till day 100.

PART III
Economic Impact

CHAPTER FIVE

DOES THE 21ST CENTURY'S FIRST GREAT WORLDWIDE ECONOMIC DEPRESSION LIE AHEAD?

Jack Rasmus

Economists generally distinguish between what they call "normal" recessions and "great recessions"—as well as between both normal, great and what's called an economic depression. All three forms of capitalist economic contractions share certain characteristics in common, but are distinguished by certain fundamental differences as well.[1]

By all accounts, after four months of economic collapse—March 2020 through June 2020—the U.S. economy is clearly now mired in another Great Recession once again. And it appears the current 2020 Great Recession 2.0 is far worse than the 2008–09 prior Great Recession event. Moreover, the odds are greater today than in 2008 that the current 2.0 contraction may evolve into the first Great Depression of the 21st century.

Great recessions are worse than "normal" recessions in the depth and duration of their economic decline. They are also anterooms to Great Depressions. They may be prevented from evolving into bona fide depressions; or they may fail to be contained, deteriorate further, and eventually transform into a Great Depression. They are thus highly unstable events.

So how does today's Great Recession 2.0 compare on the spectrum of U.S. capitalist crises and collapse over the past century? And will it be prevented from further deteriorating? By all indications thus far, the chances of the latter are growing. What happens in the second half of 2020 will determine its trajectory—and whether it is successfully contained or morphs into the first Great Depression of the 21st century!

---

1 For an in-depth and detailed explanation of how normal recessions, great recessions, and bona fide depressions differ, both quantitative and qualitative, see Jack Rasmus, *Epic Recession: Prelude to Global Depression* (Pluto Books, 2010), chapters 1–3.

A SPECTRUM OF CAPITALIST CRISES

The Great Depression of the 1930s decade began as a Great Recession in 1929–30 that collapsed further into a Great Depression after 1930. In contrast, the Great Recession of 2008–09 was successfully contained and prevented from evolving into a Great Depression—albeit at great longer term cost to the stability of the capitalist system itself over the subsequent decade. So what can be said of the current crisis? How is it similar or different from 2008–09? And what is the likelihood of a repeat of the 1930s?

It remains yet to be seen, after only four months from March through June 2020, what the future trajectory of today's Great Recession of 2020 may be: containment or further deterioration. The odds favor the latter, however, for seven reasons:

- Today's 2020 collapse comes on the heels of a weak U.S. and global economy in 2019, in contrast to the much stronger U.S. and global real economy in 2007.

- The current collapse has occurred much faster; it has also already contracted five times deeper compared to 2008–09. In just four months, March to June, the U.S. economy has contracted somewhere around 25%–30% in U.S. GDP terms.[2] In 2008–09 the decline was no more than 6%.

- Today's U.S. collapse occurs with more than 90% of other world economies similarly in deep recession—compared to 60% in 2008–09. This time there won't be any China and emerging markets economic boom, as occurred in 2009–10, to put a floor under the collapse of the U.S., Europe, and Japan by stimulating global trade.

- Governments' policy responses to stimulate their economies will prove even less effective this time around compared to 2008–09 due to a decade of accelerating income inequality, low productivity and business real investment, widespread wage and incomes stagnation of working classes, collapse of social safety nets, record budget deficits and tens of trillions of dollars of debt run-up by business, households, and governments alike.

- The COVID-19 overlay is continuing to depress the economy still further, with no sign thus far of its moderating; in fact, today at mid-year signs are growing of an even worse second wave of mass

---

2 Initial estimates for the second quarter and the first half of 2020 will begin to appear publicly in late July 2020, and a more thorough estimate in August.

infections and hospitalizations with all the negative consequences for the U.S. economy and recovery.

- The growing political instability—especially in the USA—has a great potential to negatively impact both consumer and business expectations that would further dampen household spending and business real investing. Political instability and uncertainty becomes itself a negative economic force.

- Finally, there's the very large wild card looming on the horizon in the somewhat longer term. Should recovery lag or falter, a combination of the preceding six factors may cause the volume and rate of defaults and bankruptcies (business, consumer, and even state-local governments) in the U.S. economy to overwhelm the U.S. banking system once again, leading to a financial crash. This in turn will exacerbate still further the decline in the real, non-financial side of the U.S. economy, possibly descending into the first Great Depression of the 21st century.

These seven great forces are emerging from deep within the current economic crisis and have yet to play themselves out. But any one of them, and certainly any combination, is capable of pushing the already fragile U.S. real economy into an even deeper contraction in the coming months.

THE 1930S: A GREAT RECESSION MORPHS INTO A GREAT DEPRESSION

Historically, it is not well understood by economists that 1929–30 began as a Great Recession and only after 18 months began to morph into an actual Great Depression.

A stock market crash in October 1929 precipitated and accelerated a sharper decline in manufacturing and construction that had already slowly begun to develop even before October. The faster decline of manufacturing and construction that followed after the October 1929 stock market crash had not yet spilled over to the rest of the U.S. economy. Unemployment rose to around 10% in 1930. But banks were not to begin collapsing for another 15 months, more than a year later, in December 1930. It was only when a series of increasingly severe banking crashes began to occur—in December 1930, in 1931, 1932, and March 1933—that the U.S. economy, "ratchet-like," fell off a series of cliffs, plunging ever deeper into the Great Depression, only hitting a trough in summer 1933.

Thereafter the road to recovery took seven years of stop-go, partial recoveries then relapses. In 1933–34 the banks were bailed out, and a pro-business policy called the National Recovery Act was introduced to benefit businesses but not wages and employment. The non-bank real economy rebounded (not recovered) modestly but failed to attain a sustained recovery. In 1935 the Roosevelt New Deal fiscal spending programs succeeded in partially stimulating the economy and generated some sustained recovery. However, the New Deal was prematurely repealed in part by a Republican dominated Congress and conservative U.S. Supreme Court in 1937–38. The result was a relapse into depression once again. Restoration of the New Deal programs in 1938 restored the track to sustained recovery, although slowly. In 1940–41 an acceleration of U.S. war preparation spending provided a much needed second push for recovery, which was fully attained by 1942, as the U.S. government share of total GDP spending rose to 40% of GDP from less than 20%, even during the peak years of the New Deal.

2008–09: A GREAT RECESSION IS SUCCESSFULLY CONTAINED

Unlike the 1929–30 period, the 2008–09 events illustrate how a Great Recession was contained, averting a slide into a bona fide Great Depression.

In both periods, a crash in the financial sector provided the catalyst. While in 1929 a financial crash precipitated a decline in the real, non-financial economy, in 2008 the financial markets responsible were the housing markets and what were called the derivatives markets (i.e. credit default swaps or CDSs). Together these interacted and resulted in a collapse first of several investment banks, then of the quasi-government financial institutions associated with the housing market, Fannie Mae and Freddie Mac. The financial crash quickly accelerated to impact mortgage companies and banks which had overextended in providing mortgages. The financial crisis culminated in September 2008 with the collapse of the investment bank, Lehman Brothers, that had over-invested in subprime mortgages and the giant insurance company, AIG, that had over-written CDS insurance contracts on Lehman Brothers that it couldn't pay for. A general banking crisis and freeze of lending by the banks to all companies, non-financial as well as financial, followed. The banking crash thus brought down the "real" economy. Mass layoffs followed, peaking at 600,000+ per month through late 2008 and into early 2009.

The banks and financial system were quickly bailed out and stabilized. In mid–2009 the U.S. central bank, the Federal Reserve, quickly provided trillions of dollars in emergency funds to the banking system and lowered interest rates to near zero—unlike in 1930–32 when the Federal Reserve failed to bail out the banks and eventually allowed 17,000 U.S. banks to fail.

The Federal Reserve would continue to provide free money to the banks to the tune of $5.5 trillion over the next seven years, 2009–16, and to hold rates at near zero. By 2010, banks had been bailed out but they continued to be subsidized for years thereafter by the Federal Reserve by keeping rates near zero and providing banks with further trillions of dollars of virtually free money. The trillions of dollars of free money found its way from the U.S. banks to non-bank businesses and investors and to U.S. multinational corporations expanding offshore.

The Fed's allocation of more than $5 trillion in virtually free money to banks and investors was processed by an annual distribution of money to U.S. corporations over the next seven years at the rate of $800 billion a year, which these utilized in the form of stock buybacks, dividend payouts, and other corporate to shareholder distributions. This historic massive distribution of more than $5 trillion by the U.S. central bank, the Fed, contributed significantly to the accelerating wealth concentration among corporations and wealthiest 1% households in the USA from 2010 to 2016.

With most of the Bank bailout money now going to fuel corporate mergers & acquisitions, offshore investing by U.S. multinational corporations, and creating asset price bubbles in stocks and other financial assets, the real non-financial economy was starved of money capital for investing in the U.S. real economy and fared less well in the following years. The financial sector of the U.S. economy in effect "crowded out" job-creating real investment in the real economy.

In contrast to the more than $5 trillion pumped into the U.S. banking system and private investors by the Federal Reserve from 2009 through 2015, the non-financial real economy was provided with only a $787 billion fiscal stimulus in January 2009 by Obama's economic recovery program.

This proved insufficient as a stimulus, not only due to its insufficient magnitude but because of its composition as well—with only about $600 billion in business tax cuts and subsidies going to state & local governments. Both business and state governments in turn then largely hoarded the stimulus at first and then spent it very slowly, if at all. This failed fiscal stimulus accounted for much of the weak and protracted recovery of the real economy after 2009—in contrast to the massive, immediate and continued bail out of the banks and investors by the Federal Reserve over the same post-2009 period.

Unlike the quick recovery of banks and investors, the real economy struggled to obtain a sustained recovery. Economic growth in GDP on average annually was only 60% of a normal post-recession recovery. It took six years just to recover jobs lost since 2008, which didn't occur until late 2015. Real wages stagnated at best for most of the U.S. work force over the same period. A typical legacy of great recessions is always a weak real economy recovery, very slow job restoration, and wage stagnation. The 2008–09 was thus no different.

The trajectory of the post-2008 collapse was a short, shallow recovery followed by similar relatively short periods of anemic growth. The U.S. economy stalled, almost falling into subsequent recessions, on two occasions in the winters of 2012 and 2015. Europe and Japan fared worse. Europe stumbled into a second, double dip recession in 2011–13 and Japan slipped in and out of short recessions on three separate occasions after 2009.

Near economic stagnation, and short economic relapses, for an extended period for another 5–6 years was thus the defining characteristic of the period of from June 2009 through 2015—i.e. the first Great Recession in the 21st century. A second banking crash did not follow the real economy's decline of 2008–09. The Great Recession of 2008–09 was thus prevented from transforming into a bona fide Great Depression, such as occurred in 1931.

The weak recovery of the real economy, 2010–16, was achieved at the great cost of a weak jobs recovery, stagnant wages for most, low real business investment and productivity, and growing income inequality in favor of the financial-banking sector and wealthiest 1% investor households—all of which would eventually come at a price when the 2020 crisis erupted.

2020 Phase 1: The Second Great Recession

The current 2020 crash of the real economy in the USA dwarfs the 2008-09 first Great Recession. Since late February 2020, the U.S. economy has contracted more than four times faster than it did in 2008–09. In the latter case the contraction took 19 months for U.S. GDP to decline by 6%. In 2020 U.S. GDP faced a similar decline in just the first quarter, January–March 2020. Official forecasts for the second quarter 2020, April thru June 2020, are for the U.S. economy to contract by another astounding 30%–40%: The Federal Reserve bank's districts of Atlanta and New York provide GDP prediction services for the economy.[3]

The combined economic decline for the entire first six months of 2020 will likely range from 20% to 25% of U.S. GDP. That's a loss of about $5 trillion in GDP terms— in just four months, compared to 19 months in 2007–09; and four to five times deeper than that which occurred in 2008–09.

Another pair of key sources indicating the severe dimensions of the current second quarter collapse are the Purchasing Managers Indexes (PMIs) for manufacturing and for services. An index number of 50 indicates stagnation: no growth in manufacturing and/or services but no contraction either. A number above 50 indicates growth of the economy in these sectors; below 50 indicates a contraction or recession in activity. PMIs for both manufacturing and services plummeted in March and April to record lows in the 30s range, and, while rising as in the April–June second quarter, both PMIs are still below 50, indicating a continued contraction of both manufacturing and services.

---

3 The Atlanta Fed currently predicts a -41.9% contraction of the U.S. economy, on top of the 6%. The New York Fed is forecasting a -30.5% decline.

It is thus a myth that the U.S. economy is growing once again in June. It is just not falling as fast as it had in March–May.

Another way to envision the special severity of the current 2020 Great Recession is that more than 90% of countries globally are accompanying the USA in the decline—compared to 60% in 2008–09, making the current contraction even more global in character than was 2008–09—occurring not only faster but also steeper.

According to June 2020 latest forecasts of the global economy by the World Bank (WB) and the International Monetary Fund (IMF), the volume of world trade is projected to decline by double digit percentages throughout 2020. The World Bank predicts a -13.4% fall in 2020; the IMF, 12%.[4] Both sources see a -5% fall in global GDP—something that has never occurred before in modern record keeping. Both the IMF and World Bank forecast the USA, Europe, and advanced economies will contract by 8%–10% for the entire year, 2020—about double that of the 2008–09 Great Recession![5]

However, that optimistic forecast of 8%–10% for the U.S. and other advanced economies assumes a successful fiscal-policy implementation in the second half of 2020 as well as the absence of a second COVID-19 surge in the coming months—neither of which appear likely to happen.

The World Bank's -5% and -8% best case forecasts include the assumption there is no second COVID-19 wave and no premature reopening of the U.S. and other economies. If either happens, "then we will begin talking about depression-level growth and policy responses."[6] Of course both had already begun to occur by late June 2020. The World Bank added that its best case -5% contraction (and -8% for USA) is further dependent on sufficiently strong government fiscal stimulus as well as on no resumption of the global trade war.

It further warns that should these assumptions prove real, then that "will almost certainly be followed by a solvency (financial) crisis, particularly among small firms in the retail, leisure and hospitality sectors."[7]

U.S. Federal Reserve chair Jerome Powell has more or less echoed the World Bank's conditional optimistic forecast, noting that much depends on the U.S. economy reopening without a second COVID-19 wave. While Trump and company continue to spin the V-shaped recovery scenario, Fed chairman Powell

---

4 World Bank, *Global Economic Prospects* (June 2020) and International Monetary Fund, *World Economic Outlook Update* (June 2020).

5 So-called "normal" recessions average a decline of 2–3% and last, on average, only six to nine months in comparison.

6 World Bank, *Global Economic Prospects* (June 2020), Chapter 1, "Pandemic, Recession: The Global Economy in Crisis."

7 Ibid.

and other Federal Reserve governors have been consistently warning that is not on the horizon. Appearing before Congress in mid-May 2020 Powell made it plain that the United States faces a long overall recovery...likely not before the end of 2021.[8] European Central Bank chair Christine Lagarde has echoed Powell's warning, pointing out "we're not going to return to the ex-ante status quo" and that global trade will be "significantly reduced."[9]

Another big factor among the noted "seven" forces that could potentially drive the U.S. economy deeper into recession is the adequacy of a U.S. government fiscal stimulus response to the current crisis.

First, Congress passed two small fiscal spending bills of $100 billion and $75 billion, targeting reimbursements to hospitals; neither were designed as general economic stimulus bills. Then in March 2020, the U.S. Congress passed the dubiously-termed CARES ACT, amounting to about $2.2 trillion. It included three business lending programs: for small, medium and large businesses, totaling $1.45 trillion, to which a further $310 trillion was quickly added to what was called the Payroll Protection Program (PPP), for small business loans.

To this approximately $1.8 trillion in business loans, convertible to cash grants if the business borrower used 70% to maintain the wages of its employees—was added another $500 billion in direct subsidies to workers in the form of expanded unemployment benefits and one-time supplemental income checks of $1,200 per adult and $600 per dependent for no more than two dependents.

In addition to the loans/grants and unemployment/supplement checks were $650 billion in tax cuts in the CARES ACT. This is seldom referenced in the media, and are virtually all business- and investor-targeted, leaving less than 3% of the total to be provided to households earning less than $100,000 a year in annual income. Featured tax cuts include a payroll retention tax credit, temporary business payroll tax deferment, net operating loss corporate tax averaging, faster depreciation write-offs, and a larger business loss allowance.

Summed up, the CARES ACT and its predecessors provided a fiscal stimulus—at least on paper—of $1.8T in business loans/grants, $500 billion to workers and families, $650 billion in business tax cuts, and about two hundred billion in direct subsidies to hospitals and health care deliverers. Or about $3.2 trillion total.

If it is assumed all the $3.2 trillion actually entered the U.S. economy as a stimulus by the end of June, then the stimulus as a percent of U.S. GDP amounts to about 11% of GDP. But it didn't. As of end of June 2020, only about half that has actually been spent. So the stimulus is only 5.5% of GDP. In other words, about the same 5.5% as in 2009, for an economy in 2020 that has contracted five

---

8 Lauren Fedor, "Powell Warns the U.S. recovery could take until the end of 2021," *Financial Times,* May 18, 2020, p. 1.

9 Christine Lagarde, *Financial Times,* June 27, 2020, p.2.

times faster and five times deeper! And if 5.5% was insufficient to stimulate the real economy in 2009 (in contrast to the Fed's successful $5 trillion bailout of the financial side of the economy), then the 5.5% fiscal stimulus embodied in the CARES Act will certainly prove insufficient for real economic recovery as well in 2020!

In short, the fiscal stimulus as of midyear 2020 is woefully inadequate to ensure a sustained recovery of the U.S. economy in 2020—let alone anything resembling a V-shape recovery.

As of June 30, 2020 the $500 billion in unemployment benefits and income checks has been spent already. There is no further stimulus effect for the coming 3rd quarter. Only $517B of the $660 billion small business PPP program has been loaned out. No more than $100 billion of the $500 billion allocated for loans for big businesses has been loaned. And the additional $600 billion for loans for medium sizes businesses, called the "Main Street" program, has yet to lend anything.

Congress never intended the CARES ACT as a fiscal stimulus bill but rather as a "mitigation" effect, to put a floor under the collapsing economy to prevent it from plummeting even further than it has. Rather, Congress, or at least the U.S. House of Representatives, intended it to be followed up by a subsequent, true fiscal stimulus package. This package was introduced by the U.S. House in May and is called the "HEROES ACT." But at this writing, this actual fiscal stimulus is being held up by Mitch McConnell and the Republican Senate, who are opposed to further stimulus in the form of continued unemployment benefits and income checks, the former of which expires on July 31, 2020.

Nor are McConnell and Republicans interested in adding more to the large and medium size corporations' $1.1 trillion loans allocated by the CARES ACT. Neither large or medium corporations have taken up the loans. $1 trillion is still allocated but not being used. Even $135 billion of the small business PPP program is still not taken up. The question is why, if the economy has contracted so sharply? The answer is that big businesses are already bloated with cash they've been accumulating since January 2020. They don't need the loans and don't want them, if they come with the condition of using 70% to maintain their workers' wages.

The cash-bloated U.S. big corporations have accumulated a cash war chest of at least $3 trillion. In January–February they quickly drew down their bank credit lines by hundreds of billions of dollars and issued record levels of corporate bonds, raising another more than $1.3 trillion in March–May, more than in all of 2019. They suspended hundreds of billions of dollars in their dividend payouts to shareholders and, in some cases, sold off their minority equity (stock) ownerships in other companies to gather in more cash. They issued more stock of their own, and cut facilities and wages in the shutdown. Bloated with cash, they have had no need of the CARES ACT loans, and Republicans McConnell & Co. know this.

Their main constituency of big business, bankers and investors don't need their further financial assistance.

What the Senate Republicans have been proposing in negotiations on the HEROES bill is to convert the money spent on unemployment insurance after July 31 to a direct wage subsidy to employers. Instead of issuing unemployment checks to workers, they propose issuing checks to their employers to pay their wages instead of the employers having to pay them wages out of their revenues and profits. Another provision proposed is more tax cuts for business: a permanent payroll tax cut, more capital gains tax cuts, and more tax cuts for business expenses.

With an election in just months, it is highly unlikely any further significant fiscal stimulus will be forthcoming this summer—with ominous consequences for achieving a sustained economic recovery in 2020.

When combined with a reopening of the domestic economy which is intensifying a second COVID wave underway, and with a continuing decline in the global economy and therefore global trade, and given the likely end of extended unemployment benefits come July 31, 2020, it is increasingly likely the U.S. economy will deteriorate further in the second half of 2020. Making matters worse, after July a wave of renter evictions and mortgage payment defaults is expected, further intensifying the negative economic effects in the U.S.

In addition, the reopening of the U.S. economy will not result in a full and rapid return of jobs and therefore of wage income and consumption. Household credit is also tightening, reducing potential consumption as well. Employers are calling back workers selectively and carefully, with many re-employed with fewer hours to be worked. Uncertain of the recovery, businesses will not return to robust investing and production expansion; households, uncertain of future employment prospects, will not return to prior levels of spending either.

But it will appear as if recovery has begun in the 3rd quarter as GDP recovers moderately. It is not impossible for any economy to continue to contract at 30% every quarter. A modest 5–10% "rebound"—not recovery—is likely in the 3rd quarter simply as the economy reopens, even if only partially. Similarly, some of the current 40 million plus jobless will return to work. Politicians will hype the GDP and jobs data to spin it as a "recovery."

But a mere rebound is not a recovery.

2020 PHASE 2: GREAT RECESSION OR GREAT DEPRESSION?

It remains to be seen whether the 20th century's second Great Recession, now in its fourth month and still early in its trajectory—in just Phase 1 thus far—will be contained. The alternative scenario is a failed containment and a subsequent descent into the first true Great Depression of the 21st century in 2021–22. It's inherent in the nature of a Great Recession to be unstable. It either moderates or it intensifies and morphs into a Great Depression. For the latter to happen, however, a major financial system crash must occur—i.e. the seventh "wild card" force noted above.

Thus far the U.S. central bank, the Federal Reserve Bank, has undertaken historic and unprecedented action to forestall a financial crash of the banking system. In the first Great Recession, the Fed bailed out the banks to the tune of more than $5 trillion. In the current crisis, it has pre-emptively bailed out the banks with more than $3 trillion thus far, and promised "whatever it takes" in additional virtual free money capital injections, should the banks need it. A pre-emptive bail out of the banking system has never before occurred in U.S. history, but is underway today.

The Fed is pre-bailing out non-financial corporations for the first time as well. That too has never occurred in U.S. economic history. Trillions of dollars more are being allocated by the Fed to buy the bonds of corporations directly. Even derivatives of corporate bonds, called "Exchange Traded Funds" (ETFs). Even junk bonds of corporations. This massive corporate bond buying program by the Fed is designed to throw trillions of dollars at corporations in order to offset the waves of corporate defaults expected to come. Defaults and bankruptcies will mean banks that provided the companies with loans will have to assume their corporate debt when they default. That could lead to bank insolvencies and a banking crash in turn. So the Fed is flooding both banks to have sufficient cash to absorb the coming defaults as well as the potentially defaulting corporations. It is an historic experiment in monetary policy. And it is uncertain whether the even historic money injections will succeed in preventing the waves of defaults that are likely to be coming.[10]

The areas of major corporate defaults expected are not just the obvious travel, leisure and hospitality, and big box retail companies. Defaults are already spreading as well in the fracking energy industry, in commercial properties (malls, office buildings, hotels, theme parks, etc.), and soon in local governments and agencies.

All Great Recessions are characterized by mutually amplifying negative effects between financial cycles and real economic cycles. In 2008 a major financial instability event precipitated and exacerbated the subsequent steep contraction of the U.S. real economy from October 2008 through June 2009. Today, in 2020, the real side of the economy has contracted even more severely first. It remains to be seen whether and when that real contraction might precipitate a subsequent

---

10 For the evolution of central bank policies in the last forty years, in particular the U.S., and why central banks like the Fed are engaging in ever-increasing desperate policy initiatives, see Jack Rasmus, *Central Bankers at the End of Their Ropes: Monetary Policy and the Coming Depression* (Clarity Press, 2017).

financial crash in turn. Should that occur, the feedback effects on the real economy will intensify, driving the real economy even further into contraction—and into a possible Great Depression.

The economic jury is still out and will remain so for months as to whether the Fed's historic massive pre-emptive bailout of both banks and non-bank corporations can succeed in preventing a bona fide descent into depression. The failure of fiscal policy will be decided much sooner, well before the November 2020 elections. A failure of central bank monetary policy, should it occur, will likely be sometime in 2021.

In the interim, the trajectory of the U.S. economy will be more W-shaped—as is the case in all Great Recessions. While V-shape recoveries are more frequent in normal recessions, it appears capitalist economies no longer undergo normal recessions, with contractions of only three to six months and GDP declines of only 1–3%. Capitalism in the 21st century is more prone to major crises, like Great Recessions and Great Depressions. The mutual amplifying effects of financial cycles and real cycles, and the growing financialization of capitalism, are likely the cause of this phenomenon of growing mutual cycle amplification and more intensified Great Recessions.[11]

Much of the trajectory of the U.S. economy in the second half of 2020 and beyond depends on the response of fiscal and monetary policy both this year and in 2021, after the November 2020 national U.S. elections. Will Congress continue to fail to provide sufficient fiscal stimulus, as it did in 1929–32? Will the Federal Reserve's March–June 2020 even more massive—and this time pre-emptive bank bailout—successfully forestall a banking crash in 2021?

Other key questions impacting the economic trajectory include whether the reopening of the U.S. economy now underway significantly exacerbates the COVID-19 negative effects on the economy. Rising infections and hospitalizations will discourage and dampen further both business investment, job recalls, and household consumption, and lead to further layoffs. What will happen with global trade and other economies' recoveries?

Political instability events should not be discounted as well. A growing direct conflict between two wings of the U.S. capitalist elite and their political constituencies has been assuming constitutional forms as well as grass roots protests and conflicts between their supporters. It is not impossible that the upcoming November 2020 elections will result in an intensification of these conflicts and a general political and constitutional crisis not seen since the 1850s. The economic fallout of that would be severe.

---

11 For a discussion of financialization and mutual cycle effects, see chapters 11–13 and 19 in Jack Rasmus, *Systemic Fragility in the Global Economy* (Clarity Press, 2016).

The most likely scenario for the U.S. economy in 2020–21, is an extended, weak and unstable economic recovery—not to be confused with a temporary "rebound" over the summer—that will take years to unfold.

The trajectory and scenario of the current Great Recession 2.0 is therefore strongly in favor of a W-shape recovery at best, in the shorter run, with the possibility of a descent into the first great worldwide economic depression of the 21st century in the intermediate to longer run.

What Lies Ahead?

The U.S. economy at mid-year 2020 is at a critical juncture. What happens in the next three months will likely determine whether the current Great Recession 2.0 continues to follow a W-shape trajectory—or drifts over an economic precipice into an economic depression. With prompt and sufficient fiscal stimulus targeting U.S. households, minimal political instability before the November 2020 elections, and no financial instability event, it may be contained. No worse than a prolonged W-shape recovery will occur. But should the fiscal stimulus be minimal (and poorly composed), should political instability grow significantly worse, and a major financial instability event erupt in the U.S. (or globally), then it is highly likely a descent to a bona fide economic depression will occur.

The prognosis for a swift economic recovery is not all that positive. Multiple forces are at work that strongly suggest the early summer economic "rebound" will prove temporary and that a further decline in jobs, consumption, investment, and the economy is on the horizon.

A Second Wave of Job Losses

Through mid-June to mid-July, the COVID-19 infection rate, hospitalization rate, and soon the death rate, have all begun to escalate once again. Daily infections consistently now exceed 60,000 cases—i.e. more than twice that of the earlier worst month of April 2020. Consequently, states are beginning to order a return to more sheltering in place and shutdowns of business, especially retail, travel, and entertainment services. The direction of events cannot but hamper any initial rebound of the economy, let alone generate a sustained economic recovery.

Exacerbating conditions, a second wave of job layoffs is clearly now emerging—and not just due to economic shutdowns related to the resurging virus. Reopening of the U.S. economy in June resulted in 4.8 million jobs restored for that month, according to the U.S. Labor Department. That number included, however, no fewer than 3 million service jobs in restaurants, hospitality, and retail establishments. These are the occupations that are now being impacted again with layoffs, as States retrench once more due to the virus resurgence underway. But there's a new development as well: A second jobless wave is now emerging in addition to the renewed layoffs due to shutdowns not only of the resumed service and retail occupations, but reflecting longer term and even permanent job layoffs across various industries.

Household consumption patterns have changed fundamentally and permanently in a number of ways due to both the virus effect and the depth of the current recession. Many consumers will not be returning soon to travel, to shopping at malls, to restaurant services, to mass entertainment or to sport events at the levels they had, pre-virus.

In response, large corporations in these sectors have begun to announce job layoffs by the thousands. Two large U.S. airlines—United and American—have announced their intention to lay off 36,000 and 20,000, respectively, including flight attendants, ground crews, and even pilots. Boeing has announced a cut of 16,000, and Uber, in just its latest announcement, a cut of 3,000. Big box retail companies like JCPenneys, Nieman Marcus, Lord & Taylor, and others are closing hundreds of stores with a similar impact on what were formerly thousands of permanent jobs. Oil & gas fracking companies like Cheasepeake and 200 other frackers now defaulting on their debt are laying off tens of thousands more. Trucking companies like YRC Worldwide, the Hertz car rental company, clothing & apparel sellers like Brooks Brothers, small–medium independent restaurant and hotel chains like Krystal, Craftworks—all are implementing, or announcing permanent layoffs by the thousands as well.

Reflecting this, since mid-June new unemployment benefit claims have continued to rise weekly at a rate of more than 2 million—with about 1.3 million receiving regular state unemployment benefits plus another 1 million independent contractors, gig workers, self-employed receiving the special federal government unemployment benefits. The latter group's numbers are rising rapidly since mid-June.

As of mid-July no fewer than 33 million are receiving unemployment benefits, with another 6 million having dropped out of the labor force altogether and no longer even being counted as unemployed. Unemployment therefore remains at what will likely be a chronically high number, at around 40 million—with about 25% of the U.S. labor force unemployed—as renewed service-retail sector layoffs, plus new permanent layoffs, both loom on the horizon.

Added to the growing problem of renewed service layoffs and the 2nd wave of permanent layoffs in the private sector is the growing likelihood of significant layoffs in the public sector, as states and cities facing massive budget deficits are forced to lay off several millions of the roughly 22 million public sector workers in the U.S.. This potential public employee layoff wave will accelerate and occur sooner, should Congress in summer 2020 fail to bail out the states and cities whose budgets have been severely impacted by the collapse of tax revenues while facing escalating costs of dealing with the health crisis. Estimates as of last May are that the states and cities will need $969 billion in bailout funding this summer—roughly two-thirds for the states and the rest for cities and local governments.

The resurgence of layoffs from all these sources is a sure indicator that the economy's rebound—let alone recovery—is in trouble. Rising joblessness means less wage income for households and therefore less consumption and, given that consumption is 70% of the economy, a slowing of the rebound and recovery. Problems in consumption in turn mean business investment suffers as well, further slowing the economy and recovery. Exacerbating the decline in personal income devoted to consumption due to unemployment is the evidence that even those fortunate enough to return to work after spring 2020's economic shutdown are doing so increasingly as part time employed—which means less wage income for consumption compared to the pre-COVID period before March 2020.

Overlaid on these negative prospects for employment, consumption, business investment is the intensification of economic crisis-related problems.

Rent Evictions, Child Care & Education Chaos

There is an imminent crisis in rents affecting tens of millions. At the peak in April, it is estimated that roughly one-third of the 110 million renters in the U.S. economy had stopped making rent payments due to the COVID-related shut-downs of the economy. The CARES ACT, passed in March, provided forbearance on rental payments, although perhaps as many as 20 states failed to enforce it. That forbearance directive expires at the end of July, with as many as 23 million rent evictions projected in coming months. A major housing crisis is thus brewing, as well as the second wave of job layoffs.

A combined education–child care crisis is about to occur almost simultane-ously. The K-12 public education system is approaching chaos, as school districts plan to introduce remote learning on a major scale in order to deal with the renewed COVID-19 infection and hospitalization wave. The heart of the crisis is that tens of millions of U.S. working class families dependent on two paychecks to survive economically cannot afford to accommodate school district practices for remote learning—especially for young children in the K-6 grade levels. Even if such fam-ilies could afford to pay for expensive childcare, the current U.S. childcare system is far from being able to accommodate them. Many minority and working class households, moreover, lack the computers and networking equipment, or even the requisite skills to set it up, to enable their children participate in remote learning.

Several forces are driving the shift to remote learning: school district fears of liability actions by parents if children become ill, the significant cost of ensuring disinfected classrooms, the lack of classroom space to allow distance learning on site, and the growing concern of teachers regarding their own exposure to infection. At least 1.5 million public school teachers are over age 50 and have health conditions that put them at greater risk of serious infection, should they attend closed-in classroom environments.

The child care plus K-12 education crisis will likely erupt within months on a major scale. Chaos in education is around the corner.

This fall, higher education—colleges and universities—will also experience chaos of their own kind. While distance learning will not be as serious an implementation problem as it will in K-12 levels, costs from the pandemic will force many smaller, private colleges into bankruptcy, consolidation or closure. Public colleges' funding problems will require them to sharply reduce available services. Remote education will create a two-tier system of higher education—educational services delivered remotely and those of a more traditional nature on campus; or a hybrid of both.

However, demand for higher education services will likely decline sharply in the short term, during which higher education will experience a devastating decrease in tuition and other sources of college revenues. Some estimates show a third of freshmen plan to take what's called a "gap year": i.e., accept entrance but not attend for a year. That's a massive revenue loss. Some estimates foresee a 15%–30% decline in new student attendance, with another 5%–10% decline in transfer students, and a similar decline of 5%–10% in continuing students. In addition, attendance by international students, the "cash cow" for most colleges, would have declined sharply due to the Trump administration's new rules, had they not been rescinded.

Still other developments will sharply reduce college revenues. Students forced to attend classes via remote learning will demand lower tuition. One can expect a wave of legal suits as students seek to "claw back" full tuition expenses. Other secondary sources of college revenues—from fees, on-campus room and board, endowment earnings and gifts, and sports revenues—also spell a looming revenue crunch.

A wave of college consolidations and closures is inevitable. And with student loan debt at $1.6 trillion it is unlikely that the federal government will introduce new aid through that channel. Nor will States increase their subsidization of public colleges, given the severe state budget deficits on the horizon.

In short, the economic crisis is about to assume more socio-economic dimensions and character: rent, childcare, education chaos will soon overlay the continuing unemployment problem and worsening recession. Social and political discontent, frustration, and anxiety are almost certainly to rise in turn in coming months as a consequence.

Global Recession & Sovereign Debt Defaults

The weakness of the global economy is yet another factor likely to ensure the U.S. economy's W-shape trajectory. As noted previously, with 90% of other countries in recession, global demand for U.S. exports will remain weak or declining. In addition, global supply chains have also been severely disrupted by the health crisis, or even broken, and will not be restored soon. The global economy is suffering from deep problems of both demand and supply. This too is a unique historical event. Never before have demand and supply problems occurred congruently. Together, they increase the potential for a global depression.

Commodity producing economies have been hard hit, especially oil and metal producing countries. Many were in a recession well before the COVID health crisis. Global trade in general had stagnated, registering little to no growth in 2019, for the first time since modern records were kept. Many countries had over-extended their borrowing, expanding their sovereign debt loads during the last decade. This was money capital borrowed largely from western banks and capital markets (i.e. shadow banks).

Now, with global trade flat and declining, and prices for their export goods deflating in price as well, these debt-extended countries cannot earn sufficient income from exports in order to pay the principal and interest on their debt. As a result, several countries in the worst shape may soon default on their debt payment to western banks, hedge funds, private equity firms, and so on. Debt defaults potentially mean the same western financial institutions that loaned the funds now experience financial crises in turn. In such a manner, financial instability events abroad are often transmitted to the domestic U.S. economy through its banking system. It would not be the first time, moreover, that foreign bank crashes have spilled over the U.S. and rest of the world economy and in the process significantly exacerbated a recession already underway.

Theoretically, countries experiencing severe sovereign debt crises could borrow from the International Monetary Fund. However, the IMF has nowhere near the funds to accommodate multiple large sovereign defaults that occur simultaneously. Nor is it likely that the U.S. and Europe will increase the IMF's funding to enable it to do so. Once it becomes clear the IMF cannot handle a crisis of such potential dimensions, the global capitalist economy will slip even further toward global depression.

The further deterioration now already occurring in economic relations between the U.S. and China may also potentially impact the Great Recession in the U.S., and ensure its continued W-Shape recovery. Trump's trade pact with China signed December 2019 has proven thus far a colossal failure. The president declared at the deal's signing it would mean $150 billion in China purchases of U.S. goods in 2020—especially farm products, oil & gas, and manufactured goods.

At mid-year, China has purchased only $5 billion of the agreed $40 billion in farm products and only $14 billion of $85 billion in U.S. manufactured goods. Trump's promised $150 billion was never agreed to by China, even before the COVID pandemic struck the U.S. economy in 2020. China had never agreed to a dollar value of purchases of U.S. exports but announced it would purchase based on conditions in 2020–21. Trump's $150 billion was typical Trump misrepresentation of a deal never made. At best China would purchase perhaps $40 billion in agricultural goods—i.e. about the level of its purchases before Trump launched a trade war against it in March 2018. Failing to deliver his exaggerated public promise in 2020 Trump turned on China and further embraced his anti-China hardline advisors on trade and other matters. The former "trade war" with China will likely transform now, in the wake of COVID, into a broader economic war with China. Furthermore, the deterioration of relations with China, set in motion by the current recession and the collapse of global trade, shows signs of spilling over to other political and even military affairs.

Permanent Industry Transformation

The COVID health crisis is accelerating the transformation of entire industries and sectors of the economy, U.S. and global. As noted above, household consumption patterns are already changing fundamentally and will continue as changed even after the health crisis passes. Entire industries will shrink as a consequence. Company consolidations and downsizing are inevitable in airlines, cruise lines, and even public land transport. So too will companies fail, consolidate and restructure in the hospitality, leisure and hotel industries, in mall-based retail establishments, inside entertainment (movies, casinos, etc.) to name but the obvious. Sports and public entertainment companies are struggling to redefine their business models and how they bring their "product" to the public for consumption. Even education—public and private—is undergoing a radical shift. Not so obvious is similar fundamental change in oil & energy industries, and later as well in manufacturing as supply chains are slowly returned to the U.S. economy.

Not only will these changes significantly (and often negatively) impact employment levels and wage incomes, but business practices as well. Already businesses are instituting new cost cutting practices under the pressure of the health crisis and shutdowns. These practices will become permanent. And since much of the practices and cost cutting will focus on workers' pay and benefits, more of what economists call "long term structural unemployment" will result—in addition to the current "cyclical unemployment" occurring due to the current recession.

An historic consequence of the current Great Recession precipitated by the COVID-19 health crisis is the accelerating introduction underway of what some call the Artificial Intelligence revolution. AI is about cost-cutting. It's about new data accumulation, data processing and statistical evaluation, to allow software machines to make decisions previously made by human beings. AI will eliminate millions of low level decision-making by workers in both services and manufacturing. A 2017 report by the business consulting firm, McKinsey, predicted no less than 30% of all workers' occupations will be severely impacted by AI by the end of the present decade. 30% of jobs will either disappear or have their hours reduced significantly. That means less wage income and less consumption still.

The important linkage to the current Great Recession 2.0 is that the introduction of AI by businesses will now speed up. What McKinsey formerly predicted for the late 2020s decade will now take place by mid-decade. The economic consequences for the next generation of U.S. workers, the late Millennials and the GenZers will be serious, to say the least. After decades of the permeation of low-pay, low-benefits, "contingent" part-time and temp jobs since the 1990s, after the impact of the 2008–09 crash and aftermath on employment, after the acceleration of "gig" jobs with the *Uberization* of the capitalist economy since 2010, and after the even more serious negative economic effects of the current Great Recession 2.0, the tens of millions of U.S. workers entering the labor force today and in coming years will have to face the transformation of another 30% of all occupations. The future does not portend very well for the 70 million millennials and GenZers. U.S. neoliberal economic policies and the Great Recession 2.0 is accelerating the long-term structural unemployment crisis of both the U.S. and the global capitalist economy.[12]

Return of Fiscal Austerity

The U.S. federal budget deficit under Trump averaged more than a trillion dollars annually during his first three years in office. The federal national debt at the end of 2019 was $22.8 trillion. As of July 2020 it has risen to $26.5 trillion—and rising. Earlier projections in March were that it would increase by $3.7 trillion in 2020. That has already been exceeded. So, too, will projections for 2021, or another $2.1 trillion. The deficit and debt will likely rise to more than $4 trillion in this fiscal year and another $3 trillion in 2021. That means the current national debt within 18 months will reach $30 trillion. And that's not counting the debt level rise for state and local governments, already $3 trillion; nor the debt carried on the U.S. central bank, the Federal Reserve, balance sheet which is scheduled to rise another $3 trillion at minimum.

---

12 For a more detailed analysis of the effects of AI and other technologies on 21st century U.S. capitalist policy see Jack Rasmus, *The Scourge of Neoliberalism: U.S. Economic Policy from Reagan to Trump* (Clarity Press, 2020), chapters 8 and 9.

The point of presenting these statistics is that the U.S. elites, sooner or later, will introduce a major austerity program. It will likely come later in 2021. And it will make little difference whether the administration that time is headed by Democrats or Republicans. It will come and it will target social security, Medicare, Medicaid, Obamacare, education, housing, transport and other social programs.

The first Great Recession provides a historical precedent. Obama's recovery program in January 2009 provided for $787 billion in stimulus. But the joint Republican-Democrat austerity agreement introduced in August 2011 took back nearly twice that stimulus, or $1.5 trillion, in 2011–13. That austerity contributed significantly to the W-shape recovery from the 2008–09 economic crash and contraction—i.e. the first Great Recession. With the current deficit surge of $6 trillion to date, likely to increase to $9 to $10 trillion, the U.S. economic elites will no doubt pursue a new austerity regime at some point within the next few years. That austerity will, like its predecessor, ensure at best a W-shape recovery typical of Great Recessions. At worst, it may prove the final event that pushes the U.S. economy into another Great Depression.

Financial Instability

Those who deny that the U.S. and global economy have already entered a second Great Recession offer the argument that the 2008–09 crash and recession was caused by the banking and financial crash of 2008–09, and therefore, since there has not yet been a financial crash, the economy at present is not in another Great Recession. But they are wrong.

Great Recessions are always associated with a financial crisis, but that crisis need not precede the deep contraction of the real, non-financial economy. The COVID-19 pandemic has played the role of a financial crash in driving the real economy into a contraction that is both quantitatively and qualitatively worse than a "normal" recession. Furthermore, a subsequent banking system–financial crash is not impossible in the coming months, although not yet likely in 2020.

The preconditions for a financial crisis are in development. It won't be precipitated by a residential mortgage crisis, as in 2007–08. But there are several potential candidates for precipitating a financial crash once again. Here are just a few:

- The commercial property sector in the U.S. is in deep trouble. Commercial property includes malls, office buildings, hotels, resorts, factories, and multiple tenant apartment complexes. Many incurred deep debt obligations as they expanded after 2010 or just kept operating by accruing more high cost debt when they were unprofitable. Today they are unable to continue servicing (i.e. paying principal and interest) on their excessive debt load. Many have begun the process of default and chapter 11 bankruptcy reorganization. Banks and investors hold much of the commercial property debt that will never be repaid. Excess derivatives (credit default swaps) have been written on the debt. A debt crisis and wave of defaults and bankruptcies in 2020–21 in the commercial property sector could easily precipitate a subprime mortgage–like debt crisis as occurred in 2008–09. And derivatives obligations could transmit the crisis throughout the banking system—as it did in 2009. Regional and small community banks in the U.S. are particularly vulnerable.

- The oil and gas fracking industry, where junk bond and leverage loan debt had already risen to unstable levels by the advent of the COVID crisis. The collapse of world oil and gas prices—which began before the COVID-19 impact and continues—will render drillers and others unable to generate the income with which to service their debt. Already more than 200 companies in this sector are in default and bankruptcy proceedings. Again, regional banks that financed much of the expansion of fracking in Texas, the Dakotas, and Pennsylvania will be impacted severely by the defaults. Their financial instability could easily spread to other sectors of banking and finance in the U.S.

- State and local governments, should Congress fail to appropriate sufficient bailout funding in its next round of fiscal spending in July 2020. State and local governments are capable of default and bankruptcy—unlike the Federal government, which is not. The U.S. has a long history of state defaults associated with the onset of Great Depressions. This time around, state financial instability will quickly spill over to public pension funds, and from public to private pensions, and from there to the municipal bond markets with which state and local governments raise revenue by borrowing to fund deficits.

- Global sovereign debt markets, as previously noted. Defaults on massive debt accumulated since 2010 by many countries could result in serious contagion effects on the private banking systems of the advanced economies, including the U.S., Europe, and Japan. Should the IMF fail to contain a chain of sovereign debt crises that could follow in the wake of the current Great Recession, a chain reaction of defaults across emerging market economies in particular has the potential to precipitate a global financial crisis.

History shows that financial crises often originate from unsuspected corners of the economy. The above candidates are the "known unknowns." There may also lurk in the bowels of the capitalist global financial system still more "unknown unknowns"—i.e., what are sometimes called "black swan" events.

Political Instability

The U.S. and other countries are on new ground in terms of potential political instability. The piecemeal curtailment of democratic and civil rights has been progressing at least since the mid-1990s. In the 21st century it has been accelerating, both in the U.S. and across the globe. Recent years have seen a growing public confrontation between contending wings of the capitalist elites and their political operatives. Institutions of even limited capitalist democracy are under attack and atrophying. And now political instability is growing as well at both the institutional and grass roots levels. One should not underestimate the potential for even more intense political confrontation among elites, or between segments of the U.S. population itself, from having a negative impact on the current economic crisis and 2nd Great Recession. A Trump "October Surprise" or a November 2020 constitutional crisis are no longer beyond the realm of the possible, but even likely.

The expectations of both households and business may serve as transmission mechanisms propagating political instability into more economic and financial instability. Political instability has the effect of freezing up business investment and therefore employment recovery. It has the further effect of causing households to hoard what income they have and raise the savings rate—at the expense of consumption. It also leads to government inaction on the policy necessary to provide stimulus for recovery.

On a global front, political instability may even assume a global dimension. History in general, and U.S. history in particular, reveals that U.S. presidents seek to divert public attention from domestic economic and social problems by provoking foreign wars. Targets for U.S. attack, in the short term, are Iran and Venezuela—especially the latter, which is more susceptible to U.S. military action. But tomorrow, in 2021 and after, it could well be Russia (Ukraine or Baltics U.S. provocations), North Korea (a U.S. attack on its nuclear facilities) or China (a U.S. naval confrontation in the South China sea)—irrespective of the unlikely success of such ventures.

Like another financial-banking crash, a major political instability event—domestic or foreign—could easily send an already weak U.S. economy struggling in the midst of a Great Recession into the abyss of the first Great Depression of the 21st century.

Overall, the future looks grim.

CHAPTER SIX

HOW AN "ACT OF GOD" PANDEMIC IS DESTROYING THE WEST:

THE U.S. IS SAVING THE FINANCIAL SECTOR, NOT THE ECONOMY

Michael Hudson

Before juxtaposing the U.S. and alternative responses to the coronavirus's economic effects, I would like to step back in time to show how the pandemic has revealed a deep underlying problem. We are seeing the consequences of Western societies painting themselves into a debt corner by their creditor-oriented philosophy of law. Neoliberal anti-government (or more accurately, anti-democratic) ideology has centralized social planning and state power in "the market," meaning specifically the financial market on Wall Street and in other financial centers.

At issue is who will lose when employment and business activity are disrupted. Will it be creditors and landlords at the top of the economic scale, or debtors and renters at the bottom? This age-old confrontation over how to deal with the unpaid rents, mortgages and other debt service is at the heart of dealing with today's virus pandemic as large and small businesses, farms, restaurants and neighborhood stores have fallen into arrears, leaving businesses and households—along with their employees who have no wage income to pay these carrying charges that accrue each month.

This is an age-old problem. It was solved in the ancient Near East simply by annulling these debt and rent charges. But the West, shaped as it still is by the legacy of the Roman Empire, has left itself prone to the massive unemployment, business closedowns and resulting arrears for these basic costs of living and doing business.

Western civilization distinguishes itself from its Near Eastern predecessors in the way it has responded to "acts of God" that disrupt the means of support and leave debts in their wake. The United States has taken the lead in rejecting the path by which China, and even social democratic European nations have prevented the coronavirus from causing widespread insolvency and polarizing their economies. The U.S. coronavirus lockdown is turning rent and debt arrears into an opportunity to further impoverish the indebted economy and transfer mortgaged property and its income to creditors.

There is no inherent material need for this fate to occur. But it seems so natural and even inevitable that, as Margaret Thatcher would say, There Is No Alternative.

But of course there is, and always has been. However, resilience in the face of economic disruption always has required a central authority to override "market forces" to restore economic balance from "above."

Individualistic economies cannot do that. To the extent that they have a strong state, they are not democratic but oligarchic, controlled by the financial sector in its own interest, in tandem with its symbiotic real estate sector and monopolized infrastructure. That is why every successful society since the Bronze Age has had a mixed economy. The determining factor in whether or not an economic disruption leaves a crippled economy in its wake turns out to be whether its financial sector is a public utility or is privatized from the debt-strapped public domain as a means to enrich bankers and money-lenders at the expense of debtors and overall economic balance.

China is using an age-old policy common ever since Hammurabi and other Bronze Age rulers promoted economic resilience in the face of "acts of God," given that, unless personal debts, rents and taxes that cannot be paid are annulled, the result will be widespread bankruptcy, impoverishment and homelessness. In contrast to America's financialized economy, China has shown how natural it is for society simply to acknowledge that debts, rents, taxes and other carrying charges of living and doing business cannot resume until economic normalcy is able to resume.

Near Eastern Protection of Economic Resilience in the Face of Acts of God

Ancient societies had a different logic from those of modern capitalist economies. Their logic—and the Jewish Mosaic Law of Leviticus 25, as well as classical Greek and Roman advocates of democratic reform—was similar to modern socialism. The basic principle at work was to subordinate market relations to the needs of society at large, not to enrich a financial *rentier* class of creditors and absentee landowners. More specifically, the basic principle was to cancel debts that could not normally be paid, and prevent creditors from foreclosing on the land of debtors.

All economies operate on credit. In modern economies bills for basic expenses are paid monthly or quarterly. Ancient economies operated on credit during the crop year, with payment falling due when the harvest was in—typically on the threshing floor. This cycle normally provided a flow of crops and corvée labor to the palace, and covered the cultivator's spending during the crop year. Interest typically was owed only when payment was late.

But bad harvests, military conflict or simply the normal hardships of life frequently prevented this buildup of debt from being paid. Mesopotamian palaces had to decide who would bear the loss when drought, flooding, infestation, disease or military attack prevented the payment of debts, rents and taxes. Seeing that this was an unavoidable fact of life, rulers proclaimed amnesties for taxes and these various obligations incurred during the crop year. That saved smallholders from having to work off their debts in personal bondage to their creditors and ultimately to lose their land.

For these palatial economies, resilience meant stabilization of fiscal revenue. Letting private creditors (often officials in the palace's own bureaucracy) demand payment out of future production threatened to deprive rulers of crop surpluses and other taxes, and corvée labor or even service in the military. But for thousands of years, Near Eastern rulers restored fiscal viability for their economies by writing down debts, not only in emergencies but more or less regularly to relieve the normal creeping backlog of debts.

These Clean Slates extended from Sumer and Babylonia in the 3rd millennium BC to classical antiquity, including the neo-Assyrian, neo-Babylonian and Persian Empires. They restored normal economic relations by rolling back the consequences of personal and agrarian debts—avoiding bondage to creditors, and loss of land and its crop yield. From the palace's point of view as tax collector and seller of many key goods and services, the alternative would have been for debtors to owe their crops, labor and even liberty to their creditors, not to the palace. So cancelling debts to restore normalcy was simply pragmatic, not utopian idealism as was once thought.

The pedigree for "act-of-God" rules specifying what obligations need not be paid when serious disruptions occur goes back to the laws of Hammurabi c. 1750 BC. Their aim was to restore economic normalcy after major disruptions. §48 of Hammurabi's laws proclaim a debt and tax amnesty for cultivators if Adad the Storm God has flooded their fields, or if their crops fail as a result of pests or drought. Crops owed as rent or fiscal payments were freed from having to be paid. So were consumer debts run up during the crop year, including tabs at the local ale house and advances or loans from individual creditors. The ale woman likewise was freed from having to pay for the ale she had received from palace or temples for sale during the crop year.

Whoever leased an animal that died by an act of god was freed from liability to its owner (§266). A typical such amnesty occurred if the lamb, ox or ass was eaten by a lion, or if an epidemic broke out. Likewise, traveling merchants who were robbed while on commercial business were cleared of liability if they swore an oath that they were not responsible for the loss (§103).

It was realized that hardship was so inevitable that debts tended to accrue even under normal conditions. Every ruler of Hammurabi's dynasty proclaimed a Clean Slate, when military or other disruptions occurred during their reign, cancelling personal agrarian debts (but leaving normal commercial business loans intact) upon taking the throne. Hammurabi did this on four occasions.[1]

Bronze Age rulers could not afford to let such bondage and concentration of property and wealth to become chronic. Labor was the scarcest resource, so a precondition for survival was to prevent creditors from using debt leverage to obtain the labor of debtors and appropriate their land. Rulers therefore acted to prevent creditors from becoming a wealthy class seeking gains by impoverishing debtors and taking crop yields and land for themselves.

By rejecting such alleviations of debts resulting from economic disruption, the U.S. economy is subjecting itself to depression, homelessness and economic polarization. It is saving stockholders and bondholders instead of the economy at large. That is because today's *rentier* interests take the economic surplus in the form of debt service, holding labor and also corporate industry in bondage. Mortgage debt is the price of obtaining a home of one's own. Student debt is the price of getting an education to get a job. Automobile debt is needed to buy a car to drive to the job, and credit-card debt must be run up to pay for living costs beyond what one is able to earn. This deep indebtedness makes workers afraid to go on strike or even to protect working conditions, because being fired is to lose the ability to pay debts and rents. So the rising debt overhead serves the business and financial sector by lowering wage levels while extracting more interest, financial fees, rent and insurance out of their take-home pay.

DEBT DEFLATION AND THE TRANSITION FROM FINANCE CAPITALISM TO AN AUSTERITY ECONOMY

By injecting $10 trillion into the financial markets (when Federal Reserve credit is added to U.S. Treasury allocation), the CARES act enabled the stock market to recover all of its 34 percent drop (as measured by the S&P 500 stocks) by June 9, even as the economy's GDP was still plunging. The government's new money creation was not spent to revive the real economy of production and consumption, but at least the financial One Percent was saved from loss. It was as

---

1 I provide a detailed history of Clean Slate acts from the Bronze Age down through Biblical times and the Byzantine Empire in *"... and forgive them their debts"* (ISLET 2018).

if prosperity and living standards would somehow return to normal in a V-shaped recovery.

But what is "normal" these days? For 95 percent of the population, their share of GDP had already been falling ever since the Obama Depression began with the bank bailout in 2009, leaving an enormous bad-debt overhead in place. The economy's long upswing since World War II was already grinding to an end as it struggled to carry its debt burden, rising housing costs, health care and related monthly "nut."[2]

This is not what was expected 75 years ago. World War II ended with families and businesses rife with savings and with little debt, as there had been little to buy during the wartime years. But ever since, each business cycle recovery has started with a higher ratio of debt to income, diverting more revenue from businesses, households and governments to pay banks and bondholders. This debt burden raises the economy's cost of living and doing business, while leaving less wage income and profit to be spent on goods and services.

The virus pandemic has merely acted as a catalyst, ending the long postwar boom. Yet even as the U.S. and other Western economies begin to buckle under their debt overhead, little thought has been given to how to extricate them from the debts and defaults that have accelerated as a result of the broad economic disruption.

The "business as usual" approach is to let creditors foreclose and draw all the income and wealth over subsistence needs into their own hands. Economies have reached the point where debts can be paid only by shrinking production and consumption, leaving them as strapped as Greece has been since 2015. Rejecting debt writedowns to restore social balance was implanted at the outset of modern Western civilization. Ever since Roman times it has become normal for creditors to use social misfortune as an opportunity to gain property and income at the expense of families falling into debt. Blocking the emergence of democratic civic regimes empowered to protect debtors, creditor interests have promoted laws that force debtors to lose their land or other means of livelihood to foreclosing creditors or sell it under distress conditions and still have to work off their debts.

In times of a general economic disruption, giving priority to creditor claims leads to widespread bankruptcy. Yet it violates most peoples' ideas of fairness and distributive justice to evict debtors from their homes and take whatever property they have if they cannot pay their rent arrears and other charges that have accrued through no fault of their own. Bankruptcy proceedings will force many businesses and farms to forfeit what they have invested to much wealthier buyers. Many small businesses, especially in urban minority neighborhoods, will see years of

---

2 I provide the details in *Killing the Host: How Financial Parasites and Debt Destroy the Global Economy* ((SLET, 2015).

saving and investment wiped out. The lockdown also forces U.S. cities and states to cope with plunging sales- and income-tax revenue by slashing social services and depleting their pension funds savings to pay bondholders. Balancing their budgets by privatizing hitherto public services will create monopoly rents and new corporate empires.

These outcomes are not necessary. They also are inequitable. Instead of being a survival of the fittest and the most efficient economic solutions, they are a victory for the most successfully predatory. Yet such results are the product of a long-pedigreed legal and financial philosophy promoted by banks and bondholders, landlords and insurance companies who reject economy-wide debt relief. They depict writing down debts and rents owed to them as unthinkable. Banks claim that forgiving personal and business rents would lead absentee landlords to default on their mortgages, threatening bank solvency. Insurance companies claim that to make their policy holders whole would bankrupt them.[3] So something has to give: either the population's broad economic interests, or the vested interests insisting that labor, industry and the government must bear the cost of arrears that have built up during the economic shutdown.

As in oligarchic Rome, financial interests in today's world have gained control of governments and captured the political and regulatory agencies, leaving democratic reformers powerless to suspend debt service, rent arrears, evictions and depression. The West is becoming a highly centrally planned economy, but its planning center is Wall Street, not Washington or state and local governments.

RISING REAL ESTATE ARREARS PROMPT A MORTGAGE BAILOUT

Canada and many European governments are subsidizing businesses to pay up to 80 percent of employee wages even though many must stay home. But for the 40 million Americans who haven't been employed during the closedown, the prospect is for homelessness and desperation. Already before the crisis about half of Americans reported that they were living paycheck to paycheck and could not raise $400 in an emergency. When the paychecks stopped, rents could not be paid, nor could other normal monthly living expenses.

---

3 Lawsuits are exploding over the role of insurance companies supposed to protect business from such interruptions. See Julia Jacobs, "Arts Groups Fight Their Insurers Over Coverage on Virus Losses," *The New York Times*, May 6, 2020, which reports that "insurance companies have issued a torrent of denials, prompting lawsuits across the country and legislative efforts on the state and federal levels to force insurers to make payments. The insurance industry has argued that…fulfilling all of these requests would bankrupt the industry."

America is seeing the end of the home ownership boom that had endowed its middle class with property steadily rising in price. For buyers, the price was rising mortgage debt, as bank credit was the major factor in raising property prices. (A home is worth however much a bank will lend against it.) For non-whites, to be sure, neighborhoods were redlined against racial minorities. But by the early 2000s, banks began to make loans to black and Hispanic buyers, but usually at extortionately high interest rates and stiffer debt terms. America's white home buyers now face a fate similar to that which has long been imposed on minorities: debt-inflated purchase prices for homes so high that they leave buyers strapped by mortgage and compulsory insurance payments, with declining public services in their neighborhoods.

When mortgages can't be paid, foreclosures follow. That causes declines in the proportion of Americans that own their own homes. That home ownership rate already had dropped from about 58 percent in 2008 to about 51 percent at the start of 2020. Since the 2008 mortgage-fraud crisis and President Obama's mass foreclosure program that hit minorities and low-income buyers especially hard, a more landlord-ridden economy has emerged as a result of foreclosed properties and companies bought by speculators and vast absentee-owner companies like Blackstone.

Many businesses that closed down did not pay the landlords, realizing that if they are held responsible for paying full rents that accrued during the shutdown, it would take them over a year to make up the payment, leaving no net earnings for their efforts. That was especially the case for restaurants with compulsory limited "distance" seating and other stores obliged to restrict the density of their customers. Many restaurants and other neighborhood stores decided instead to go out of business. For hotels standing largely empty, some 19 percent of mortgage loans had fallen into arrears already by May, along with about 10 percent of retail stores.[4]

The commercial real estate sector owes $2.4 trillion in mortgage debt. About 40 percent of tenants did not pay their rents for March, April and May, from restaurants and storefronts to large national retail markets. A moratorium on evictions put them off until August or September 2020. But in the interim, quarterly state and local property taxes were due in June, which also was when the annual federal income-tax payment was owed for the year 2019, having been postponed from April in the face of the shutdown.

The prospective break in the chain of payments by landlords to their banks may be bailed out by the Federal Reserve, but nobody can come up with a scenario whereby the debts owed by non-elites can be paid out of their debtors'

---

4 Conor Dougherty and Peter Eavis, "In Commercial Real Estate, the Domino Effect Escalates," *The New York Times*, June 9, 2020.

own resources, any more than they were rescued from the junk-mortgage frauds that left over-mortgaged homes (mainly for low-income victims) in the wake of Obama's decision to support the banks and mortgage brokers instead of their victims. In fact, it takes a radical scenario to see how state and local debt can be paid as public budgets are thrown into limbo by the virus pandemic.

THE FISCAL SQUEEZE FORCES GOVERNMENTS TO PRIVATIZE PUBLIC SERVICES AND ASSETS

Since 1945, the normal Keynesian response to an economic slowdown has been for governments to run budget deficits to revive the economy and employment. But that can't happen in the wake of the 2020 pandemic. For one thing, tax revenue is falling. Governments can create domestic money, of course, but the U.S. government quickly ran up a $2 trillion deficit by June 2020 simply to support Wall Street's financial and corporate markets, leaving a fiscal squeeze when it came to public spending into the real economy. Many U.S. states and cities have laws obliging them to balance their budgets. So public spending into the real economy (instead of just into the financial and corporate markets) had to be cut back.

Facing the loss of sales taxes from restaurants and hotels, income taxes, and property taxes from landlords not receiving rents, U.S. states and localities are having a huge tax shortfall that is forcing them to cut back basic social services and infrastructure. New York City mayor de Blasio has warned that schools, the police and public transportation may have to be cut back unless the city is given $7 billion. The CARES act passed by the Democratic Party in control of the House of Representatives made no attempt to allocate a single dollar to make up the widening fiscal gap. As for the Trump administration, it was unwilling to give money to states voting Democratic in the presidential or governorship elections.

The irony is that just at the time when a pandemic calls for public health care, political pressure for that abruptly stopped. Logically, the virus might have been expected to have become a major catalyst for single-payer public health care, not least to prevent a wave of personal bankruptcy resulting from high medical bills. But hopes were dashed when the leading torch bearer for socialized medicine, Senator Bernie Sanders, threw his support behind Joe Biden and other opponents for the presidential nomination instead of focusing the primary elections on what the future of the Democratic Party would be. The Democrats decided to focus the 2020 U.S. election merely on the personality of which candidate would impose neoliberal policy: Republican Donald Trump, or his opponent running simply on a platform of "I am not Trump."

Both candidates—and indeed, both parties behind them —sought to downsize government and privatize as much of the public sector as possible, leaving administration to financial managers. Past government policy would have restored prosperity by public spending programs to rebuild the roads and bridges, trains and subways that have fallen apart. But the fiscal squeeze caused by the economic shutdown has created pressure to Thatcherize America's crumbling transportation and urban infrastructure—and also to sell off land and public enterprises, basic urban health, schools—and at the national level, the post office. Fiscal budgets are to be balanced by selling off this infrastructure, in lucrative Public-Private Partnerships (PPPs) with financial firms.

The neoliberal rent-extractive plan is for private capital to buy monopoly rights to repair the nation's bridges by turning them into toll bridges, to repair the nation's roads and highways by making them toll roads, to repair sewer systems by privatizing them. Schools, prisons, hospitals and other traditionally public functions—even the police—are to be privately owned security-guard agencies and managed for profit—on terms that will provide interest and capital gains for the financial sector. It is a New Enclosures movement seeking monopoly rent much as landlords extract land rent.

Having given $10 trillion dollars to support financial and mortgage markets, neoliberals in both the Republican and Democratic parties announced that the government had created so large a budget deficit as a result of bailing out the banking and landlord class that it lacked any more room for money creation for actual social spending programs. Republican Senate leader Mitch McConnell advised states to solve their budget squeeze by raiding their pension funds to pay their bondholders.

For many decades, public employees accepted low wage growth in exchange for pensions. Their patient choice was to defer demands for wage increases in order to secure good pensions for their retirement. But now that they have worked at stagnant wages for many years, the money ostensibly saved for their pensions is to be given to bondholders. Likewise, at the federal level, pressure was renewed by both parties to cut back Social Security, Medicare and Medicaid, with Obama's 2010 Simpson-Bowles Commission on Fiscal Responsibility and Reform to reduce the deficit at the expense of retirees and the poor.

In sum, money is being created to fuel the financial sector and its stock and bond markets, not to increase the economy's solvency, employment and living standards. The coronavirus pandemic did not create this shift, but it catalyzed and accelerated the power grab, not least by pushing public-sector budgets into crisis.

IT DOESN'T HAVE TO BE THIS WAY

Every successful economy has been a mixed public/private economy with checks on the financial sector's power to indebt society in ways that impoverish it. Always at issue, however, is who will control the government. As American and European industry becomes more debt ridden, will they be oligarchic or democratic?

A socialist government such as China's can keep its industry going simply by writing down debts when they can't be paid without forcing a closedown, bankruptcy and the loss of assets and employment. The world thus has two options: a basically productive public financial system as in China, or a predatory financial system as in the United States.

China can recover financially and fiscally from the virus disruption because most debts ultimately are owed to the government-based banking system. Money can be created to finance the material economy, labor and industry, construction and agriculture. When a company is unable to pay its bills and rent, the government doesn't stand by and let it be closed down and sold at a distressed price to a vulture investor.

China has an option that Western economies do not: It is in a position to do what Hammurabi and other ancient Near Eastern palatial economies did for thousands of years: write down debts so as to keep the economy resilient and functioning. It can suspend scheduled debt service, taxes, rents and public fees from having to be paid by troubled areas of its economy, because China's government is the ultimate creditor. It need not contend with politically powerful bankers who insist that the economy at large must lose, not themselves. The government can write down the debt to keep companies in business, and also their employees. That's what socialist governments do.

The underlying problem is finance capitalism. Its roots lie at the heart of Western civilization itself, rejecting the "circular time" permitting economic renewal by Clean Slates in favor of "linear time" in which debts are permanent and irreversible, without public oversight to manage finance and credit in the economy's overall long-term interest.

It often is easier to get rich in such times of disaster and need than in times of normal prosperity. While the U.S. economy polarizes between creditors and debtors, the stock market anticipates fortunes being made quickly from the insolvency of business with assets and property to be grabbed. Coupled with the Federal Reserve's credit creation to support the financial and real estate markets, asset prices are soaring (as of June 2020) for companies that expect to get even richer from the widespread distress to come in autumn 2020 when evictions and foreclosures ae scheduled to begin again.

In that respect, the coronavirus's effect has been to help defeat the financial sector's enemy, governments strong enough to regulate it. The fiscal squeeze resulting from widespread unemployment, business closedowns, rent and tax arrears is being seized upon as a means of dismantling and privatizing government at the federal, state and local levels, at the expense of the citizenry at large.

CHAPTER SEVEN

CHINA'S ECONOMY OF PEACE

Peter Koenig

When China sneezes, the West does more than catch a cold. It roars with anger. China has become a threat to western aggression, abuse and wasteful lifestyle. China bashing by the West, predominantly the U.S. and some of her allies, knows no end. The corona crisis is just one of the fabricated and convenient reasons.

THE CORONA CRISIS

Many people strongly suspect that the new coronavirus, with its name mutating from SARS-2-2019, or 2019-nCoV to SARS-CoV-2, and with the disease itself finally termed COVID-19 by WHO, did not originate in China, though the first outbreaks were reported in Wuhan (pop. 11 million), Hubei Province. Most probably Patient Zero contracted it in the United States. We may never know for sure. The U.S.-Western–paid propaganda machine keeps accusing China, with no solid argument, of having mishandled the coronavirus, and especially of having been secretive about it, instead of immediately informing WHO and the rest of the world, so other countries could prepare for it.

What may be true, however, is that the corona pandemic has been instrumentalized as part of a plan that goes back possibly decades, far prior to the present corona pandemic. But let's concentrate on more recent indications of its existence—the "2010 Rockefeller Report." This report spelled out a program that starts in 2020 with a corona pandemic. It would start in China and in no time, it would engulf the entire globe. That initial phase is called "The Lockstep Scenario."

The final goal, per the report, is global government, also called the New World Order or the One World Order (NWO/OWO). The financial and political elite, some of whom are at times visible, at times underground, often regarded as key components of what is referred to as the Deep State, have for decades contemplated and planned for the NWO/OWO. This is projected to happen via the destruction of society as we know it, using lockdowns, total population control, vaccination, and ultimately leading to massive population reduction. Reading the report—the scariest parts of it, like the "Lockstep Scenario," can still be found on the internet as of June 2020—itself inspires fear. People in fear can easily be manipulated. It also lowers people's immune level which seems to be all part of the plan. Could such a monstrous, vast undertaking possibly succeed?

Yet it is now evident that a globally coordinated event has indeed occurred. A pandemic, a very light one at that, hardly deserving the term—has engulfed the entire globe within weeks—and shortly thereafter most of the countries of the world were on lockdown. Under the guise of a purported pandemic, havoc has been wreaked around the world, wiping out as of yet inestimable chunks of the global economy, creating misery, hardship, despair, famine and death. All that within the first five months of 2020! Such a comprehensive outcome is practically impossible to have happened naturally. So, it must have been helped.

The precursor to this oppressive endgame is the 1989 Washington Consensus—an agreement, or a *consensus,* of the (Western) world's foremost financial institutions, the U.S. Federal Reserve (FED), the International Monetary Fund (IMF), and the World Bank (WB), to submit civilization to the plague of neoliberalism—an extreme form of everything-goes capitalism, with no rules, no regulations—a freestyle turbo-market economy with privatization of everything. It started with massive programs by the IMF and WB of so-called "structural adjustment" loans for developing countries whose "conditionalities" were designed to tailor their economies to Western needs. This kind of financial enslavement was already tried by the two Bretton Woods Institutions in the 1980s. The Washington Consensus merely confirmed their concept.

At the time of this writing, we are in the first stages of the Lockstep Scenario. It includes a global shutdown of everything, to protect humanity from an invisible enemy, a coronavirus, now called COVID-19. It includes, also, an enormous and unprecedented media fear campaign, preparing the global population for global vaccination, which seems to be Bill Gates' raison d'être. Since he and GAVI (Global Alliance for Vaccines and Immunization), which the Gates Foundation created, fund more than half of WHO's budget, WHO also supports this vaccination craze. In our neoliberal western world, conflicts of interest are no longer an issue.

Vaccination is a multi-multi-billion-dollar business, especially since it needs to be repeated every year, as the coronavirus tends to mutate like the different flu viruses mutate, at least once a year, justifying a new vaccine every year—even though virologists and medical doctors have been saying for years that flu vaccination has, on average, a 30% to 60% effectiveness, vaccination may also have nefarious side effects, including allergies, high fever dizziness, respiratory difficulties and—yes—autism.

A global COVID-19 vaccination also offers an opportunity to inject along with the vaccine a nano-chip which can be uploaded with all personal identification data, from health records to bank accounts. A universal digital ID is also a Bill Gates promoted idea, to be implemented by Agenda ID2020, another Bill Gates creation.

Universal ID as part of Agenda ID2020 was incorporated in 2016 in the UN's Sustainable Development Goals (SDG); it is SDG 16.9 (*by 2030 provide legal identity for all including birth registration*).[1] Agenda 2030 is officially the target date for reaching the 17 Sustainable 1 Development Goals (SDG). It is also the target date for the New or One World Order becoming fully operational.

Foreseen under this monstrous plan is a fully digitized human life. This comes with digital money, already promoted for the financial banking oligarchy by WHO's Director General, Dr. Tedros Adhanom Ghebreyesus, a close friend of Bill Gates. It was widely reported in the UK that WHO had claimed cash was transmitting coronavirus.[2] The media message was: digital is more hygienic. Contrary to physical cash, it does not transmit diseases.

Trials with digital money have already been going on for years in Nordic countries, where entire department stores only accept electronic money. A digital payment system works towards total control of every citizen's move—and provides an opportunity for the authorities to monitor people's bank accounts. Digital money is easily traceable. It's possible that in future, your bank account details may be uploaded on the nano-chip under your skin.

Already today in China, more than 90% of monetary transactions are carried out electronically by Ali-Pay, WeChat and others. But, so far, cash has not been banned anywhere in China. The Government of China is currently preparing the rolling out of an international blockchain-based crypto-currency.[3]

To make this plan of a digitized world work, a strong system of electromagnetic radiation is needed. Hence, the invention and introduction of 5G (Fifth Generation) technologies, also called the "internet of things." One marvels at the description of the forthcoming robotic capacities of 5G, like self-driven cars, refrigerators that tell you when you run out of beer and remind you when your medical cabinet is out of your essential medication.

---

1 United Nations, "#Envision2030 Goal 16: Peace, Justice and Strong Institutions," https://www.un.org/development/desa/disabilities/envision2030-goal16.html.

2 While WHO contended its words had been misrepresented, the widespread publicity had more impact than the subsequent disclaimer. See Meera Jagannathan, "World Health Organization: 'We did NOT say that cash was transmitting coronavirus,'" MarketWatch, March 9, 2020, https://www.marketwatch.com/story/who-we-did-not-say-that-cash-was-transmitting-coronavirus-2020-03-06.

3 See below, "China's New Monetary System," for more details.

Nobody, so far, has told us that the utmost purpose of 5G is controlling us, our moves, purchases, the 'likes and the dislikes' of goods and services—every step we take, every penny we spend and every word we say or write is being surveilled and registered. The latter is already the case today. The ultimate plan is to control our minds, to remotely orient them towards specific objectives our superiors want us to pursue. It will be a very much refined version of what is today called MK-Ultra, a mind control technique pursued by the CIA in the 1960s.

Corona/COVID-19 History

When the coronavirus first hit China in Wuhan, Hubei Province, towards the end of 2019, China was on her guard, remembering SARS (Severe Acute Respiratory Syndrome) of 2002/2003. SARS hit Hong Kong first in November 2002 and then in 2003 spread to China and to the rest of the world. SARS was basically over by mid-2003. It has caused worldwide about 8,400 infections and about 800 deaths. Already questions were raised as to whether the SARS virus was "manufactured" to affect specifically the Chinese genome. This may be not far-fetched if one looks at the statistics of registered cases: Mainland China 5327; Hong Kong 1755; Taiwan 671; Singapore 206—a total of 7959, out of 8437 registered cases, About 95% were people of Chinese ethnicity. All or most of the other cases, predominantly in Canada, Vietnam and the United States, are likely also to be traced to people with Chinese DNA.

Being aware of this, China's labs tested the new / old coronavirus and came to the conclusion that it was a mutation of SARS—likely also directed to the Chinese DNA. With the ongoing trade war initiated by Washington to destabilize China, the prospect that it was designing a virus that predominantly attacked Chinese people was not an unrealistic fear. In reaction China immediately locked down the city of Wuhan with its 11 million people along with the entire Hubei Province of about 50 million people.

Other cities followed later. China reacted fast with widespread quarantines and countrywide lockdowns, meaning that 60% to 80% of all manufacturing and construction stopped—and people stayed home. The Chinese are known as extremely disciplined, and they trust their government. This paid off. For China the pandemic peaked about the end of April—and as at mid-June 2020, China reports no new cases.

On June 8, 2020, China, with a population of 1.4 billion people, has reported a total of 84,634 confirmed cases and 4,645 deaths. In comparison, the United States, with a total population of 330 million, has registered about 1.9 million cases and almost 110,000 deaths. Globally, there have been about 7 million confirmed cases of COVID-19, including about 401,000 deaths, according to WHO. This in theory is a death to infection rate of 5.7%. How trustworthy are these statistics, the basis for which is different in almost every country? In the U.S., the Covid-accounting practices vary from state to state.

In a peer reviewed article in the prestigious *New England Journal of Medicine* (NEJM), Dr. Anthony Fauci, head of the National Institute of Allergy and Infectious Diseases (NIAID), one of 27 agencies forming the U.S. National Institute of Health (NIH), said in the article's core statement, "This suggests that the overall clinical consequences of COVID-19 are ultimately more similar to those of a severe seasonal influenza (with a lethality of about 0.1%) or pandemic influenza (similar to those of 1957 and 1968) than to a disease like SARS or MERS, which had lethalities of 9 to 10% and 36% respectively."

All these figures have to be taken with a lot of caution. Not all statistics use the same methods of counting. The overall belief is that the infection as well as the death accounting was inflated—some say vastly inflated—mostly for political purposes and for fear-mongering. People in fear can easily be manipulated, especially when it comes to administering vaccines. It is also recognized that people living in fear have lowered immune system protection. All of which facilitates the total control agenda of the deep state super elite that calls the shots behind the scenes.

Unfortunately, it cannot be said that the peak has been reached in all parts of the world. For example, in South America and the Global South, where fall and winter are about to begin—the typical flu season—a new corona wave may emerge. In Europe, while most countries are easing their overall social distancing and contact restrictions with a view to normalizing life, some are still hesitant to open borders without quarantining visiting foreigners.

President Trump has accused China and WHO of not having been transparent, of having hidden Covid information from the rest of the world, resulting in the rest of the world, particularly the U.S., being unable to prepare in a timely manner for the outbreak. Citing the same reasoning, President Trump has also exited WHO membership. This timescale has been proved to be untrue, and is pure China bashing with the intent to discredit China, an up and coming economic super power, with the rest of the world. China is already second to the U.S. and unstoppable in overpassing the U.S. within the next three to maximum five years. More importantly, the Chinese Yuan, backed by a solid economy and by gold—not fiat currency like the U.S.-dollar and the euro—may soon replace the U.S. dollar as the world's chief reserve currency. When that happens, it may mark the end of dollar hegemony, the dollar dictatorship that has so far been used to "sanction" dissenting countries, one after the other—totally illegally according to international law, destroying national economies and people's livelihoods. That will be highly welcomed by most countries of Mother Earth. While Washington will not miss an opportunity to belittle China, it will be to no avail. China is already looking to markets in different directions with different monetary policies.

Irrespective of whether China and WHO informed Trump, clearly other U.S. interested parties were well ahead of the curve. On October 18, 2019, the Johns Hopkins Institute for Health, together with the Bill and Melinda Gates Foundation (BMGF) and the World Economic Forum (WEF—the club of elitists that meets every January in Davos, Switzerland to decide the fate of the world—so they wish) sponsored Event 201 in New York City. One of the main purposes of the event was a computer simulation of a corona pandemic. Per their simulation, the pandemic produced 65 million deaths in the span of 18 months, and as a byline wiped out more than 30% of the stock market, caused untold bankruptcies and created unfathomable unemployment. The simulation predicted a socioeconomic holocaust unheard of in human history, vastly surpassing the Great Depression of 1929–33. Participating in the Event 201, were, among others, representatives of the World Bank, WHO, UNICEF, the U.S. and the Chinese CDC (Centers for Disease Control and Prevention) and other important players.

A few weeks later, the first coronavirus case, alias COVID-19, was discovered in Wuhan, where it allegedly was transmitted by a bat to a human in a wet market, a contention that is now widely disputed. The reality is that the U.S. and all those aware of the Rockefeller Report and participating in the Event 201 simulation, knew that a pandemic was imminent.

A few months later at the WEF (January 21–24, 2020), a meeting at which Dr. Tedros, the DG of WHO, also participated, it was decided that this corona outbreak should be called a "pandemic." On January 30, 2020, WHO declared it a Public Health Emergency of International Concern (PHEIC). At that time there were only about 150 confirmed cases outside of China. On March 11, WHO characterized COVID-19 as a pandemic.

By late February, early March, the pandemic surged and started to spread to other countries, first to Europe, Italy and Spain, but also France and Germany and to the U.S. and worldwide. It is widely assumed that after the COVID-19 strand that affected China, other mutated versions of the coronavirus (was it originally laboratory mutated, is the question) hit the rest of the world.

There are also as of yet unproven allegations that the rolling out of 5G—the intense electromagnetic fields (EMF)—may have an impact on COVID-19, especially affecting the respiratory capacity of certain more vulnerable people.

The Global Economic Impact

The worldwide economic impact is hardly predictable at this stage. In the U.S., in early June 2020, an additional 1.5 million people filed for unemployment benefits; 25% of U.S. families are considered food-insecure; and the FED predicts unemployment in the U.S. may reach 50% by the end of the year. The International Labor Office (ILO) says that global unemployment may reach 2 billion within the next few months. The meltdown of assets has hardly begun.

A peak in bankruptcies may not be seen for the next three to six months, and the consequences will be disastrous: more unemployment, more precariousness, more misery and despair, leading to suicide and massive famine. The World Food Program predicts hundreds of millions of people will be affected by famine and maybe tens of millions, possibly reaching hundred million, may die from hunger and famine-related diseases. The present average annual death rate from hunger per year is around 9 million.

In the same four or five months that a majority of the world will have slipped into poverty, some into extreme destitution, the crust of the elite, the billionaires, have gotten richer, much richer. They have added almost 300 billion more to their fortune—thanks to Covid-19. This is the largest wealth gain by billionaires in a comparable time span in recorded history.

In a recent presentation to China, the IMF has predicted a global GDP decline for 2020 of 3%, (later adjusted to –5%), and a slight growth for 2021. In the author's opinion, the decline will be more likely in the neighborhood of 10% in 2020—with a slight recovery, but still in the negative growth range for 2021. For the U.S. the IMF predicted a decline of 5.4% for 2020—and a just above zero growth rate in 2021. Chinese authorities predict China's growth for 2020 between 3% and 3.5%. The IMF presented three different projection scenarios, two of which included a second corona wave, either later in 2020 or in 2021.

China's Recovery from COVID-19

In China the economic impact was also stark, with close to 80% of all manu-facturing and construction work suddenly halted. This made the Chinese economy plunge by about 30% in the first three months of the year. Since China is virtually the supply chain for the rest of the world, especially for the West, the impact of the Chinese lockdown was mostly felt by the West, where suddenly merchandise, spare parts and, foremost on the minds of many, medical supplies were missing. China supplies about 80% of medicines and medical equipment and 90% of anti-biotics to the west, including ingredients for manufacturing the medication.

The Chinese lockdown lasted from January 23 to April 8, 2020, some 72 days. Once China relaunched their economic activities they recovered fast. China has a "trick"—called public banking. There are more than 4,000 public banking or financing institutions throughout China. They target sectors and regions that need fast recovery and job creation with special conditions, with low or no interest. If loan repayments are delayed or fail altogether, it's not a drama. The point is public banks do not work for shareholders—there aren't any. They work for the local economy and the local people.

If a sector or a region or both at times needs grants or subsidies for their recovery, job creation and construction of infrastructure that will pay off in the medium-or long-term future, so be it. Public banks do not go broke, as Western observers would like to have you believe, they have their lines of credit with the People's Bank of China (PBC), China's central bank. They fulfill a public utility's role for the national and local economy, for the well-being of the people.

China could have served as a model for the West. But it takes confidence in government intentions, discipline and coordination, not dictatorship, lies, fear and propaganda blame-casting against others. The public in the west faced chaotic and often contradictory statements and recommendations from the foremost health authorities. First the facemasks are on, then they are off, then it's maybe, under certain circumstances... WHO is a champion in such inconsistencies. Even the most obedient citizens lose trust in the authorities.

And then there are the systemic issues. In the West, the economy is in the hands of private banking and often of semi-privatized central banks. In the United States, the FED is an entirely private institution acting as a central bank. Private for-profit banking doesn't usually invest where its most needed from a socioeconomic point of view, but rather where the profit projections are good. It's a component of the economic policy called neoliberalism that works basically without any rules, investing where the profit margins are the highest—and keeping the shareholders happy—irrespective of the service or disservice they may provide for the community.

In the West, policy benefits for the community and social development of the people is of lesser importance. This depends on the "trickle-down" effect which already in the late sixties and early seventies, as the World Bank itself had concluded, didn't work. Now, after the Washington Consensus and its super-imposed neoliberal dogma, this wise World Bank recognition of the seventies that investments at the grassroots level serve the communities and in the medium to long run serve the entire national economy, is conveniently forgotten. Neoliberalism has no major interest in the national economy, only in instant *private* profit—as instant as possible. That's why recovery in the U.S. and Europe will be much slower, possibly more chaotic and may bring even more societal imbalance and injustice.

CHINA'S RECOVERY FROM WESTERN DOMINATION

In 1949, under Chairman Mao Zedong, China rose literally from the ashes. The century of imperial domination, or as the Chinese call it, the Hundred Years of National Humiliation, encapsulates the intervention and subjugation of the Chinese Empire by western powers, the Russian Empire and Japan between 1839 and 1949. This period included calamitous wars suffered by China: the First and the Second Opium Wars (1839–1842 and 1856–1860)—to the Brits; the Sino-French War (1884–1885); and the Sino-Japanese War

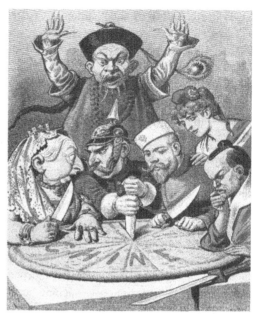

Henri Meyer, "China—the cake of kings and of emperors." French political cartoon from 1898. (Bibliothèque Nationale de France)

(1937–1945), where the Communist Party of China (CPC) joined forces with its opposition, the western supported government of the Republic of China, led by the Kuomintang (KMT) and finally defeated the Japanese invasion.

After the KMT-CPC joint defeat of the Japanese, the civil war between these rival parties that was lingering on and off since 1927, called the *War of Liberation,* resumed from 1945 to 1949. The Communist Party won and declared on October 1, 1949 the People's Republic of China (PRC). The KMT, under Chiang Kai-shek retreated to Taiwan, where he claimed to represent the official China, until on October 25, 1971, a UN Resolution recognized the People's Republic of China (PRC) as "the only legitimate representative of China to the United Nations." As of this day, no end to the Chinese civil war has been officially declared, and there are still some 15 countries, including the Holy See, recognizing Taiwan as the official representative of China (May 2020).

These are just a few of the battles and conflicts China has fought against colonial powers, all of whom were intent on plundering China's riches. China's defense was relentless, but all at an enormous cost. The Chinese also call the civil war between 1945 and 1949 the war of the Communist Revolution. Indeed, the Communist Revolution began officially under Chairman Mao on October 1, 1949 and—as the dynamics between China and the West attest—the War of Liberation is still ongoing.

The pre-1949 wars and conflicts devastated China, leaving it literally in ashes, ravaged by extreme poverty, famine, diseases, and dysfunctional social and institutional infrastructure and education. Mao launched a two-part revolution. The Great Leap Forward (1958–1962) was to rebuild China from an agrarian economy into an industrialized communist society. Western infiltrations attempted to bring about "regime change"—including the usual atrocities as we recognize them to this day. As an instance, Western "agents" along with Chinese opposition, disrupted and sabotaged food supplies, resulting in the so-called Great Chinese Famine (1959–1961).

With ideas of a Great Chinese Communist nation unperturbed, Chairman Mao proceeded with the Chinese Cultural Revolution (1966–1976). The objective was to consolidate Chinese communist values and to purge the Chinese Revolution from foreign interventions. Also, and equally important, Mao wanted to make China an autonomous country, self-sufficient in health, food and education, the three pillars of a truly sovereign nation, with an independent and self-determined monetary policy. This is key for an independent economy to prosper. China started gradually and cautiously opening her borders in the mid-1970s to 1980s, thoughtfully building up foreign relations and foreign trade, including foreign investments.

From this compressed history of China and China's revolution emerges a simple but important principle for an national economy to recover and rebuild itself as an autonomous economy: *Local production for local consumption with local money and local public banks, backed by a state-owned central bank that designs local monetary policies to develop the local economy, benefitting the local population.*

When a reasonable level of self-sufficiency of the Three Pillars (health, food and education) was reached, it was felt to be prudent to open up for selective foreign trade. Their historical experience led the Chinese to beware of globalization, which in its massive dimensions is largely to blame for the devastating destruction COVID-19 was able to wreak.

China has again applied this simple principle to recover from the corona crisis. Within months of the corona peak and descending curve, China has been recovering quickly, with its borders largely closed. Gradual reopening may happen in the second half of 2020. The West could learn a lesson, by concentrating on the domestic market by using public banking as a public utility enabling the local economy to blossom again, before embarking on massive foreign trade—as if nothing had happened. And foreign trade should never be massive, just sufficient to allow for an equilibrium of societal well-being. Primarily, consume locally what the local production—agriculture, manufacturing, services—can provide.

What has happened—a mammoth destruction of the world economy—has left untold misery behind. But the silver lining is the opportunity to reset and rethink the Western lifestyle, its consumerism, waste-economy, environmental degradation…all of which is largely linked to globalization where corporate profit-driven doctrines and consumerism drive and define our civilization's values.

By the end of 2020, China is expected to be back to "speed," meaning, to have surmounted the economic interruption and COVID decline. Indeed, there is no intent to go back to a 12% annual GDP growth rate. China's aim is to grow moderately and horizontally rather than vertically. The West will try, if at all possible, to revert to its corporate and finance-driven vertical growth model, typical for a private profit-maximizing economy. Growth and pillage of natural resources are embedded in that system.

China calls her new growth model, "quality growth," putting emphasis on attaining, as much as possible, an economic equilibrium between the regions, their peoples and their cultures. Public banking is ideal. It creates growth that eventually allows all people to "live well," while observing the protection of natural resources and, foremost, of Mother Earth. It means development of local social services and infrastructure to optimize the people's potential to auto-develop—to create their own market and interchange with neighbors—living in harmony.

Endless creation, avoiding conflicts for the benefit of all, is a basic Tao principle which is practiced on a daily basis in China. This simple belief is applied internally as well as in China's foreign policy. No aggression. It is also part of rebuilding after a catastrophe.

The Belt and Road Initiative or the New Silk Road

In April 2013, China embarked on a new mammoth economic development scheme, unheard of in human history, that may span the world in the course of the 21st Century, the *Belt and Road Initiative* (BRI). It is a peaceful approach to a world in "equilibrium"—where trade means equal benefits for all, and where economic development means guidance to becoming socioeconomically autonomous peoples and nations.

The BRI, also called the New Silk Road, is based on a 2,100-year-old trade route between the Middle East and Eastern Asia, called the Silk Road. It wound its ways across the huge landmass Eurasia to the most eastern parts of China. It favored trading, based on the Taoist philosophy of harmony and peaceful coexistence—trading in the original sense of the term, an exchange with "win-win" outcomes, both partners benefiting equally.

Today, in the Western world, we have lost this concept. The terms of trade are always imposed by the "stronger" partner, the West, or Global North, versus the poorer Global South—the south where most of the natural resources are lodged.

Mother Earth's assets have been and are coveted by the west—or north—for building and maintaining a lifestyle in luxury, abundance and waste. This trend has lasted for centuries of western colonialism: Exploitation, loot, esclavisation and rape of entire peoples of the Global South by the Global North.

The New Silk Road, or BRI, is Chinese President Xi Jinping's brainchild. It's based on the same ancient Silk Road principles, adjusted to the 21st Century, building bridges between peoples, exchanging goods, research, education, knowledge, cultural wisdom, peacefully, harmoniously and "win-win" style. On 7 September 2013, Xi presented BRI at Kazakhstan's Nazarbayev University. He spoke about "People-to-People Friendship and Creating a better Future." He referred to the Ancient Silk Road of more than 2,100 years ago, that flourished during China's Western Han Dynasty (206 B.C. to 24 A.D.).

Referring to this epoch of more than two millenniums back, Xi Jinping pointed to the history of exchanges under the Ancient Silk Road, saying, "they had proven that countries with differences in race, belief and cultural background can absolutely share peace and development as long as they persist in unity and mutual trust, equality and mutual benefit, mutual tolerance and learning from each other, as well as cooperation and win-win outcomes." President Xi's vision may be shaping the world of the 21st Century. Since 2017, enshrined in China's Constitution, *BRI has become the flagship for China's foreign policy.*

Already today BRI has investments involving more than 120 countries and 40 international organizations—and is growing in Asia, Africa, Europe, the Middle East and the Americas. BRI is a multi-trillion investment scheme, for transport routes on land and sea, for the construction of industrial and energy infrastructure and energy exploration, as well as for trade among connected countries. Unlike the World Trade Organization (WTO), BRI is encouraging nations to benefit from their comparative advantages. In essence, BRI is trying to develop mutual under-standing and trust among member nations, allowing for free capital flows, a pool of experts and access to a BRI-based technology database.

At present, BRI's closing date is foreseen for 2049 which coincides with new China's 100th Anniversary. The size and likely success of the program indicates, however, already today that it will most probably be extended way beyond that date. It is worth noting, though, that not until 2019, six years after its inception, did BRI become a news item in the West. Remarkably, for six years BRI was effectively ignored by the western media, in the hope it may go away. But in-stead, many European Union members have already subscribed to BRI, including Greece, Italy, France, Portugal—and more will follow, as the temptation to partic-ipate in this projected socioeconomic boom is overwhelming.

Germany, the supposed economic leader of Europe, is mulling over the pros and cons of participating in BRI. The German business community, like businesses throughout Europe, is strongly in favor of lifting U.S.-imposed sanctions and reconnecting with the East, in particular with China and Russia. But official Berlin is still with one foot in the White House—with the other trying to appease the German and European world of business. This balancing act is in the long run not sustainable and certainly not desirable.

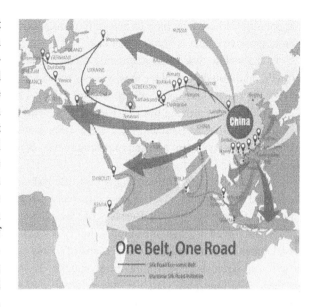

One Belt, One Road

BRI is already actively involved in at least half of the EU member countries.

To deflect attention from their participation in BRI, the European Union, basically run by NATO and intimately linked to Washington, has initiated its own "Silk Road," attempting to connect Asia with Europe through Japan. The EU and Japan have signed a "free trade agreement" which includes a compact to build infrastructure, in sectors such as energy, transport and digital devices. The purpose is to strengthen economic and cultural ties between the two regions, boosting business relations between Asia and Europa. It is an obvious effort to compete with or even sideline China's BRI. It is, however, equally obvious that this effort will fail. Usually initiatives taken in bad faith are not successful. Non-belligerent China is unlikely to challenge this EU-Japan competitive approach.

In another approach to counter BRI, the U.S. Overseas Private Investment Corporation (OPIC), Australia's Department of Foreign Affairs and Trade (DFAT), and the Japan Bank for International Cooperation (JBIC), launched on November 4, 2019 the *Blue Dot Network* (BDN), an initiative supposedly run entirely by private actors, funded by private banking, and intended to bring together governments, the private sector, and civil society "to promote high-quality, trusted standards for global infrastructure development in an open and inclusive framework."

It is not clear how the BDN will interact with or counteract BRI. Anything run entirely by the private sector, especially western private banking, is not a good omen for the country their "development effort" touches. Such investment objectives are primarily shareholder profits, not socioeconomic development benefiting the countries where they plan to invest. No competition for China's BRI. Again, non-aggressive China is unlikely to react.

China's New Silk Road is creating a multipolar world, fostering economic growth, distributed in a balanced way, so as to prioritize development opportunities for the under-developed areas of western China, eastern Russia, Central Asia, Central Europe—reaching out to Africa and the Middle East, Latin America, as well as to South East Asia and the Pacific. BRI is already actively building and planning some six to ten land and maritime routes, connecting Africa, the Middle East, Europe and South America.

The expected multi-trillion-dollar equivalent dynamic budget is expected to be funded by China largely, but not exclusively, by the Asian Infrastructure and Investment Bank (AIIB), by Russia—and by all the countries that are part of BRI and involved in singular or multi-country projects. This revolutionary global development scheme will require trillions of yuans and dollars for investments. It will also be generating trillions in revenues over time, to be shared with BRI partners. The long-term return on these massive investments which will affect people's wellbeing is an exponential multiple of the original investments and cannot be limited to numerical economics, as such social benefits cannot be defined by linear accounting.

Implementing BRI, or the New Silk Road, is itself the realization of a positive vision of the interaction of nations: peaceful interconnectivity, joint infrastructure and industrial development, as well as joint management of natural resources. For example, BRI may help with infrastructure and management advice resolving or preventing conflicts on *transboundary water resources*. There are some 263 transboundary lake and river basins, covering almost half the earth's surface and involving some 150 countries. In addition, there are about 300 transboundary aquifers serving about 2 billion people who depend on groundwater. China calls the New Silk Road Initiative "a bid to enhance regional connectivity and embrace a brighter future."

CHINA'S NEW MONETARY SYSTEM

"Endless creation" is a movement of dynamic activities that flows like a river, avoiding and circumventing obstacles, promoting a harmonious cohabitation with different nations. China has been confronted throughout its 70 years of Revolution with aggression, threats, military encirclements, denigrations and insults by the West. China's response has always been a polite reaction, not counterattack, applying the Tao principle of

Skillful soldiers
Are not easily provoked;
Skillful conquest of opponents
Does not require battle;
Skillful employer
Become humble.....

This is known as
Living congruently with the universe.....
(excerpts of Tao 68)

China is attacked by the U.S. on various fronts, among them initiating a seemingly endless trade war despite the fact that the West, in particular the U.S., depends on the China supply chain for maintaining her living in comfort; attacking China's currency, the yuan, as it climbs rapidly toward taking a key role in international reserves; disrupting international sea routes in the South China Sea and occupying the South China Sea against international law; encircling China with a myriad of military bases; and—as is highly probable—launching a bio-war (or bio-wars) against China. Let alone the countless sanctions, most of them based on China's transactions in western currencies, predominantly the U.S. dollar.

When President Trump referred with visible anger to what he calls China's "mismanagement" of the corona crisis, he was simply using a new pretext to defame China to the world for something he knows has no basis, but is merely a further iteration of the old-new China bashing hardline being pushed by his administration. On May 14, he said in a Fox Business News interview, referring to the CDC February offer of assistance to Wuhan, "I'm very disappointed in China.... We asked to go over [to help] and they said no. They didn't want our help. And I figured that was OK because they must know what they are doing. So, it was either stupidity, incompetence or deliberate."

These are strong and unsubstantiated words, since there has never been an accusation against China clearly documenting precisely how China mismanaged the COVID-19 outbreak and is supposedly responsible for the COVID crisis in the U.S. Rather, it is in the U.S. where real mismanagement of the coronavirus response is taking place, as evident in the corruption, conflicts of interest (particularly pharma-interests, competing private vaccine company interests), warp speed development of untested vaccines, and falsification of corona statistics (falsifying death certificates, paying hospitals for declaring any patient a COVID-patient, even if many of them aren't, and for using ventilators, though it is widely known that ventilators are causing death in 60% to 80% of patients).

It seems increasingly probable that the virus was created in a U.S. bioweapons lab from where it escaped deliberately or by accident, that patient zero was in the U.S., and that the virus was brought to China in one way or another. President Trump must know it. He also must know that this pandemic had been prepared by long in advance, all the way back at least to the *2010 Rockefeller Report* with its "Lockstep Scenario."

Donald Trump must also know about *Event 201* of October 18, 2020, that took place in New York City, sponsored by the Johns Hopkins University's School of Health and co-funded by Gates, WEF, CDC and other interested players, and that the key event of *Event 201* was a simulation of a corona pandemic that produced in the simulation 65 million deaths in 18 months, plunged the stock market by more than 30%, created untold bankruptcies and unfathomable unemployment and misery.

Trump's China bashing has nothing to do with China's "mismanagement" of the corona epidemic, but rather with China's bold move to step further away from the dollar-economy, by:

First, using the yuan and local currencies to boost trade among the ASEAN+3 countries (Association of Southeast Asian Nations—Brunei, Cambodia, Indonesia, Laos, Malaysia, Myanmar, the Philippines, Singapore, Thailand, and Vietnam; plus 3—Japan, South Korea and China). Future monetary transactions will use the China-designed CIPS (Cross-Border Interbank Payment System), avoiding the dollar-controlled SWIFT payment scheme, to prevent U.S. interference in international monetary transactions—and also counter the United States' threat to cut off Chinese supply chains.

The U.S. cutting off its Chinese supply chains is, of course, sheer bluff, as the vast majority of U.S. industries depend in one way or another on deliveries from China. These U.S. supply chains will not be swiftly replaced, leaving the U.S. facing the possibility of suddenly standing there with an empty cup.

In the first quarter of 2020, ASEAN countries became China's largest trading partner with 15.1% of its trade, outpacing the European Union (EU). Trade with South Korea and Japan amounted to another 13.7%, bringing the total close to 30%. Adding China's trade with Russia, another at least 15%, is getting close to a 50% tipping point where China's closest partners may abandon commercial transactions in U.S. dollars.

Second, by launching a new People's Bank of China controlled blockchain-based crypto-currency for international trade, thereby further circumventing the U.S.-dollar and SWIFT controlled international money transfer system which makes all transactions vulnerable to U.S. interference and sanctions. China's new cyber-money, e-RMB (*Ren Min Bi,* meaning People's Money), or Yuan, is currently being tested in several Chinese cities, including Shenzhen, Suzhou,

Chengdu, and Xiong'an. In these cities it has almost universal acceptance, i.e. for salary payments, public transportation, food and most retail shopping.

Commodity pricing, today mostly dollarized, will be quoted by China in yuan and traded in crypto-yuan. Yuan pricing for commodities, such as gold, crude oil and iron ore, has already started. As China is recovering from the pandemic more quickly than the rest of the world, relatively high-returning yuan-denominated investments and commodity assets will become more attractive.

The non-interference factor of a Chinese Central Bank-backed crypto-currency to avoid U.S. sanctions may prompt many countries to gradually and quietly divest their dollar holdings into Chinese yuan.

When about 50% of world trade and world reserves are denominated in yuan, the worldwide dollar hegemony may be no more. It may be displaced by the yuan.

Several leaders of countries were killed for attempting to replace the dollar for trading with other currencies: Saddam Hussein, for his intent to use the euro for trading Iraq's hydrocarbon riches, and Libya's Gadhafi who, when he wanted to introduce the Gold-Dinar as a Pan-African trading currency, thereby freeing Africa from western monetary slavery, was literally lynched by NATO on 20 October 2011, at the initiative of Hillary Clinton with the strong support of then French President Sarkozy. This western monetary stranglehold on Africa prevails as of this day—a new-old kind of colonization that nobody in the western mainstream reports on.

Once the new e-RMB (yuan) has been successfully tested locally it will be launched internationally. While China's new cyber-currency internationalization will make the yuan even more attractive among trading partners and also as a reserve currency, China may simultaneously divest its huge reserves of U.S. Treasury bonds (about U.S. $1.2 trillion) to purchase assets abroad, paid for in U.S. dollars. The Belt and Road investments may serve as a suitable vehicle to reduce dollar holdings at home.

In the current high corona debt-crisis around the world, especially in the Global South, China may also consider a program of Debt Jubilee (debt forgiveness) to the poorest partner countries, which may already be, or potentially become, future Belt and Road associates.

Since October 2016, the Renminbi (Chinese yuan) has been part of a 5-currency basket at the IMF that constitutes its Special Drawing Rights (SDR), the world's ultimate virtual reserve currency. The present SDR share distribution is U.S. dollar 41.73%, euro 30.93%, Chinese yuan 10.92%, Japanese yen 8.33% and the British pound 8.09%. This currency allocation to the SDR is disproportionate with regard to the economic strength of the respective countries, especially China, the world's second largest economy, rapidly moving towards first place.

China may want to vigorously renegotiate with the IMF her currency proportion in the SDR, as well as call for a review of country quotas which by now
are out-of-line with member countries' present economic weight. An IMF capital
increase is overdue. The IMF capital base today is SDR 477 billion (U.S. $677
billion). In addition, there is the temporary New Arrangement to Borrow (NAB)
which in January 2020 has been doubled to SDR365 billion (U.S. $475 billion), a
total resource-base of about U.S. $1.15 trillion. Yet, the IMF already foresees U.S.
$1 trillion as required for additional corona debt lending and debt forgiveness.
Since the NAB is only a temporary arrangement, a quota increase and review, i.e.
a proper adjustment for China's economy, is also more than overdue.

A quota adjustment in favor of China and the corresponding adjustment of
the yuan's proportion in the SDR basket would further enhance China's currency
vis-à-vis the rest of the world. This, coupled with an incorruptible cryptocurrency
controlled by China's Central Bank and backed by gold, would be a formidable
reserve currency that most countries would like to hold as their chief reserve
asset. This, of course, is what Washington is afraid of. It would clearly endanger
and probably crush the global U.S.-dollar hegemony. Some 20 years ago the U.S.
dollar accounted for more than 90% of all reserve assets in nations' treasuries
around the globe. Today, that percentage has shrunk to less than 60% and is fading
rapidly. The decline of the U.S. dollar as a world reserve currency means that
the U.S. dollar hegemony is fading. This is inadmissible for the U.S. In order to
prevent the Yuan from taking a lead role in countries' reserve coffers, Washington
along with the major western allies are considering to abandon the key reserve
role of the dollar and replacing it with some kind of an SDR, in which the dollar
would maintain a prominent role, but its Ponzi-scheme characteristics would no
longer be openly visible.

The world would be a better place for it.

The current China bashing with guilt for COVID-19 is pretty similar to the
real reason for the 2018–2019 U.S.-China trade war, initiated by President Trump.
It too, had the objective of ruining the yuan's reputation in the world financial
arena. To no avail. Washington eventually quietly and unceremoniously lost the
conflict over trade. Despite Trump's loud declarations to the contrary, the U.S.
needs China much more than vice-versa.

Under President Xi Jinping's leadership, China is enhancing relations with
Asian markets, i.e. the ASEAN countries, plus Japan and South Korea, to detach
Asia even further from western, still dollar-dominated markets.

Members of the SCO (Shanghai Cooperation Organization) are also markets China is already engaged in. The SCO, in addition to China and most of the
Central Asian countries, includes Russia, India and Pakistan, with Iran waiting for

imminent admission. Others, like Malaysia and Mongolia, are in observer status and also slated to become SCO members in due course.

The combination of SCO and ASEAN–plus 3 amounts to more than half the world population and accounts for more than a third of the world's economic output. This is a formidable global "market share"—and will likely increase with every atrocity—military and economic—that Washington is committing around the globe.

With her new eventually internationalized crypto-currency, China is well on her way to fully dedollarize, and displace the United States as the world's financial and economic hegemon.

CHINA'S VISION FOR THE FUTURE

China has been following a peace philosophy throughout her 70-years Revolution, often against challenging situations, especially in the last decade with almost permanent aggressions of one kind or another by the United States and its coopted allies in Europe. No wonder the West does not seek Peace. Peace is bad for business. War is good and profitable, as such prominent mainstream journals as those of the *Washington Post* have voiced repeatedly in their op-ed columns.

The motto of non-aggression and peace prevails in China's foreign policy as key principle. There is no indication that China will depart from this belief which has brought China internal stability, international recognition—and has made China over the last decades into one of the world's foremost economies, as well as a leader in technological and environmental advances. Yes, despite this, it faces constant Western chastising for pirating western technology and destroying the environment. Such demonization is little but a propaganda tool to deviate the world's attention from western capitalist disasters around the world.

China's vision for the future started with Chairman Mao Zedong's victory of the civil war, also called the War of Liberation (1945–1949), over Chiang Kai-shek, the leader of the Kuomintang (KMT), and the head of the Republic of China. Chairman Mao led China through a two-part revolution, *The Great Leap Forward* (1958–1962) and the *Cultural Revolution* (1966–1976). These 27 years since 1949 were fraught with constant Western interference to break the Revolution's back and imposed a huge cost on China. To no avail. Mao cleaned China from foreign interference and led her to national autonomy in health, education and food—ready for gradually opening up to foreign trade and investments.

As a consequence, Mao's revolutions are often portrayed by the West as failures, the usual western tarnishing the success of other nations, of other socioeconomic systems, in order to hide its own disastrous failures. From a Chinese perspective, Mao's Revolutions drastically improved the public education and health system, eradicated endemic deadly diseases inherited from the

Western-dominated colonial and KMT times—and, foremost, eradicated poverty. As of today, almost a billion people have been lifted out poverty. Alleviation of poverty was an emphasis under both of Mao's revolutions. These revolutions also taught valuable lessons to Chinese scholars and future leaders—and dramatically advanced China towards food self-sufficiency, which she reached by 2018.

After Mao's death in 1976, his successor, Deng Xiaoping, led China through a far-reaching economic reform that included elements of a market economy always kept, however, under central government control—a principle that is maintained as of today. Deng called the new Chinese economic model *"socialism with Chinese characteristics,"* a concept that is ongoing. He helped develop China into the world's fastest-growing economy, improving the lives of hundreds of millions of citizens. Deng also masterminded the return of Hong Kong from a UK colony to China in 1997, and Macau from Portugal in 1999. The transition was completed by Deng's successor, Jiang Zemin.

Deng retired in 1992. His successor, Jiang Zemin, opened China further for foreign investments and trade, meeting with President Clinton on a U.S. visit in 1997. Jian followed a non-confrontational foreign policy like his predecessors, strengthened relations with Western partners, especially the United States—and maintained at home an economic annual growth of at least 8%. This led to an explosion of wealth, but also initially to its less than optimal distribution, with most of it concentrated along China's eastern shores, risking conflicts with the lesser developed Chinese "hinterland."

Hu Jintao followed Jiang Zemin as China's leader from 2002 to 2012. Hu, with his Premier, Wen Jiabao, and his Vice-President, Xi Jinping, continued the policy of economic growth and development, achieving more than a decade of double-digit growth, while shifting the economy gradually to non-consumption growth, towards socioeconomic equality, towards a "Harmonious Socialist Society." During Hu's rule China increased its influence in Africa and Latin America, laying the groundwork for future closer relationships with these regions. Hu was also known for shared and consensus-based leadership. Hu was succeeded in 2013 by Xi Jinping.

China, the second largest world economy in absolute terms, is now number one measured by purchasing power parity (PPP), meaning that China's purchasing power for a basket of essential goods and services is the strongest in the world, having surpassed the U.S. in 2017.

The vision for a free, prosperous and equitable China continues under President Xi Jinping. Xi is a lawyer, chemical engineer, philosopher—and visionary. In September 2013, Xi renewed the ancient Silk Road of 2,100 years back, into the new Belt and Road Initiative, to be addressed in further detail below.

Notably, during the 19th National Congress in 2017, BRI was included in the Chinese (CPC) Constitution as an amendment to promote the BRI's objective of "shared interests" and "shared growth" which are major political objectives for China. This amendment to the Constitution requiring the pursuit of international cooperation through a multifaceted socioeconomic development endeavor is unique in China's history.

"THE FUTURE IS IN THE EAST."

So goes one of the western progressive axioms, and by the East is mostly meant China, Russia, most of Central Asia; now all represented by the Shanghai Cooperation Organization (SCO), or the Shanghai Pact. SCO is a Eurasian political, economic, and security alliance, the creation of which was announced on June 15, 2001 in Shanghai, by the leaders of China, Kazakhstan, Kyrgyzstan, Russia, Tajikistan, and Uzbekistan. The Pact was signed in June 2002 and entered into force in September 2013. SCO's headquarters are in Beijing.

Today, the SCO counts eight members (China, India, Kazakhstan, Kyrgyzstan, Pakistan, Russia, Tajikistan, Uzbekistan). Iran, Malaysia and Mongolia are on a "waiting list," on the verge of becoming members. Turkey, already a dialogue partner, is increasingly trying for SCO access, either through association or membership –despite the conflict it may create with Turkey's NATO partners, mainly the U.S. Clearly, were Turkey to join the SCO, its exit from NATO would be imminent—and disastrous for NATO, perhaps the stumbling block that would bring NATO to an end—especially since popular anti-NATO pressure from Italy to Germany, Greece, Spain and Portugal is steadily growing. Turkey is also the most strategically located NATO partner between East and West, between Europe and Asia, controlling the Bosporus, access to the Black Sea.

The SCO is called the alliance of the east and is considered a security pillar. The powerhouse SCO is overlaid by the Eurasian Economic Union (EAEU). Its members are located in central and northern Asia, and include Armenia, Belarus, Kazakhstan, Kyrgyzstan and Russia. The treaty was formally established in January 2015.

This block of eastern countries and associations is seeking, against all odds, a multi-polar world. This is a big challenge, given the current socioeconomic disequilibrium, but feasible with mutual respect and a will to cooperate, to apply the forces of synergy and solidarity, as is inherent in the Belt and Road approach. The stakes are high. As Russia's Foreign Minister, Mr. Lavrov pointed out during the 74th UN General Assembly, in September 2019: "The West ignores reality by trying to prevent the formation of a multi-polar world by imposing its narrow 'liberal' rules on others." But, he added, "Western dominance is on the wane, 'we're liberals so everything's allowed' just isn't working anymore." These words are the basis for a strong pillar and union of eastern associations.

China's economy has registered during the past decades a phenomenal economic growth, at times exceeding 12% per year. In 2019 it was purposefully reduced to about 6%, so as to allow a better distribution of the growth benefits, and also spread wealth more horizontally to create greater equality of wellbeing. The Chinese call it *"quality growth."*

In figures and facts:

China's GDP measured in U.S.-dollars amounted to $14.2 trillion (nominal; 2019 est.), which corresponds to $27.3 trillion in Purchasing Power Parity (PPP; 2019 est.). This corresponds to U.S. $10,153 / capita, in nominal term (2019 est.), or to U.S. $19,520 / capita measured by PPP (2019 est.).

Compare this with the U.S. GDP of U.S. $21.345 trillion in nominal terms (2019 est.) and $64,767 per capita (2019 est.)

EXAMPLES OF ECONOMIC EFFICIENCY

New Airport in Beijing: In only four years China built by far the world's largest airport in Beijing, Daxxin International Airport. It was ready for China's 70th Birthday on October 1, 2019, when it was inaugurated by President Xi Jinping. It has been operational since the week after inauguration. This airport, an architectural wonder, covers some 700,000 m² (almost 100 football fields) and carries passengers by fast train in 20 minutes to the center of Beijing. It is expected to accommodate in 2021 already 45 million passengers and can easily be expanded to receive and serve 100 million passengers as the need requires. This airport is a sign that China is capable of realizing extraordinary achievements—it signals a visionary future.

China's Rapid Urbanization: When in 2017, Beijing was faced with a housing shortage for low-wage migrant workers, they built 100,000 low-rent apartments in twelve months. The speed of China's infrastructure development, the rapid urbanization, providing millions of new subsidized housing units for migrant workers, is a model that has worked and is being replicated throughout China. In fact, China has been building homes for a million people–the entire housing stock of San Francisco—every month since 1950. This policy aims at and creates wellbeing among the workers, among the people—and is at the same time a solid tool for China's economic development—and people's wellbeing. China's successful and rapid housing development is being closely watched by Australia, as her major cities, Sydney and Melbourne face similar problems.

Trade: China has been the world's largest exporter of goods since 2009. Official estimates suggest Chinese exports amounted to about $2.1 trillion in 2017. Since 2013, China has also become the largest trading nation in the world.

The total annual value of the country's exports equates to approximately $1,500 for every Chinese resident.

China is also a significant importer and accounts for about 10% of total global imports, i.e., about U.S. $1.7 trillion, leaving China as a net exporter with a trade surplus of about U.S. $400 billion.

Monetary Policy: China's Yuan, is a solid currency, backed by China's economy and by gold. In 2017 the Yuan was admitted in the International Monetary Fund's (IMF) basket of reserve currencies, which constitute the SDR—or special Drawing Rights. This has been addressed in China's New Monetary System, above.

Future Economic Growth: China will most likely keep to a "modest" growth rate, around 5% to 7%, concentrating on horizontal distributive growth, with a focus on improved public wellbeing for all, universal access to affordable housing, public transportation, rural higher education, as well as internal cultural exchange and harmonization. Two areas of economic development, merit being singled out: Artificial Intelligence (AI) and Environmental Improvement.

Artificial Intelligence (AI). China plans putting considerable resources into research, for example into AI. In 2017, the State Council (CCP) issued a "Next Generation Intelligence Development Plan," including a U.S. $ (equivalent) 2.1 billion AI industrial park. By 2025 the State Council predicts China to be a leader in AI research and predicts that China's AI core industry will be worth some U.S. $60 billion, amounting to about U.S. $700 billion equivalent, when accounting for related industries. By 2030, the State Council expects China to be the global leader in development of AI.

Environmental Improvement. China has made leaps in improving her environment, by far exceeding efforts of western countries. China's environmental policies are developing BRI at home and abroad in shades of green. New parks with trees and recreation areas are emerging in every major city in China. According to an expert at the School of Regulation and Global Governance of the Australian National University, Beijing has improved its air quality by 30% in the last five years.

A study by the University of Chicago demonstrates that Chinese cities have reduced the concentrations of fine particulates on average by 32% between 2014 and 2018. The Chinese people and government are devoting utmost importance to protecting the environment and the ecosystem. Green development makes for improved public health but is also attractive for investments.

China has a three-year "green" plan to improve air quality and tighten regulations. Further, the government is accelerating the electrification of vehicles, and has pledged that by 2030 all new cars will be powered by electricity. The government is also tackling drinking water quality and shortages as well as improving urban and rural sanitation. These are longer-term propositions. Cost estimates for China's overall environmental programs are not readily available but may easily reach into hundreds of billions of U.S.-dollar equivalents over a ten-year period.

CONCLUSION

Gradually, the SCO and associated countries are detaching themselves from the western dollar-based fiat system. In terms of trading, the SCO countries, mainly China, control most of the Asian markets, even making rapid inroads into Japan, and are evermore present in Latin America and Africa. Before long Europe may see the light and turn eastwards. It would be a wise decision. Dealing first within the confines of the huge Eurasian landmass, then including the Middle East and parts of Africa, has been the logical trajectory of trading since the Ancient Silk Road, more than 2,000 years ago.

China has a great visionary future that began more than 70 years ago and was enhanced seven years ago with President Xi Jinping's launching of the Belt and Road Initiative. BRI will continue spanning the globe for the next at least 50 to 100 years, spreading development in a multi-polar world, stressing equality and wellbeing for all.

A further bright side of this initiative is the Chinese philosophy of non-aggression, of diplomacy to resolve conflicts and of promoting peaceful economic coexistence and development around the globe.

China's determination to develop with an Economy of Peace, a "green" economy, an economy of distributive and quality growth that emphasizes equality and inclusion, is a landmark model for the world to embrace. It is a model to construct a *Community with a Shared Future for Mankind.*

CHAPTER EIGHT

A DISEASE DEADLIER THAN COVID-19: GLOBAL CAPITALISM IN CRISIS

William I. Robinson

If there's one thing the coronavirus made clear it is that, if we are to have any hope of resolving the dire problems that plague humanity, from ecological collapse, to war, poverty, inequality and disease, we have to collectively confront across borders the powers that be in the world capitalist system and their control over the means of our existence. From U.S. President Donald Trump's criminal ineptitude in addressing the pandemic, to the multi-trillion-dollar bailouts for capital, the threat to survival that billions of precarious workers faced as the global economy plunged, and the overwhelming of woefully underfunded and collapsing public health systems, the pandemic laid bare how it cannot be left to our rulers to resolve the crisis of humanity.[1]

The pandemic brought home the extent to which the fate of any one community on the planet is now bound up inextricably with that of humanity as a whole. What appeared as a localized virus in Wuhan quickly spread to just about every country and community in the world, leading to the lockdown of several billion people and prompting what some called the greatest crisis since World War II. The economic meltdown triggered by the virus underscored how dependent we all are now on the globally integrated production, financial, and service system, controlled as it is by the transnational capitalist class (TCC) and its political agents in capitalist states around the world.

These agents were quick to blame the meltdown on the virus as stock markets and global commerce went into free fall starting in March 2020. But the economic calamity it unleashed was a chronicle foretold. The bug was but the spark that ignited the combustible of a global economy that had never fully recovered from the 2008 financial collapse and has been teetering on the brink of renewed crisis ever since. The pundits of global capitalism had deluded themselves into believing that

---

1 On the crisis of global capitalism, see William I. Robinson, *Global Capitalism and the Crisis of Humanity* (New York: Cambridge University Press, 2014).

all was well. But the underlying structural causes of the 2008 debacle, far from being resolved, had become steadily aggravated. Frenzied financial speculation, unsustainable debt, the plunder of public finance, an overinflated tech sector, and state-organized militarized accumulation[2] kept the global economy sputtering along in recent years in the face of chronic stagnation and concealed its underlying instability. The pandemic will pass but the crisis of global capitalism is here to stay and has become more acute in the wake of COVID-19.

Capital wasted no time in endeavoring to shift the burden of the crisis and the sacrifice that the pandemic imposes onto the working and popular classes. For this purpose, it could count on capitalist state power. Many governments turned to massive new bailouts of capital with only very modest relief, if at all, for the working classes. The U.S. government injected several billion dollars into Wall Street banks, as the White House promised from the start that its response to the pandemic was "centered fully on unleashing the power of the private sector,"[3] meaning that capitalist profit would come first and would shape the response to the emergency. In late March 2020 it passed a $2 trillion stimulus package, the single biggest component of which was a giveaway to corporations along with smaller amounts for relief to the unemployed and poor families. In Europe, the EU and member governments approved similar stimulus packages,[4] as did the Chinese government.[5] Most governments around the world approved packages that involved the same combination of fiscal stimulus, corporate bailout, and modest public relief, if at all provided.[6]

---

2 On militarized accumulation, see William I. Robinson, *The Global Police State* (London: Pluto Press, 2020). For a synopsis, see William I. Robinson, "Accumulation Crisis and Global Police State," *Critical Sociology,* 2018 (accessed March 31, 2020), http://revolutionary-socialism.com/wp-content/uploads/2018/05/Robinson-2018-Accumulation-Crisis-Global-Police-State1.pdf.

3 "Remarks by President Trump, Vice President Pence, and Members of the Coronavirus Task Force in Press Conference," White House home page, March 13, 2020 (accessed April 1, 2020), https://www.whitehouse.gov/briefings-statements/remarks-president-trump-vice-president-pence-members-coronavirus-task-force-press-conference-3/.

4 See, e.g., "How Major Economies are Trying to Mitigate the Coronavirus Shock," *Financial Times*, March 30, 2020 (accessed April 1, 2020), https://www.ft.com/content/26af5520-6793-11ea-800d-da70cff6e4d3.

5 "China Signals Ramped-Up Stimulus as Coronavirus Impact Widens," *Bloomberg News*, March 27, 2020 (accessed April 1, 2020), https://www.bloomberg.com/news/articles/2020-03-27/china-pledges-to-raise-fiscal-deficit-ratio-sell-special-debt.

6 The most comprehensive country-by-country summary was provided by the International Monetary Fund in late March (no exact date for posting), accessed April 1, 2020, https://www.imf.org/en/Topics/imf-and-covid19/Policy-Responses-to-COVID-19.

There were no mass bailouts for the billions of poor precarious workers who face daily struggles for survival. The International Labor Organization estimated in April 2020 that some 200 million people worldwide would lose their jobs as a result of the virus,[7] although some considered this a significant underestimate. Some one billion children worldwide were affected by school closures. Hundreds of millions of transnational and internal migrants and refugees faced the virus with no access to any health infrastructure. Prisoners in overcrowded jails the world over, the homeless, and those in war zones were sitting ducks for the virus. As the worst of the pandemic passes and long-term economic depression sets in, the TCC will take advantage of long-term mass unemployment and job insecurity to attempt to enhance its class power over labor through further discipline and austerity. The capitalist crisis unleashed by the coronavirus, it would seem, may be even more deadly for impoverished workers than the virus itself.

But this crisis is not just economic, or structural. It is also a political crisis of state legitimacy and capitalist hegemony. Crises are times of rapid social change and open up the possibility of pushing society in many different directions, depending on the outcome of battles among contending social and class forces. Any popular outcome to these battles will depend on how the oppressed and exploited around the world may come together in united struggle. The gravest danger is that in the face of mass struggle unleashed by the crisis the ruling classes will use the pandemic and its aftermath as a smokescreen to consolidate a global police state.[8] Before we turn to this danger and to the prospects for struggle from below let us analyze the structural dimension of the crisis.

GLOBAL CAPITALISM'S STRUCTURAL CRISIS

All the telltale signs of what political economists refer to as an overaccumulation crisis have been present for some time. Capitalist globalization and neoliberal austerity since the late 1970s has pushed the global working and popular classes onto the defensive and shifted the global balance of class forces in favor of transnational capital following the period of mass struggles in the 1960s and 1970s. But globalization also aggravated capitalism's most fundamental contradiction, overaccumulation. This refers to a situation in which enormous amounts of capital are built up but without productive outlets for reinvestment. This capital then becomes stagnant. By liberating emergent transnational capital from national constraints, globalization undermined redistributive programs that had attenuated

---

7 International Labor Organization, "Almost 25 Million Jobs Could be Lost Worldwide as a Result of COVID-19," March 18, 2020 (accessed April 1, 2020), https://www.ilo.org/global/about-the-ilo/newsroom/news/WCMS_738742/lang--en/index.htm.

8 Robinson, *The Global Police State.*

capitalism's inherent tendency towards social polarization. The result has been an unprecedented sharpening of inequality that has fueled overaccumulation.

As is now well known, the level of global social polarization and inequality now experienced is unprecedented. In 2018, the richest one percent of humanity controlled more than half of the world's wealth while the bottom 80 percent had to make do with just 4.5 percent.[9] Such inequalities end up undermining the stability of the system as the gap grows between what is (or could be) produced and what the market can absorb. The extreme concentration of the planet's wealth in the hands of the few and the accelerated impoverishment and dispossession of the majority meant that transnational capital had increasing difficulty in finding productive outlets to unload the enormous amounts of surplus it had accumulated. The more global inequalities expand, the more constricted is the world market and the more the system faces a structural crisis of overaccumulation. If left unchecked, the expanding social polarization results in crisis—in stagnation, recessions, depressions, social upheavals and war.

Overaccumulation originates in the circuit of capitalist production, yet it becomes manifest in the sphere of circulation, that is, in the market, as a crisis of overproduction or underconsumption. Over the past few years there has been a rise in underutilized capacity and a slowdown in industrial production around the world[10] As the productive economy stagnates, capitalists have turned to financial speculation. This surplus of accumulated capital with nowhere to go is without precedent. Transnational corporations recorded record profits during the 2010s at the same time that corporate investment declined[11] Worldwide corporate cash reserves topped $12 trillion in 2017,[12] more than the foreign exchange reserves of the world's central governments.

In the wake of the Great Recession of 2008 the U.S. Federal Reserve undertook a whopping $16 trillion in secret bailouts to banks and corporations from

9 Oxfam (London), *Wealth: Having it all and Wanting More*, Oxfam, accessed March 31, 2020, http://policy-practice.oxfam.org.uk/publications/wealth-having-it-all-and-wanting-more-338125.

10 Eric Toussaint, "No, The Coronavirus is not Responsible for the Fall in Stock Prices," *MR Online*, March 4, 2020 (accessed March 31, 2020), https://mronline.org/2020/03/04/no-the-coronavirus-is-not-responsible-for-the-fall-of-stock-prices/.

11 "The Problem with Profits," *The Economist,* May 26, 2016 (accessed March 31, 2020), https://www.economist.com/leaders/2016/03/26/the-problem-with-profits.

12 *Nikkei Asian Review*, "Asia's Multinationals are Hoarding Cash Like Never Before," September 16, 2017 (accessed March 31, 2020), https://asia.nikkei.com/Economy/Asia-s-multinationals-are-hoarding-cash-like-never-before.

around the world.[13] But then the banks and institutional investors simply recycled the trillions of dollars they received into new speculative activities in global commodities markets, in cryptocurrencies, and in land around the world, fueling a new global "land grab." As opportunities have dried up for speculative investment in one sector the TCC simply turned to another sector to unload its surplus. As a result, the gap between the productive economy and fictitious capital grew into an enormous chasm. In 2018, for example, the gross world product or the total value of goods and services, stood at some $75 trillion whereas the global derivatives market was estimated at a mind-boggling $1.2 quadrillion.[14] This accumulation of fictitious capital gave the appearance of recovery. But it only offset the crisis temporally into the future while in the long run exacerbating the underlying problem.

In addition to speculation, mounting government, corporate, and consumer debt have driven growth. Consumer credit has served the dual purpose of class pacification and of generating demand even as real incomes have dropped for the immiserated majority subject to austerity and ever more precarious forms of employment. In countries around the world, consumer debt was higher on the eve of the pandemic that it has been for all of postwar history. State and corporate debt also reached breaking points. The global bond market—an indicator of total government debt worldwide—surpassed $100 trillion in 2017, while total global debt reached a staggering $215 trillion in 2016.[15] Worldwide corporate debt has soared to $75 trillion, up from $32 trillion in 2005, while corporations have issued $13 trillion in bonds, more than twice the bond debt on the eve of the 2008 collapse.[16] A default on consumer, state, or corporate debt will set off a further chain reaction in the downward plunge of the global economy.

In sum, financial speculation, pillaging the state, and debt-driven growth were "fixes" that could not address the underlying structural conditions that triggered the 2008 financial collapse. The massive concentrations of transnational finance capital destabilized the system as global capitalism ran up against the limits of

---

13 General Accounting Office (GAO), "Federal Reserve System: Opportunities Exist to Strengthen Policies and Processes for Managing Emergency Assistance" (Washington, D.C.: GAO-11-696, July 2011).

14 J.B. Maverick, "How Big is the Derivatives Market," *Investopedia*, January 22, 2018 (accessed March 31, 2020), https://www.investopedia.com/ask/answers/052715/how-big-derivatives-market.asp.

15 David Scutt, "Global Debt Has Hit an Eye-Watering $215 Trillion," *Business Insider,* April 4, 2017 (accessed March 31, 2020), http://www.businessinsider.com/global-debt-staggering-trillions-2017-4?&platform=bi-androidapp.

16 Paul Wiseman, Bernard Condon, and Cathy Bussewitz, "Corporate Debt Loads a Rising Risk as Virus Hits Economy," *AP News*, March 11, 2020 (accessed March 2020), https://apnews.com/7cd0108d79c6b4f1ee2e6ec5fc3a2275.

these fixes. The global economy was a ticking time bomb. All that was needed was something to light the fuse. That came in the form of the coronavirus.

MILITARIZED ACCUMULATION: THE GLOBAL WAR ECONOMY

But beyond financial speculation, debt-driven growth, and pillaging state finances, the TCC turned to another mechanism to sustain accumulation in the face of stagnation, what I have termed militarized accumulation.[17] Savage global inequalities are politically explosive and to the extent that the system is simply unable to reverse them or to incorporate surplus humanity it turns to ever more violent forms of containment to manage immiserated populations. As popular discontent has spread in recent years, the dominant groups have imposed systems of mass social control, repression and warfare—from mass incarceration to deadly new modalities of policing and omnipresent systems of state and private surveillance—to contain the actual and the potential rebellion of the global working class and surplus humanity.

The ruling groups will turn to expanding the global police state as the aftermath of the pandemic aggravates the structural crisis and leads to a further breakdown of capitalist hegemony. Militarized accumulation refers to how the global economy is becoming ever more dependent on the development and deployment of systems of warfare, social control, and repression, apart from political considerations, simply as a means of making profit and continuing to accumulate capital in the face of stagnation. As the crisis intensifies, militarized accumulation may take over as primer driver of the global economy. The so-called wars on drugs and terrorism, the undeclared wars on immigrants, refugees and gangs (and poor, dark-skinned, and working-class youth more generally), the construction of border walls, immigrant detention centers, prison-industrial complexes, systems of mass surveillance, and the spread of private security guard and mercenary companies, have all become major sources of profit-making and they will become more important to the system as economic depression sets in.

The events of September 11, 2001 marked the start of an era of permanent global war in which logistics, warfare, intelligence, repression, surveillance, and even military personnel are more and more the privatized domain of transnational capital. The criminalization of surplus humanity activates state-sanctioned repression that opens up new profit-making opportunities for the TCC. The Pentagon budget increased 91 percent in real terms between 1998 and 2011, while worldwide, total defense outlays grew by 50 percent from 2006 to 2015, from $1.4

---

17 William I. Robinson, "Beyond the Economic Chaos of Coronavirus is a Global War Economy," *Truthout*, March 23, 2020 (accessed April 1, 2020), https://truthout.org/articles/beyond-the-economic-chaos-of-coronavirus-is-a-global-war-economy/.

trillion to $2.03 trillion, although this figure did not take into account hundreds of billions of dollars in "homeland security" spending. In the decade from 2001 to 2011 military industry profits nearly quadrupled.[18] Led by the United States as the predominant world power, military expansion in different countries has taken place through parallel, and often conflictive, processes, yet all show the same relationship between state militarization and global capital accumulation. Worldwide, official state military outlays in 2015 represented about three percent of the gross world product of $75 trillion.

But militarized accumulation involves vastly more than activities generated by state military budgets. There are immense sums involved in state spending and private corporate accumulation through militarization and other forms of generating profit through repressive social control that do not involve militarization *per se*. The various wars, conflicts, and campaigns of social control and repression around the world involve the fusion of private accumulation with state militarization. In this relationship, the state facilitates the expansion of opportunities for private capital to accumulate through militarization, such as by facilitating global weapons sales by military-industrial-security firms, the amounts of which have reached unprecedented levels. Global weapons sales by the top 100 weapons manufacturers and military service companies increased by 38 percent between 2002 and 2016.[19]

The U.S.-led wars in Iraq and Afghanistan precipitated the explosion in private military and security contractors around the world deployed to protect the TCC and global capitalism. Beyond the United States, private military and security firms have proliferated worldwide and their deployment is not limited to the major conflict zones in the Middle East, South Asia, and Africa. In his study, *Corporate Warriors*, Singer documents how private military forces (PMFs) have come to play an ever more central role in military conflicts and wars. "A new global industry has emerged," he noted. "It is outsourcing and privatization of a

---

18 For this data, see William I. Robinson, "Global Capitalist Crisis and Trump's War Drive," *Truthout*, April 19, 2017 (accessed March 2020), http://www.truth-out.org/opinion/item/40266-global-capitalist-crisis-and-trump-s-war-drive, and "Global Homeland Security and Public Safety Market Report 2019—Market is Expected to Grow from $431 Billion in 2018 to $606 Billion in 2014," *CISION PR Newswire*, February 6, 2019 (accessed March 31, 2020), https://www.prnewswire.com/news-releases/global-homeland-security--public-safety-market-report-2019---market-is-expected-to-grow-from-431-billion-in-2018-to-606-billion-in-2024-at-a-cagr-of-5-8-300790827.html.

19 Aude Fleurant, Alexandra Kuimova, Nan Tian, Pieter D. Wezeman, and Seimon T. Wezeman, "The SIPRI Top 100 Arms-Producing and Military Services Companies," *Stockholm International Peace Research Institute* (SIPRI), 2017 (accessed March 13 2020), https://www.sipri.org/sites/default/files/2017-12/fs_arms_industry_2016.pdf.

twenty-first century variety, and it changes many of the old rules of international politics and warfare. It has become global in both its scope and activity."[20]

Beyond the many based in the United States, PMFs come from numerous countries around the world, including Russia, South Africa, Colombia, Mexico, India, the EU countries, and Israel. PMF clients include states, corporations, land-owners, non-governmental organizations, even the Colombian and Mexican drug cartels. By 2018, private military companies employed some 15 million people around the world, deploying forces to guard corporate property, provide personal security for TCC executives and their families, collect data, conduct police, para-military, counterinsurgency and surveillance operations, carry out mass crowd control and repression of protesters, manage prisons, run private detention and interrogation facilities, and participate in outright warfare.[21]

The private security (policing) business is one of the fastest growing eco-nomic sectors in many countries and has come to dwarf public security around the world. The amount spent on private security in 2003, the year of the invasion of Iraq, was 73 percent higher than that spent in the public sphere, and three times as many persons were employed in private forces as in official law enforcement agencies. There were an outstanding 20 million private security workers world-wide in 2017, and the industry was expected to be worth over $220 billion by 2020. In half of the world's countries, private security agents outnumber police officers.[22]

Meanwhile, criminalization of the poor, racially oppressed, immigrants, refugees and other vulnerable communities is the most clear-cut method of accumulation by repression. This type of criminalization activates "legitimate" state repression to enforce the accumulation of capital, whereby the state turns to private capital to carry out repression against those criminalized. There has been a rapid increase in imprisonment in countries around the world, led by the United States, which has been exporting its own system of mass incarceration. The global prison population grew by 24 percent from 2000 to 2018.[23] This carceral state

20 P.W. Singer, *Corporate Warriors: The Rise of the Privatized Military Industry* (Ithaca: Cornell University Press, 2003), 69.

21 William Langewiesche, "The Chaos Company," *Vanity Fair*, March 18, 2014 (accessed March 31, 2020), http://www.vanityfair.com/news/business/2014/04/g4s-global-security-company.

22 Niall McCarthy, "Private Security Outnumbers the Police in Most Countries Worldwide," *Forbes*, August 31, 2017 (accessed March 31, 2020), https://www.forbes.com/sites/niallmccarthy/2017/08/31/private-security-outnumbers-the-police-in-most-countries-worldwide-infographic/#75fe283f210f.

23 Roy Walmsley, *World Prison Population List*, 12th edition (Institute for Criminal Policy Research, 2018), accessed March 31. 2020, http://www.prisonstudies.org/sites/

opens up enormous opportunities at multiple levels for militarized accumulation. Worldwide there were in the early 21st century some 200 privately operated prisons on all continents and many more "public-private partnerships" that involved privatized prison services and other forms of for-profit custodial services such as privatized electronic monitoring programs. The countries that were developing private prisons ranged from most member states of the EU, to Israel, Russia, Thailand, Hong Kong, South Africa, New Zealand, Ecuador, Australia, Costa Rica, Chile, Peru, Brazil, and Canada.

Every phase in the war on migrants and refugees has become a wellspring of profit making, from private, for-profit detention centers and the provision of services inside public detention centers such as healthcare, food, phone systems, to other ancillary activities of the deportation regime, such as government contracting of private charter flights to ferry deportees back home, and the equipping of armies of border agents. In the United States, the border security industry was set to double in value from $305 billion in 2011 to some $740 billion in 2023.[24] In Europe, the refugee crisis and the European Union's program to "secure borders" has provided a bonanza to military and security companies providing equipment to border military forces, surveillance systems and IT infrastructure. The budget for the EU public-private border security agency, Frontex, increased a whopping 3,688 percent between 2005 and 2016, while the European border security market was expected to nearly double, from some $18 billion in 2015 to approximately $34 billion in 2022.[25]

When the health emergency comes to an end we may be left with a global economy even more dependent on this militarized accumulation than before the virus hit, and with the threat that the ruling groups will turn to war. Historically wars have pulled the capitalist system out of crisis while they have also served to deflect attention from political tensions and problems of legitimacy.

THE COMING UPHEAVALS: POPULAR CLASSES CONFRONT GLOBAL POLICE STATE

The crisis triggered by the pandemic has left in its wake more inequality, more political tension, more militarism, and more authoritarianism. An April

---

default/files/resources/downloads/wppl_12.pdf.

24 Michelle Chen, "The U.S. Border Security Industry Could be Worth $740 Billion by 2023," *Truthout*, October 6, 2019 (accessed March 31, 2020), https://truthout.org/articles/the-us-border-security-industry-could-be-worth-740-billion-by-2023/.

25 Mark Akkerman, *Border Wars: The Arms Dealers Profiting From Europe's Refugee Tragedy* (Amsterdam: Transnational Institute, 2014), accessed March 31, 2020, https://www.tni.org/files/publication-downloads/border-wars-report-web1207.pdf.

2020 report by the international development agency Oxfam warned that the pandemic would push an additional half a billion people into poverty, and threatened to set poor regions such as sub-Sahara Africa and the Middle East back 30 years. "Existing inequalities dictate the economic impact of this crisis," said report. "The poorest workers in rich and poor nations are less likely to be in formal employment, enjoy labor protections such as sick pay, or be able to work from home." It went on to note that women, who make up 70 percent of health workers globally and provide 75 percent of unpaid care of children, the sick, and the elderly, were at the frontline of the coronavirus response and were the hardest hit financially.[26]

Social upheaval, civil strife, and mass popular struggles will escalate in the coming months and years as the crisis deepens. The ruling groups will intensify their class warfare from above by extending the global police state to contain mass discontent from below as capitalist hegemony continues to break down. Global police state refers to three interrelated developments: 1) militarized accumulation, as a means of accumulating capital in the face of stagnation; 2) systems of mass social control and repression to contain the oppressed; and 3) the increasing move towards political systems that can be characterized as twenty-first century fascism and even as totalitarian.

Governments around the world centralized the response to the pandemic and many declared states of emergencies. Such centralized coordination was urgent to confront the health crisis. But centralization of emergency powers in authoritarian capitalist states will be used after the virus has been brought under control to contain discontent, heighten surveillance, and impose repressive social control— that is, to push forward the global police state. Military and police forces were deployed by governments around the world in response to the pandemic. Let us recall that these same governments passed draconian anti-terrorism legislation in the wake of the September 11, 2001 attacks that were used to suppress civil liberties and clamp down on political dissent.

In the United States the national guard was activated in all 50 states and the U.S. Department of Justice secretly asked Congress to suspend constitutional rights during the COVID-19 pandemic, including the suspension of habeas corpus.[27] Several states enacted laws to criminalize protest against fossil fuels

---

26 Oxfam press release, "Half a Billion People Could be Pushed into Poverty by Coronavirus, warns Oxfam," April 9, 2020 (accessed April 11, 2020), https://www.oxfam. org/en/press-releases/half-billion-people-could-be-pushed-poverty-coronavirus-warns oxfam.

27 Peter Wade, "DOJ Wants to Suspend Certain Constitutional Rights During Coronavirus Emergency," *Rolling Stone*, March 21, 2020 (accessed April 1, 2020), https://www.rollingstone.com/politics/politics-news/doj-suspend-constitutional-rights-coronavirus-970935/.

by designating them as "critical infrastructure."[28] Could martial law be far behind? Throughout Europe, thousands of soldiers were deployed to quarantined cities to patrol streets and enforce lockdowns. Even the conservative weekly, *The Economist*, felt obliged to warn that "armed forces are designed first and foremost for killing people, rather than issuing fines on street corners or delivering food to supermarkets."[29] Most EU governments declared states of emergency. In Hungary the far-right authoritarian prime minister Viktor Orban sought an open-ended state of emergency that would give him powers to bypass parliament and rule by decree.[30] One early April 2020 headline banner by the influential publication, *Foreign Policy*, declared, "Coronavirus and the Dawn of Post-Democratic Europe."[31]

From Russia, to Singapore, to South Korea, governments around the world stepped up surveillance of their populations. The Russian government demanded that the media stop publishing information on the virus that it declared to be false. The governments of Turkey, Montenegro, and Serbia carried out arrests and fined people who published information on social media that "provokes panic and jeopardizes public security."[32] The virus became a testbed for surveillance capitalism. The Italian, German, Chinese and Austrian governments, among others, put systems in place in coordination with the giant tech corporations as the disease spread to analyze smartphone data so as to determine to what extent populations were complying with the lockdown.[33] The Tunisian government deployed

---

28 Tal Axelrod, "Three States Push Criminal Penalties for Fossil Fuel Protests Amid Coronavirus," *The Hill*, March 27, 2020 (accessed April 1, 2020), https://thehill.com/policy/energy-environment/489960-three-states-push-criminal-penalties-for-fossil-fuel-protests-amid.

29 *The Economist*, "Armies are Mobilizing Against the Coronavirus," March 23, 2020 (accessed April 1, 2020), https://www.economist.com/international/2020/03/23/armies-are-mobilising-against-the-coronavirus.

30 Shaun Walker and Jennifer Rankin, "Hungary Passes Law That Will Let Orban Rule by Decree," *The Guardian*, March 30, 2020 (accessed April 1, 2020), https://www.theguardian.com/world/2020/mar/30/hungary-jail-for-coronavirus-misinformation-viktor-orban.

31 Paul Hockenos, "Coronavirus and the Dawn of Post-Democratic Europe," *Foreign Policy*, March 31, 2020 (accessed April 1, 2020), https://foreignpolicy.com/2020/03/31/hungary-orban-coronavirus-europe-democracy/.

32 Maria R. Sahuquillo, Silvia Blanco, Macarena Vidal Liy, "Democracia en Cuarentena por Coronavirus," *El Pais* (Spain), March 30, 2020 (accessed April 1, 2020), https://elpais.com/internacional/2020-03-30/democracia-en-cuarentena-por-coronavirus.html.

33 Simon Chandler, "Coronavirus Could Infect Privacy and Civil Liberties Forever," *Forbes*, 23 March 23, 2020 (accessed April 2, 2020), https://www.forbes.com/sites/simonchandler/2020/03/23/coronavirus-could-infect-privacy-and-civil-liberties-forever/#6d224468365d.

robocops to patrol streets. In the Philippines, the authoritarian president Rodrigo Duterte issued shoot to kill orders for anyone defying the stay-at-home lockdown.

In India, the government declared a state of emergency and mandatory confinement to home. But hundreds of millions of precarious and informal workers who had no choice but to starve or leave home to scrape by were met with brutal and humiliating police violence, scenes of which were caught on televisions cameras and social media recordings and aired around the world. Tens of millions more migrant workers were caught by the lockdown far away from their villages. With public transportation shut down, they were forced to endure pitiless state repression as they marched hundreds of kilometers to get home.

Honduras provided a case study in how the ruling groups used the health emergency to legitimate an escalation of state repression. The dictatorial regime, put into power by a U.S.-backed coup d'état in 2009, ordered a nation-wide lockdown enforced by the Honduran military and police. The lockdown included the suspension of numerous constitutional guarantees, including freedom of expression, freedom of movement, and freedom from arbitrary detention. Hundreds of arrests, some of them of known political dissidents, were carried out in the first few days of the order.

Emblematic of what took place throughout the Global South, a life and death situation spread across Honduras with the closure of street markets and road-side vendors. Some 60 percent of all Hondurans live in poverty, and a full 70 percent are employed in the informal sector. Just as in other countries around the world, confinement at home was simply not possible for this impoverished majority. The repressive lockdown meant that millions faced starvation, unable to go out in search of food, assistance, or other survival activities without risking state military and police repression. The government used emergency funds to politicize food packages doled out to supporters of the ruling National Party. In several municipalities, bullets, tear gas, and arrests met residents who took to the streets to demand relief.[34]

There has been a rapid political polarization in global society since 2008 between an insurgent far-right and an insurgent left. The crisis will animate far-right and neofascist groups that have surged in many countries around the world. They

---

34 For details on the Honduran case, see various entries at the web page of the U.S-based Honduras Solidarity Network, http://www.hondurassolidarity.org/. See also, statement released by the Committee to Protect Journalists, "Honduran Government Declares State of Emergency, Suspends Right to Free Expression," March 18, 2020 (accessed April 1, 2020), https://cpj.org/2020/03/honduran-government-declares-state-of-emergency-su.php.

will seek to capitalize politically on the calamity. But it also animated popular struggles from below.[35] At stake is the battle for the post-pandemic world.

CONCLUSION: NO RETURN TO NORMALCY

The class character of the health emergency could not be clearer. The virus did not care about the class, ethnicity or nationality of the human hosts it sought to infect but it was the poor and working classes who were unable to protect themselves from contagion. In the teaming slums of the world's megacities social distancing was a privilege that was out of reach. Millions faced death, especially in the Global South, not so much from the viral infection as from the lack of access to life sustaining services and resources. The crisis has revealed the fragility of the system, the extent of our subjugation to ruling classes that cannot be counted on to keep us safe.

These ruling classes pushed policies to exploit every aspect of the pandemic for private profit. "Never let a crisis go to waste," was how Obama's chief of staff, Rahm Emanuel, infamously put it during the 2008 financial collapse. Even if deficit spending and Keynesian stimulus remain in place for the duration of a depression, the experience of 2008 showed that governments recovered the costs of bailouts by deepening social austerity even as banks and corporations used bailout money to buy back stock and engage in new rounds of predatory activities.

Yet neoliberalism simply does not have any more reserves with which to contain financial chaos and economic implosion. The implacable drive to accumulation impedes solutions to the crisis. Renewed capitalist stability, if it can even be achieved, would require a more profound restructuring—including the rebuilding of public sectors devastated by 40 years of capitalist globalization and neoliberalism—than the agents of financial and corporate interests, along with the liberal and social democratic elite around the world, could possibly accomplish or would even want to.

Short of overthrowing the system, the only way out of the crisis is a reversal of escalating inequalities through a redistribution of wealth and power downward. That will not come without a fight. In the United States as elsewhere, in the midst of the pandemic, workers undertook a wave of strikes and protests as the virus spread to demand their safety, while tenants called for rent strikes, immigrant justice activists surrounded detention centers and demanded the release of prisoners, auto workers went out on wildcat strikes to force factories to shut down, homeless people took over homes, health care workers on the front lines demanded the

---

35 William I. Robinson, "Global Capitalist Crisis and Twenty-First Century Fascism: Beyond the Trump Hype, *Science & Society*, 83(2), 2019, accessible at my web page at http://robinson.faculty.soc.ucsb.edu/Assets/pdf/FascismbeyondTrump.pdf.

supplies they needed to do their jobs and stay safe.[36] In the aftermath of the health emergency, the social and economic crisis has the potential to awaken millions from political apathy. The ruling groups cannot but be frightened by the ongoing rumblings from below.

The pandemic underscored how the global or planetary consciousness that people have been talking about ever since globalization entered our vocabulary in the 1990s is more of a reality than ever before. As several billions of us hunkered down—although we must reiterate that billions more did not have the luxury of confinement—we stayed glued to television, internet, and social media news about the virus and its impacts around the world. We felt a new sense of connection, of community, and of solidarity with one another. We experienced as never before what Marshall McLuhan, back in 1964, dubbed the *global village*. Consciousness seemed to grow worldwide on the need for grassroots solidarity and mutual aid in the face of the pandemic.

Is it possible that we are entering a pre-revolutionary situation? The Bolshevik leader Vladimir Lenin described the symptoms of such a situation: 1) when there is a crisis in the prevailing system and it is impossible for the ruling classes to rule in the old way; 2) when the want and suffering of the oppressed classes have grown more acute than usual, and; 3) when as a consequence the masses increase their historical action. But the jump from a "revolutionary situation" to a revolutionary process requires other conditions not yet present, including a widespread belief that systemic change is possible and attainable, a revolutionary ideology and program, and organizations capable of leading the struggle for such change.

The COVID-19 pandemic marks a before-and-after turning point. We have entered into a period of mounting chaos in the world capitalist system. Short of revolution, we must struggle now to prevent our rulers from turning the crisis and its aftermath into an opportunity for them to resuscitate and deepen the neoliberal order once the dust settles. Our struggle is to push for something along the lines of a global Green New Deal as an interim program while seeking an accumulation of forces for more radical system change. Left and progressive forces must position themselves now to beat back the threat of war and the global police state and to push the coming upheavals in a direction that empowers the global working and popular classes.

---

36 Aaron Gordon, Lauren Gurley, Edward Ongweso, Jr., and Jordan Pearson, "Coronavirus Is a Labor Crisis, and a General Strike May be Next," *Vice*, April 2, 2020 (accessed April 3, 2020) https://www.vice.com/en_us/article/z3b9ny/coronavirus-general-strike?utm_source=Iterable&utm_medium=email&utm_campaign=curated_vice_daily_1023202.

PART IV
Biowarfare as Hybrid War

CHAPTER NINE

BATS, GENE EDITING AND BIOWEAPONS: RECENT DARPA EXPERIMENTS RAISE CONCERNS AMID CORONAVIRUS OUTBREAK

Whitney Webb

The emergence of a novel coronavirus in China and its subsequent spread abroad has dominated the news cycle for much of 2020 and has also upended the lives of billions around the world, resulting in major upheavals to nearly every facet of human life for a majority of countries.

As is often the case of world-altering events on this scale, there has been no small number of theories speculating about the outbreak's origin, many of which blame a variety of state actors and/or controversial billionaires. This has inevitably led to efforts to clamp down on "misinformation" related to the coronavirus outbreak from both mainstream media outlets and major social media platforms.

However, while many of these theories are clearly speculative, there is also verifiable evidence regarding the recent interest of one controversial U.S. government agency in novel coronaviruses, specifically those transmitted from bats to humans. That agency, the Pentagon's Defense Advanced Research Project Agency (DARPA), began spending millions on such research in 2018. Some of those Pentagon-funded studies were conducted at known U.S. military bioweapons labs bordering China and resulted in the discovery of dozens of new coronavirus strains as recently as April 2019. Furthermore, the ties of the Pentagon's main biodefense lab to a virology institute in Wuhan, China—where the current outbreak is believed to have begun—have been unreported in the mainstream English language media thus far.

While it remains entirely unknown as to what caused the outbreak, knowledge of the details of DARPA and the Pentagon's recent experimentation is clearly in the public interest, especially considering that the leading companies developing a vaccine to combat the coronavirus outbreak are themselves strategic allies of DARPA. Not only that, but these DARPA-backed companies are already developing controversial DNA and mRNA vaccines for this particular coronavirus strain, a category of vaccine that has never previously been approved for human use in the United States—and indeed, for a virus that itself is completely new.

Yet, given the complete societal and economic upheaval that the coronavirus outbreak has left in its wake, these vaccines are set to be rushed to market for public use, making it important for the public to be aware of DARPA's recent experiments on coronaviruses, bats and gene editing technologies, as well as their broader implications.

Examining the Recent Wuhan-Bioweapon Narrative

As the coronavirus outbreak has come to dominate headlines in recent weeks, several media outlets have promoted claims that the reported epicenter of the outbreak in Wuhan, China was also the site of laboratories allegedly linked to a Chinese government biowarfare program.

However, upon further examination of the initial sourcing for this serious claim, these supposed links between the outbreak and an alleged Chinese bio-weapons program first came from two highly dubious sources.

The first outlet to report on this claim was *Radio Free Asia*, the U.S.-government funded media outlet targeting Asian audiences that used to be run covertly by the CIA and was named by the *New York Times* as a key part in the agency's "worldwide propaganda network."[1] Though it is no longer run *directly* by the CIA, it is now managed by the government-funded Broadcasting Board of Governors (BBG),[2] which answers directly to Secretary of State Mike Pompeo, who was CIA director immediately prior to his current post at the head of the State Department.

In other words, *Radio Free Asia* and other BBG-managed media outlets are legal outlets for U.S. government propaganda. Notably, the long-standing ban on the domestic use of U.S. government propaganda on U.S. citizens was lifted in 2013,[3] with the official justification of allowing the government to "effectively communicate in a credible way" and to better combat "al-Qaeda's and other violent extremists' influence."

---

1 John M. Crewdson, "Worldwide Propaganda Network Built by the C.I.A.," *New York Times,* December 26, 1977, p. 1, https://www.nytimes.com/1977/12/26/archives/worldwide-propaganda-network-built-by-the-cia-a-worldwide-network.html.

2 Yasha Levine, "Internet privacy, funded by spooks: A brief history of the BBG," *PANDO,* March 1, 2015, https://pando.com/2015/03/01/internet-privacy-funded-by-spooks-a-brief-history-of-the-bbg/.

3 Whitney Webb, "Lifting of US Propaganda Ban Gives New Meaning to Old Song," *Mint Press News,* February 12, 2018, https://www.mintpressnews.com/planting-stories-in-the-press-lifting-of-us-propaganda-ban-gives-new-meaning-to-old-song/237493/.

Radio Free Asia's recent report on the alleged origins of the outbreak as linked to a Chinese state-linked virology center cited only Ren Ruihong, the former head of the medical assistance department at the Chinese Red Cross, for that claim. Ruihong has been cited as an expert in several *Radio Free Asia* reports on disease outbreaks in China,[4] but has not been cited as an expert by any other English-language media outlet.

Ruihong told *Radio Free Asia*:[5]

It's a new type of mutant coronavirus. They haven't made public the genetic sequence, because it is highly contagious…Genetic engineering technology has gotten to such a point now, and Wuhan is home to a viral research center that is under the aegis of the China Academy of Sciences, which is the highest level of research facility in China.

Though Ruihong did not directly say that the Chinese government was making a bioweapon at the Wuhan facility, she did imply that genetic experiments at the facility may have resulted in the creation of this new "mutant coronavirus" at the center of the outbreak.

With *Radio Free Asia* and its single source having speculated about Chinese government links to the creation of the new coronavirus, the *Washington Times* soon took it much farther in a report titled "Virus-hit Wuhan has two laboratories linked to Chinese bio-warfare program."[6] That article, much like *Radio Free Asia*'s earlier report, cites a single source for that claim, former Israeli military intelligence biowarfare specialist Dany Shoham.

Yet, Shoham does not even directly make the claim cited in the article's headline, as he only told the *Washington Times* that: "Certain laboratories in the [Wuhan] institute have *probably* been engaged, in terms of research and development, in Chinese [biological weapons], *at least collaterally*, yet *not as a principal facility* of the Chinese BW alignment [emphasis added]."

While Shoham's claims are clearly speculative, it is telling that the *Washington Times* would bother to cite him at all, especially given the key role he played in promoting false claims that the 2001 Anthrax attacks was the work of Iraq's

---

4 "China Clamps Down on Public Discussion of African Swine Flu Outbreaks," *Radio Free Asia,* September 7, 2018, https://www.rfa.org/english/news/china/outbreaks-09072018110830.html.

5 "Experts Cast Doubts on Chinese Official Claims Around 'New' Wuhan Coronavirus," *Radio Free Asia,* January 9, 2020, https://www.rfa.org/english/news/china/wuhan-outbreak-01092020133656.html.

6 Bill Gertz, "Coronavirus may have originated in lab linked to China's biowarfare program," *The Washington Times,* January 26, 2020, https://www.washingtontimes.com/news/2020/jan/26/coronavirus-link-to-china-biowarfare-program-possi/.

Saddam Hussein.[7] Shoham's assertions about Iraq's government and weaponized Anthrax, which were used to bolster the case for the 2003 invasion of Iraq,[8] have since been proven completely false, as Iraq was found to have neither the chemical or biological "weapons of mass destruction" that "experts" like Shoham had claimed.

Beyond Shoham's own history of making suspect claims, it is also worth noting that Shoham's previous employer, Israeli military intelligence, has a troubling past with bioweapons. For instance, in the late 1990s, it was reported by several outlets[9] that Israel was in the process of developing a genetic bioweapon that would target Arabs, specifically Iraqis, but leave Israeli Jews unaffected.

Given the dubious past of Shoham and the clearly speculative nature of both his claims and those made in the *Radio Free Asia* report, one passage in the *Washington Times* article[10] is particularly telling about why these claims have recently surfaced:

> "One ominous sign," said a U.S. official, "is that the false rumors since the outbreak began several weeks ago have begun circulating on the Chinese Internet *claiming the virus is part of a U.S. conspiracy to spread germ weapons. That could indicate China is preparing propaganda outlets to counter future charges the new virus escaped from one of Wuhan's civilian or defense research laboratories.*" [emphasis added]

However, as seen in that very article, accusations that the coronavirus escaped from a Chinese-state-linked laboratory is hardly a *future* charge as both the *Washington Times* and *Radio Free Asia* have already been making that claim. Instead, what this passage suggests is that the reports in both *Radio Free Asia* and the *Washington Times* were responses to the claims circulating within China that the outbreak is linked to a "U.S. conspiracy to spread germ weapons."

Though most mainstream English-language media outlets to date have not examined such a possibility, there is considerable supporting evidence that deserves to be examined. For instance, not only was the U.S. military, including its controversial research arm—the Defense Advanced Research Projects Agency

---

7 Dany Shoham, "The Anthrax Evidence Points to Iraq," *International Journal of Intelligence and CounterIntelligence* 16(1):39–68, January 2003, https://www.researchgate.net/publication/254312047_The_Anthrax_Evidence_Points_to_Iraq.

8 Julie Stahl, "Israeli Experts: Go After Saddam Hussein Before He Gets Nukes," *CNS News*, July 7, 2008, https://www.cnsnews.com/news/article/israeli-experts-go-after-saddam-hussein-he-gets-nukes.

9 "Israel's Ethnic Weapon?" *Wired*, November 16, 1998, https://www.wired.com/1998/11/israels-ethnic-weapon/.

10 Bill Gertz, *op cit.*

(DARPA)—recently funding studies in and near China that discovered new, mutant coronaviruses originating from bats, but the Pentagon also became recently interested in the potential use of bats as bioweapons.

BATS AS BIOWEAPONS

After the ongoing coronavirus outbreak centered in China spread to other countries and was blamed for a growing number of deaths, a consensus initially emerged that this particular virus, currently classified as a "novel [i.e. new] coronavirus,"[11] is believed to have originated in bats[12] and was transmitted to humans in Wuhan, China via a seafood market that also traded exotic animals,[13] though later reports discredited the market as a likely point of origin. So-called "wet" markets, like the one in Wuhan, were previously blamed for past deadly coronavirus outbreaks in China, such as the 2003 outbreak of Severe Acute Respiratory Syndrome (SARS).[14]

In addition, one preliminary study[15] on the coronavirus responsible for the current outbreak found that the receptor, Angiotensin-converting enzyme 2 (ACE2), is not only the same as that used by the SARS coronavirus, but that East Asians present a much higher ratio of lung cells that express that receptor than the other ethnicities (Caucasian and African-American) included in the study. However, such findings were preliminary and the sample size too small to draw any definitive conclusions from that preliminary data.

---

11 "Coronavirus (COVID-19)," Centers for DiseaseControl and Prevention, accessed June 6, 2020, https://www.cdc.gov/coronavirus/2019-ncov/index.html.

12 Melissa Healy, "New coronavirus spreads as readily as 1918 Spanish flu and probably originated in bats," *Los Angeles Times,* January 29, 2020, https://www.latimes.com/science/story/2020-01-29/china-coronavirus-china-likely-originated-in-bats.

13 Aylin Woodward, "Both the new coronavirus and SARS outbreaks likely started in Chinese 'wet markets.' Historic photos show what the markets looked like." *Business Insider,* February 26, 2020, https://www.businessinsider.com/wuhan-coronavirus-chinese-wet-market-photos-2020-1.

14 Robert G. Webster, "Wet markets—a continuing source of severe acute respiratory syndrome and influenza?" *The Lancet,* January 17, 2004, https://www.thelancet.com/journals/lancet/article/PIIS0140-6736(03)15329-9/fulltext.

15 Yu Zhao, Zixian Zhao, Yujia Wang, Yueqing Zhou, Yu Ma, and Wei Zuo, "Single-cell RNA expression profiling of ACE2, the putative receptor of Wuhan 2019-nCov," Cold Spring Harbor Laboratory, *bioRxiv,* January 26, 2020, https://www.biorxiv.org/content/10.1101/2020.01.26.919985v1.full.

Two years ago, media reports began discussing the Pentagon's sudden concern that bats could be used as biological weapons,[16] particularly in spreading coronaviruses and other deadly diseases. The *Washington Post* asserted that the Pentagon's interest in investigating the potential use of bats to spread weaponized and deadly diseases was because of alleged Russian efforts to do the same. However, those claims regarding Russian interest in using bats as bioweapons date back to the 1980s when the Soviet Union engaged in covert research involving the Marburg virus, research that did not even involve bats[17] and which ended with the Soviet Union's collapse in 1991.

Like much of the Pentagon's controversial research programs, the bats as bioweapons research has been framed as defensive,[18] despite the fact that no imminent threat involving bat-propagated bioweapons has been acknowledged. However, independent scientists have recently accused the Pentagon, particularly its research arm DARPA, of claiming to be engaged in research it says is "defensive" but is actually "offensive."

The most recent example of this involved DARPA's "Insect Allies" program,[19] which officially "aims to protect the U.S. agricultural food supply by delivering protective genes to plants via insects, which are responsible for the transmission of most plant viruses" and to ensure "food security in the event of a major threat," according to both DARPA and media reports.

However, a group of well-respected, independent scientists revealed in a scathing analysis of the program[20] that, far from a "defensive" research project, the Insect Allies program was aimed at creating and delivering a "new class of

---

16 Lucy Cooke, "US military is interested in bats as possible defenders against bioweapons," *Stars and Stripes,* August 15, 2018, https://www.stripes.com/news/us/us-military-is-interested-in-bats-as-possible-defenders-against-bioweapons-1.542849.

17 "The World's Most Dangerous Bioweapons," *Army Technology,* April 12, 2015, https://www.army-technology.com/features/featurethe-worlds-most-dangerous-bioweapons-4546207/.

18 The Washington Post, "How the Pentagon is planning to use bats in the battle against bioweapons," *South China Morning Post,* July 3, 2018, https://www.scmp.com/news/world/united-states-canada/article/2153562/how-pentagon-planning-using-bats-battle-against.

19 Blake Bextine, "Insect Allies," DARPA, October 4, 2018, https://www.darpa.mil/program/insect-allies.

20 Hannah Osborne, "DARPA Is Making Insects That Can Deliver Bioweapons, Scientists Claim," *Newsweek,* October 4, 2018, https://www.newsweek.com/darpa-biological-weapons-insects-scientists-warn-1152834.

biological weapon."[21] The scientists, writing in the journal *Science*[22] and led by Richard Guy Reeves, from the Max Planck Institute for Evolutionary Biology in Germany, warned that DARPA's program—which uses insects as the vehicle for horizontal environmental genetic alteration agents (HEGAAS) — revealed "an intention to develop a means of delivery of HEGAAs for *offensive purposes* [emphasis added]."

Whatever the real motivation behind the Pentagon's sudden and recent concern about bats being used as a vehicle for bioweapons, the U.S. military has spent millions of dollars over the past several years funding research on bats, the deadly viruses they can harbor—including coronaviruses—and how those viruses are transmitted from bats to humans.

For instance, DARPA spent $10 million on one project in 2018 "to unravel the complex causes of bat-borne viruses that have recently made the jump to humans, causing concern among global health officials."[23] Another research project backed by both DARPA and NIH saw researchers at Colorado State University examine the coronavirus that causes Middle East Respiratory Syndrome (MERS) in bats and camels "to understand the role of these hosts in transmitting disease to humans."[24] Other U.S. military-funded studies, discussed in detail later in this report, discovered several new strains of novel coronaviruses carried by bats, both within China and in countries bordering China.

Many of these recent research projects are related to DARPA's Preventing Emerging Pathogenic Threats, or PREEMPT program,[25] which was officially announced in April 2018. PREEMPT focuses specifically on animal reservoirs of disease, specifically bats, and DARPA even noted in its press release on the

---

21 Josh Gabbatiss, "US military plan to spread viruses using insects could create 'new class of biological weapon', scientists warn," *The Independent,* October 4, 2018, https://www.independent.co.uk/news/science/us-military-plan-biological-weapons-insect-allies-virus-crop-darpa-a8568996.html.

22 R.G. Reeves, et al., "Agricultural research, or a new bioweapon system?" *Science,* October 5, 2018,

Vol. 362, Issue 6410, 35-37, https://science.sciencemag.org/content/362/6410/35.

23 Marshall Swearingen, "MSU project to prevent bat-borne diseases wins $10 million grant," *Bozeman Daily Chronicle,* December 6, 2018, https://www.bozemandailychronicle. com/news/montana_state_university/msu-project-to-prevent-bat-borne-diseases-wins-million-grant/article_805eb8ec-763c-53ff-87da-3d9c2466cd61.html.

24 Alan S. Rudolph, "Guest Column: Wuhan Coronavirus – once again on the brink of a global health crisis, CSU researchers respond," *Colorado State University College News,* January 27, 2020, https://source.colostate.edu/wuhan-coronavirus-once-again-on-the-brink-of-a-global-health-crisis-csu-researchers-respond/.

25 "Going to the Source to Prevent Viral Disease Outbreaks," DARPA, January 4, 2018, https://www.darpa.mil/news-events/2018-01-04.

program that it "is aware of biosafety and biosecurity sensitivities that could arise" due to the nature of the research.

DARPA's announcement for PREEMPT came just a few months after the U.S. government decided to controversially end a moratorium on so-called "gain-of-function" studies involving dangerous pathogens. *VICE News* explained "gain-of-function" studies as follows:[26]

> Known as "gain-of-function" studies, this type of research is ostensibly about trying to stay one step ahead of nature. *By making super-viruses that are more pathogenic and easily transmissible,* scientists are able to study the way these viruses may evolve and how genetic changes affect the way a virus interacts with its host. Using this information, the scientists *can try to pre-empt* the natural emergence of these traits by developing antiviral medications that are capable of staving off a pandemic. [emphasis added]

In addition, while both DARPA's PREEMPT program and the Pentagon's open interest in bats as bioweapons were announced in 2018, the U.S. military—specifically the Department of Defense's Cooperative Threat Reduction Program—began funding research involving bats and deadly pathogens, including the coronaviruses MERS and SARS, a year prior in 2017.[27] One of those studies focused on "Bat-Borne Zoonotic Disease Emergence in Western Asia" and involved the Lugar Center in Georgia, identified by former Georgian government officials,[28] the Russian government[29] and independent, investigative journalist Dilyana Gaytandzhieva[30] as a covert U.S. bioweapons lab.

---

26 Daniel Oberhaus, "The US Will Fund Research to Make Pathogens Deadlier Again," *VICE News,* December 19, 2017, https://www.vice.com/en_us/article/d34vyj/the-us-will-fund-research-to-make-pathogens-deadlier-again.

27 "Science Program Review, February 8-10, 2017," U.S. Department of Defense Cooperative Threat Reduction Program, Cooperative Biological Engagement Program (DTRA CBEP), https://www.grease-network.org/content/download/5407/40323/version/1/file/2017+CBEP+SPR+Program+Book_Final.pdf.

28 "Deadly experiments: Georgian ex-minister claims US-funded facility may be bioweapons lab," *RT,* September 16, 2018 (updated April 6, 2020), https://www.rt.com/news/438543-georgia-us-laboratory-bio-weapons/.

29 "Dozens of Georgians likely killed by US toxin or bioweapon disguised as drug research – Russian MoD," *RT,* October 4, 2018 (updated April 6, 2020), https://www.rt.com/news/440309-us-georgia-toxic-bioweapon-test/.

30 Dilyana Gaytandzhieva, "US diplomats involved in trafficking of human blood and pathogens for secret military program," *Dilyana.bg,* September 12, 2018, dilyana.bg/

It is also important to point out the fact that the U.S. military's key laboratory involving the study of deadly pathogens, including coronaviruses, Ebola and others, was suddenly shut down last August after the Center for Disease Control and Prevention (CDC) identified major "biosafety lapses" at the facility.[31] The U.S. Army Medical Research Institute of Infectious Diseases (USAMRIID) facility at Fort Detrick, Maryland—the U.S. military's lead laboratory for "biological defense" research since the late 1960s—was forced to halt all research it was conducting with a series of deadly pathogens after the CDC found that it lacked "sufficient systems in place to decontaminate wastewater" from its highest-security labs and that staff failed to follow safety procedures, among other lapses.[32] It was also reported that the lab suffered two separate breaches of containment last year, but the identity of the pathogens in question remain classified. In addition, the facility contains both level 3 and level 4 biosafety labs. While it is unknown if experiments involving coronaviruses were ongoing at the time, USAMRIID has recently been involved in research borne out of the Pentagon's recent concern about the use of bats as bioweapons.[33]

The decision to shut down USAMRIID garnered surprisingly little media coverage, as did the CDC's surprising decision to allow the troubled facility to "partially resume" research late last November even though the facility was and is still not at "full operational capability."[34] The USAMRIID's problematic record of safety at such facilities is of particular concern in light of the recent coronavirus outbreak in China. As this report will soon reveal, this is because USAMRIID has a decades-old and close partnership with the University of Wuhan's Institute of Medical Virology, which is located at the epicenter of the current outbreak.

---

us-diplomats-involved-in-trafficking-of-human-blood-and-pathogens-for-secret-military-program/.

31 Heather Mongilio, "Fort Detrick lab shut down after failed safety inspection; all research halted indefinitely," *The Frederick News-Post,* April 2, 2019, https://www.fredericknewspost.com/news/health/fort-detrick-lab-shut-down-after-failed-safety-inspection-all/article_767f3459-59c2-510f-9067-bb215db4396d.html.

32 Shawna Williams, "CDC Shuts Down Army Lab's Disease Research," *The Scientist,* August 6, 2019, https://www.the-scientist.com/news-opinion/cdc-shuts-down-army-labs-disease-research-66235.

33 Boston University, "Egyptian fruit bat genome yields clues about bats' ability to harbor and transmit deadly pathogens without getting sick," *Phys.Org,* April 26, 2018, https://phys.org/news/2018-04-egyptian-fruit-genome-yields-clues.html.

34 "CDC Approves Partial Resumption of USAMRIID Select Agent Research," *Global Biodefense,* November 23, 2019, https://globalbiodefense.com/2019/11/23/cdc-approves-partial-resumption-of-usamriid-select-agent-research/.

THE PENTAGON IN WUHAN?

Beyond the U.S. military's recent expenditures on and interest in the use of bats of bioweapons, it is also worth examining the recent studies the military has funded regarding bats and "novel coronaviruses," such as that behind the recent outbreak, that have taken place within or in close proximity to China.

For instance, one study conducted in Southern China in 2018 resulted in the discovery of 89 new "novel bat coronavirus" strains that use the same receptor as the coronavirus known as Middle East Respiratory Syndrome (MERS).[35] That study was jointly funded by the Chinese government's Ministry of Science and Technology, USAID—an organization long alleged to be a front for U.S. intelligence,[36] and the U.S. National Institute of Health—which has collaborated with both the CIA and the Pentagon on infectious disease and bioweapons research.[37]

The authors of the study also sequenced the complete genomes for two of those strains and noted that existing MERS vaccines would be ineffective in targeting these viruses, leading them to suggest that one should be developed in advance. This did not occur.

Another U.S. government-funded study that discovered still more new strains of "novel bat coronavirus" was published just last year. Titled "Discovery and Characterization of Novel Bat Coronavirus Lineages from Kazakhstan,"[38] it focused on "the bat fauna of central Asia, which link China to eastern Europe" and the novel bat coronavirus lineages discovered during the study were found to be "closely related to bat coronaviruses from China, France, Spain, and South Africa, suggesting that co-circulation of coronaviruses is common in multiple bat species with overlapping geographical distributions." In other words, the coronaviruses discovered in this study were identified in bat populations that migrate between China and Kazakhstan, among other countries, and is closely related to bat coronaviruses in several countries, including China.

---

35 Chu-Ming Luo, et al., "Discovery of Novel Bat Coronaviruses in South China That Use the Same Receptor as Middle East Respiratory Syndrome Coronavirus," *Journal of Virology* 2018 Jul 1; 92(13), published online June 13, 2018, https://www.ncbi.nlm.nih.gov/pmc/articles/PMC6002729/.

36 Catherine A. Traywick, "'Cuban Twitter' and Other Times USAID Pretended To Be an Intelligence Agency," *Foreign Policy,* April 3, 2014, https://foreignpolicy.com/2014/04/03/cuban-twitter-and-other-times-usaid-pretended-to-be-an-intelligence-agency/.

37 Jeneen Interlandi, "High-Stakes Science," *Newsweek,* December 5, 2007, https://www.newsweek.com/high-stakes-science-94931.

38 Ian H. Mendenhall, et al., "Discovery and Characterization of Novel Bat Coronavirus Lineages from Kazakhstan," *Viruses,* 2019 Apr; 11(4): 356, published online April 17, 2019, https://www.ncbi.nlm.nih.gov/pmc/articles/PMC6521082/.

The study was entirely funded by the U.S. Department of Defense, specifically the Defense Threat Reduction Agency (DTRA) as part of a project investigating coronaviruses similar to MERS, such as the aforementioned 2018 study.[39] Yet, beyond the funding of this 2019 study, the institutions involved in conducting this study are also worth noting, given their own close ties to the U.S. military and government.

The study's authors are affiliated with either the Kazakhstan-based Research Institute for Biological Safety Problems and/or Duke University. The Research Institute for Biological Safety Problems, though officially a part of Kazakhstan's National Center for Biotechnology, has received millions from the U.S. government,[40] most of it coming from the Pentagon's Cooperative Threat Reduction Program.[41] It is the Kazakhstan government's official depository of "highly dangerous animal and bird infections, with a collection of 278 pathogenic strains of 46 infectious diseases."[42] It is part of a network of Pentagon-funded "bioweapons labs" throughout the Central Asian country,[43] which borders both of the U.S.' top rival states—China and Russia.

Duke University's involvement with this study is also interesting given that Duke is a key partner of DARPA's Pandemic Prevention Platform (P3) program,[44] which officially aims "to dramatically accelerate discovery, integration, pre-clinical testing, and manufacturing of medical countermeasures against infectious diseases." The first step of the Duke/DARPA program involves the discovery

---

39 *Ibid.*

40 "Scientific Research Institute for Biological Safety Problems," Facilities page produced independently by James Martin Center for Nonproliferation Studies at the Monterey Institute of International Studies and published online by NTI (Nuclear Threat Initiative), updated June 10, 2014, https://www.nti.org/learn/facilities/812/.

41 "Cooperative Threat Reduction (Nunn-Lugar) Program," Glossary entry produced independently by James Martin Center for Nonproliferation Studies at the Monterey Institute of International Studies and published online by NTI (Nuclear Threat Initiative), https://www.nti.org/learn/glossary/#cooperative-threat-reduction-nunn-lugar-program.

42 *Ibid.*

43 Alex Pasternack, "The US is building a bioweapons lab in Kazakhstan," *Salon,* August 29, 2013, https://www.salon.com/2013/08/29/the_us_is_building_a_bioweapons_lab_in_kazakhstan_newscred/.

44 "Duke DARPA Pandemic Prevent Platform (P3)," Duke Human Vaccine Institute, Duke University School of Medicine, accessed June 6, 2020, https://dhvi.duke.edu/our-programs/pandemic-preparedness/duke-darpa-pandemic-prevent-platform-p3.

of potentially threatening viruses[45] and "develop[ing] methods to support viral propagation,"[46] so that virus can be used for downstream studies."

Duke University is also jointly partnered with China's Wuhan University,[47] which resulted in the opening of the China-based Duke Kunshan University (DKU) in Kunshan in 2018. Notably, China's Wuhan University—in addition to its partnership with Duke—also includes a multi-lab Institute of Medical Virology that has worked closely with the U.S. Army Medical Research Institute for Infectious Diseases since the 1980s, according to its website.[48] As previously noted, the USAMRIID facility in the U.S. was shut down last August for failures to abide by biosafety and proper waste disposal procedures, but was allowed to partially resume some experiments late last November.

THE PENTAGON'S DARK HISTORY OF GERM WARFARE

The U.S. military has a troubling past of having used disease as a weapon during times of war. One example involved the U.S.' use of germ warfare during the Korean War,[49] when it targeted both North Korea and China by dropping diseased insects and voles carrying a variety of pathogens—including bubonic plague and hemorrhagic fever—from planes in the middle of the night. Despite the mountain of evidence and the testimony of U.S. soldiers involved in that program, the U.S. government and military denied the claims and ordered the destruction of relevant documentation.

In the post World War II era, other examples of U.S. research aimed at developing biological weapons have emerged, some of which have recently received media attention. One such example occurred this past July, when the U.S. House of Representatives demanded information from the U.S. military on its past efforts to weaponize insects and Lyme disease between 1950 and 1975.[50]

---

45 Amy Jenkins, "Pandemic Prevention Platform (P3)," Defense Advanced Research Projects Agency program information, DARPA, accessed June 6, 2020, https://dhvi.duke.edu/our-programs/pandemic-preparedness/duke-darpa-pandemic-prevent-platform-p3.

46 "Duke DARPA Pandemic Prevent Platform (P3)," *op cit.*

47 Jessica Patrick, "Duke Kunshan University closed during coronavirus outbreak in China," *WRAL.com,* updated January 25, 2020, https://www.wral.com/duke-kunshan-university-closed-during-coronavirus-outbreak-in-china/18909092/.

48 "Institute of Medical Virology," Wuhan University School of Basic Medical Sciences, accessed June 6, 2020, http://wbm.whu.edu.cn/English/Departments/Departments/Institute_of_Medical_Virology.htm.

49 Thomas Powell, "The Dirty Secret of the Korean War," CounterPunch, May 26, 2017, https://www.counterpunch.org/2017/05/26/the-dirty-secret-of-the-korean-war/.

50 Adam Forrest, "US military chiefs ordered to reveal if Pentagon used diseased insects as biological weapon," *Independent,* July 16, 2019, https://www.independent.

The U.S. has claimed that it has not pursued offensive biological weapons since 1969 and this has been further supported by the U.S. ratification of the Biological Weapons Convention[51] (BWC), which went into effect in 1975. However, there is extensive evidence that the U.S. has continued to covertly research and develop such weapons in the years since,[52] much of it conducted abroad and outsourced to private companies, yet still funded by the U.S. military. One notable example was the Pentagon's and CIA's simultaneous efforts to genetically modify anthrax to create a deadlier version of the toxin in the late 1990s and early 2000s, a project largely overseen by the privately owned Battelle Memorial Institute. In more recent years, several investigators, including Dilyana Gaytandzhieva,[53] have documented how the U.S. produces deadly viruses, bacteria and other toxins at facilities outside of the U.S.—many of them in Eastern Europe, Africa and South Asia—in clear violation of the BWC.

Aside from the military's own research, the controversial neoconservative think tank, the now defunct Project for a New American Century (PNAC), openly promoted the use of a race-specific genetically modified bioweapon as a "politically useful tool." In what is arguably the think tank's most controversial document, published in September 2000 and entitled "Rebuilding America's Defenses,"[54] there are a few passages that openly discuss the utility of bioweapons, including the following sentences:

> ...combat likely will take place in new dimensions: in space, "cyberspace," and perhaps the world of microbes...advanced forms of biological warfare that can "target" specific genotypes may transform biological warfare from the realm of terror to a politically useful tool.

Numerous members of PNAC were prominent in the George W. Bush administration, and many of its more controversial members have again risen to political prominence in the Trump administration.

---

co.uk/news/world/americas/pentagon-ticks-insects-biological-weapons-congress-bill-chris-smith-a9006701.html.

51 "Biological Weapons Convention," U.S. Department of State, https://www.state.gov/biological-weapons-convention/.

52 W. T. Whitney, "Criminal Behavior: US May be Developing Biological Weapons," *CounterPunch,* November 21, 2018, https://www.counterpunch.org/2018/11/21/criminal-behavior-us-may-be-developing-biological-weapons/.

53 Dilyana Gaytandzhieva, "The Pentagon Bio-weapons," April 29, 2018, *Dilyana. bg,* http://dilyana.bg/the-pentagon-bio-weapons/.

54 Project for a New American Century/Foreign Policy Initiative, "Rebuilding Americas Defenses," November 9, 2000, Wikipedia entry archived on Internet Archive, https://archive.org/details/RebuildingAmericasDefenses/page/n5/mode/2up.

Several years after "Rebuilding America's Defenses" was published, the U.S. Air Force published a document entitled "Biotechnology: Genetically Engineered Pathogens,"[55] which contains the following passage:

The JASON group, composed of academic scientists, served as technical advisers to the U. S. government. Their study generated six broad classes of genetically engineered pathogens that could pose serious threats to society. *These include but are not limited to binary biological weapons, designer genes, gene therapy as a weapon, stealth viruses, host-swapping diseases, and designer diseases.* [emphasis added]

Concerns about Pentagon experiments with biological weapons have garnered renewed media attention, particularly after it was revealed in 2017 that DARPA was the top funder of the controversial "gene drive" technology, which has the power to permanently alter the genetics of entire populations while targeting others for extinction.[56] At least two of DARPA's studies using this controversial technology were classified and "focused on the potential military application of gene drive technology and use of gene drives in agriculture," according to media reports.[57]

The revelation came after an organization called the ETC Group obtained over 1,000 emails on the military's interest in the technology as part of a Freedom of Information Act (FOIA) request. Co-director of the ETC Group Jim Thomas said that this technology may be used as a biological weapon:[58]

Gene drives are a powerful and dangerous new technology and potential biological weapons could have disastrous impacts on peace, food security and the environment, especially if misused. The fact that gene drive development is now being primarily funded and structured by the U.S. military raises alarming questions about this entire field.

---

55 Joel O. Almosara, *Biotechnology: Genetically Engineered Pathogens,* The Counterproliferation Papers Future Warfare Series No. 53, USAF Counterproliferation Center, Air University, Maxwell Air Force Base, Alabama, June 2010, https://apps.dtic.mil/dtic/tr/fulltext/u2/a556597.pdf.

56 Arthur Neslen, "US military agency invests $100m in genetic extinction technologies," *The Guardian,* December 4, 2017, https://www.theguardian.com/science/2017/dec/04/us-military-agency-invests-100m-in-genetic-extinction-technologies

57 "Pentagon revealed as top funder of controversial gene editing tech," *RT,* December 5, 2017, https://www.rt.com/usa/412019-pentagon-darpa-gene-drive/.

58 *Ibid.*

Though the exact motivation behind the military's interest in such technology is unknown, the Pentagon has been open about the fact that it is devoting much of its resources towards the containment of what it considers the two greatest threats to U.S. military hegemony: Russia and China.[59] China has been cited as the greatest threat of the two by several Pentagon officials, including John Rood, the Pentagon's top adviser for defense policy, who described China as the greatest threat to "our way of life in the United States" at the Aspen Security Forum last July.[60]

Since the Pentagon began "redesigning" its policies and research towards a "long war" with Russia and China,[61,62] the Russian military has accused the U.S. military of harvesting DNA from Russians as part of a covert bioweapon program,[63,64] a charge that the Pentagon has adamantly denied. Major General Igor Kirillov, the head of the Russian military's radiation, chemical and biological protection unit who made these claims, also asserted that the U.S. was developing such weapons in close proximity to Russian and Chinese borders.

China has also accused the U.S. military of harvesting DNA from Chinese citizens with ill intentions, such as when 200,000 Chinese farmers were used in

---

59 Dave Majumdar, "Pentagon: Russia and China Are America's Biggest Military Threats," *The National Interest*, February 14, 2018, https://nationalinterest.org/blog/the-buzz/pentagon-russia-china-are-americas-biggest-military-threats-24495.

60 Joel Gehrke, "Top Pentagon official: China a threat to 'our way of life in the United States,'" *Washington Examiner*, July 20, 2019, https://www.washingtonexaminer.com/policy/defense-national-security/top-pentagon-official-china-a-threat-to-our-way-of-life-in-the-united-states.

61 Aaron Mehta, "The Pentagon is planning for war with China and Russia — can it handle both?" *DefenseNews*, January 30, 2018, https://www.defensenews.com/pentagon/2018/01/30/the-pentagon-is-planning-for-war-with-china-and-russia-can-it-handle-both/

62 Michael T.Klare, "The Pentagon Is Planning a Three-Front 'Long War' Against China and Russia," *Mint Press News*, April 5, 2018, https://www.mintpressnews.com/pentagon-planning-a-three-front-long-war-against-china-and-russia/240100/.

63 Associated Press, "Pentagon denies Russia's claim that the US is running a secret biological weapons lab near border of China and Georgia," *South China Morning Post*, October 5, 2018, https://www.scmp.com/news/world/united-states-canada/article/2167058/pentagon-denies-russias-claim-us-running-secret.

64 Adam Garrie, "Putin Questions US Air Force DNA Collection From Ethnic Russians," *Mint Press News*, November 1, 2017, https://www.mintpressnews.com/putin-questions-us-air-force-dna-collection-ethnic-russians/233946/.

12 genetic experiments without informed consent.[65] Those experiments had been conducted by Harvard researchers as part of a U.S. government-funded project.

DARPA AND ITS PARTNERS CHOSEN TO DEVELOP CORONAVIRUS VACCINE

In January, the Coalition for Epidemic Preparedness Innovations (CEPI) first announced that it would fund three separate programs in order to promote the development of a vaccine for the new coronavirus responsible for the current outbreak.

CEPI—which describes itself as "a partnership of public, private, philanthropic and civil organizations that will finance and co-ordinate the development of vaccines against high priority public health threats"—was founded in 2017 by the governments of Norway and India along with the World Economic Forum and the Bill and Melinda Gates Foundation. Its massive funding and close connections to public, private and non-profit organizations have positioned it to be able to finance the rapid creation of vaccines and widely distribute them.

CEPI's January announcement revealed that it would fund two pharmaceutical companies—Inovio Pharmaceuticals and Moderna Inc.—as well as Australia's University of Queensland, which became a partner of CEPI early last year.[66] Notably, the two pharmaceutical companies chosen have close ties to and/or strategic partnerships with DARPA and are developing vaccines that controversially involve genetic material and/or gene editing. The University of Queensland also has ties to DARPA, but those ties are not related to the university's biotechnology research, but instead engineering[67] and missile development.[68]

The top funders of Inovio Pharmaceuticals include both DARPA and the Pentagon's Defense Threat Reduction Agency (DTRA).[69] The company has

---

65 "Why did OHRP SHRED informed consent documents?" Alliance for Human Resource Protection, October 25, 2003, https://ahrp.org/article-30/.

66 Mario Christodoulou, "CEPI partners with University of Queensland to create rapid-response vaccines," CEPI, January 17, 2019, https://cepi.net/news_cepi/cepi-partners-with-university-of-queensland-to-create-rapid-response-vaccines/.

67 "UCLA Engineering advance with new nanomaterials good news for next-generation electronic devices," *AAAS EurekaAlert!* University of California – Los Angeles, February 14, 2011, https://www.eurekalert.org/pub_releases/2011-02/uoc--uea021411.php.

68 Joseph Trevithick, "The United States and Australia Quietly Test Hypersonic Missiles," *TheDrive,* July 13, 2017, https://www.thedrive.com/the-war-zone/12456/the-united-states-and-australia-quietly-test-hypersonic-missiles?iid=sr-link3.

69 "Inovio Pharmaceuticals," *Crunchbase,* accessed June 6, 2020, https://www.crunchbase.com/organization/inovio-pharmaceuticals#section-funding-rounds.

received millions of dollars in grants from DARPA, including a $45 million grant[70] to develop a vaccine for Ebola. Inovio specializes in the creation of DNA immunotherapies and DNA vaccines, which contain genetically engineered DNA that causes the cells of the recipient to produce an antigen and can permanently alter a person's DNA. Inovio previously developed a DNA vaccine for the Zika virus, but—to date—no DNA vaccine has been approved for use in humans in the United States. Inovio was also recently awarded over $8 million from the U.S. military to develop a small, portable intradermal device for delivering DNA vaccines jointly developed by Inovio and USAMRIID.[71]

However, the CEPI grant to combat coronavirus may change that, as it specifically funds Inovio's efforts to continue developing its DNA vaccine for the coronavirus that causes MERS. Inovio's MERS vaccine program began in 2018 in partnership with CEPI in a deal worth $56 million.[72] The vaccine currently under development uses "Inovio's DNA Medicines platform to deliver optimized synthetic antigenic genes into cells, where they are translated into protein antigens that activate an individual's immune system."[73] The program is partnered with U.S. Army Medical Research Institute of Infectious Diseases (USAMRIID) and the NIH, among others. That program is currently undergoing testing in an undisclosed country in the Middle East.

Inovio's collaboration with the U.S. military in regards to DNA vaccines is nothing new, as their past efforts to develop a DNA vaccine for both Ebola and Marburg virus were also part of what Inovio's CEO Dr. Joseph Kim called its "active biodefense program" that has "garnered multiple grants from the Department

---

70 "Inovio Pharmaceuticals selected by DARPA to lead a $45 million program to expedite development of novel products to prevent and treat disease caused by Ebola," *MarketWatch*, April 8, 2015, https://www.marketwatch.com/press-release/inovio-pharmaceuticals-selected-by-darpa-to-lead-a-45-million-program-to-expedite-development-of-novel-products-to-prevent-and-treat-disease-caused-by-ebola-2015-04-08.

71 Inovio Pharmaceuticals, "Inovio Receives $8.14 Million Award to Support Further Development of its Commercial Skin Delivery Device," *PR Newswire*, June 10, 2019, https://www.prnewswire.com/news-releases/inovio-receives-8-14-million-award-to-support-further-development-of-its-commercial-skin-delivery-device-300864257.html.

72 Rachel Grant, "Inovio Awarded up to $56 Million from CEPI to Advance DNA Vaccines Against Lassa Fever and MERS," CEPI, April 11, 2018, https://cepi.net/news_cepi/inovio-awarded-up-to-56-million-from-cepi-to-advance-dna-vaccines-against-lassa-fever-and-mers/.

73 "CEPI to fund three programmes to develop vaccines against the novel coronavirus, nCoV-2019," CEPI, January 23, 2020, https://cepi.net/news_cepi/cepi-to-fund-three-programmes-to-develop-vaccines-against-the-novel-coronavirus-ncov-2019/.

of Defense, Defense Threat Reduction Agency (DTRA), National Institute of Allergy and Infectious Diseases (NIAID), and other government agencies."[74]

CEPI's interest in increasing its support to this MERS-specific program seems at odds with its claim that doing so will combat the current coronavirus outbreak, since MERS and the novel coronavirus in question are not analogous and treatments for certain coronaviruses have been shown to be ineffective against other strains.[75]

It is also worth noting that Inovio Pharmaceuticals was the only company selected by CEPI with direct access to the Chinese pharmaceutical market through its partnership with China's ApolloBio Corp., which currently has an exclusive license to sell Inovio-made DNA immunotherapy products to Chinese customers.[76]

The second pharmaceutical company that was selected by CEPI to develop a vaccine for the new coronavirus is Moderna Inc., which will develop a vaccine for COVID-19 in collaboration with the U.S. NIH and which will be funded entirely by CEPI. The vaccine in question, as opposed to Inovio's DNA vaccine, will be a messenger RNA (mRNA) vaccine. Though different than a DNA vaccine, mRNA vaccines still use genetic material "to direct the body's cells to produce intracellular, membrane or secreted proteins."

Moderna's mRNA treatments, including its mRNA vaccines, were largely developed using a $25 million grant from DARPA[77] and it often touts its strategic alliance with DARPA in press releases.[78] Moderna's past and ongoing research efforts have included developing mRNA vaccines tailored to an individual's unique

---

74 "Inovio Pharmaceuticals DNA Vaccine Against Ebola and Marburg Filoviruses Provides Complete Protection in Preclinical Challenge Study," *PipelineReview.com,* May 14, 2013, https://pipelinereview.com/index.php/2013051450949/Vaccines/Inovio-Pharmaceuticals-DNA-Vaccine-Against-Ebola-and-Marburg-Filoviruses-Provides-Complete-Protection-in-Preclinical-Challenge-Study.html.

75 Chu-Ming Luo, et al., "Discovery of Novel Bat Coronaviruses in South China That Use the Same Receptor as Middle East Respiratory Syndrome Coronavirus," *Journal of Virology* 2018 Jul 1; 92(13); published online June 13, 2018, https://www.ncbi.nlm.nih.gov/pmc/articles/PMC6002729/.

76 Shobhit Seth, "Inovio Inks $35M Chinese Drug License Deal (INO)," *Investopedia,* updated June 25, 2019, https://www.investopedia.com/news/inovio-inks-35m-chinese-drug-license-deal-ino/.

77 "DARPA Awards Moderna Therapeutics a Grant for up to $25 Million to Develop Messenger RNA Therapeutics™," *Moderna,* October 2, 2013, https://investors.modernatx.com/news-releases/news-release-details/darpa-awards-moderna-therapeutics-grant-25-million-develop.

78 "Moderna Announces Key 2020 Investor and Analyst Events," *Business Wire,* December 11, 2019, https://www.businesswire.com/news/home/20191211005159/en/Moderna-Announces-Key-2020-Investor-Analyst-Events.

DNA[79] as well as an unsuccessful effort to create a mRNA vaccine for the Zika Virus, which had also been funded by the U.S. government.

Both DNA and mRNA vaccines involve the introduction of foreign and engineered genetic material into a person's cells. Past studies have found that such vaccines "possess significant unpredictability and a number of inherent harmful potential hazards"[80] and that "there is inadequate knowledge to define either the probability of unintended events or the consequences of genetic modifications." Nonetheless, the climate of fear surrounding the coronavirus outbreak could be enough for the public and private sector to develop and distribute such controversial treatments due to fear about the epidemic potential of the current outbreak.

However, the therapies being developed by Inovio, Modern and the University of Queensland are in alignment with DARPA's objectives regarding gene editing and vaccine technology. For instance, in 2015, DARPA geneticist Col. Daniel Wattendorf described how the agency was investigating a "new method of vaccine production [that] would involve giving the body instructions for making certain antibodies. Because the body would be its own bioreactor, the vaccine could be produced much faster than traditional methods and the result would be a higher level of protection."[81]

According to media reports on Wattendorf's statements at the time,[82] the vaccine would be developed as follows:

> Scientists would harvest viral antibodies from someone who has recovered from a disease such as flu or Ebola. After testing the antibodies' ability to neutralize viruses in a petri dish, they would isolate the most effective one, determine the genes needed to make that antibody, and then encode many copies of those genes into a circular snippet of genetic material—either DNA or RNA, that the person's body would then use as a cookbook to assemble the antibody.

---

79 Elie Dolgin, "Unlocking the potential of vaccines built on messenger RNA," *Nature,* October 16, 2019, https://www.nature.com/articles/d41586-019-03072-8.

80 Vivian S. W. Chan, "Use of Genetically Modified Viruses and Genetically Engineered Virus-Vector Vaccines: Environmental Effects," *Journal of Toxicology and Environmental Health A* 2006 Nov; 69(21):1971-7, https://pubmed.ncbi.nlm.nih.gov/16982535/.

81 Tia Ghose, "DARPA Is Developing Human Bio-Factories to Brew Lifesaving Vaccines," *LiveScience.com,* republished on *Yahoo! News,* September 13, 2015, https://www.yahoo.com/news/darpa-developing-human-bio-factories-brew-lifesaving-vaccines-120915583.html.

82 *Ibid.*

Though Wattendorf asserted that the effects of those vaccines wouldn't be permanent, DARPA has since been promoting permanent gene modifications as a means of protecting U.S. troops from biological weapons and infectious disease. "Why is DARPA doing this? [To] protect a soldier on the battlefield from chemical weapons and biological weapons by controlling their genome—having the genome produce proteins that would automatically protect the soldier from the inside out," then-DARPA director Steve Walker (now with Lockheed Martin) said this past September of the project,[83] known as "Safe Genes."[84]

Conclusion

Research conducted by the Pentagon, and DARPA specifically, has continually raised concerns, not just in the field of bioweapons and biotechnology, but also in the fields of nanotechnology, robotics and several others. DARPA, for instance, has been developing a series of unsettling research projects that ranges from microchips that can create and delete memories from the human brain to voting machine software that is rife with problems and ripe for manipulation.[85]

Now, as fear regarding the current coronavirus outbreak persists, companies with direct ties to DARPA have been tasked with developing its vaccine, the long-term human and environmental impacts of which are unknown and will remain unknown by the time the vaccine is expected to go to market in a few months time.

Furthermore, DARPA and the Pentagon's past history with bioweapons and their more recent experiments on genetic alteration and extinction technologies as well as bats and coronaviruses in proximity to China have been largely left out of the narrative, despite the information being publicly available. Also left out of the media narrative have been the direct ties of both the USAMRIID and DARPA-partnered Duke University to the city of Wuhan and their links to virology labs in the outbreak's epicenter.

Though much about the origins of the coronavirus outbreak remains unknown, the U.S. military's ties to the aforementioned research studies and research institutions are worth detailing as such research—while justified in the

83 Russ Read, "Military wants to use gene editing to protect troops against chemical and biological weapons," *Washington Examiner,* September 23, 2019, https://www.washingtonexaminer.com/policy/defense-national-security/military-wants-to-use-gene-editing-to-protect-troops-against-chemical-and-biological-weapons.

84 Renee Wegrzyn, "Safe Genes," DARPA, accessed June 6, 2020, https://www.darpa.mil/program/safe-genes.

85 Shelly Fan, "Here's the Tech That Could One Day Track, Boost, or Erase Human Memory," *SingularityHub,* January 25, 2018, https://singularityhub.com/2018/01/25/heres-the-tech-that-could-one-day-track-boost-or-erase-human-memory/amp/.

name of "national security"—has the frightening potential to result in unintended, yet world-altering consequences. The lack of transparency about this research, such as DARPA's decision to classify its controversial genetic extinction research and the technology's use as a weapon of war, compounds these concerns. While it is important to avoid reckless speculation as much as possible, it is the opinion of this author that the information in this report is in the public interest and that readers should use this information to reach their own conclusions about the topics discussed herein.

CHAPTER TEN

BIOWARFARE AS ECONOMIC WARFARE

Claudio Peretti

What is war? Typically it is killing and damaging the enemy, so that they will accept to be governed and exploited by the victor. In the past, the defeated populations were made slaves, forced to work for their owners. In that period labor was only provided by humans and animals, so to achieve a comfortable lifestyle for their own populations, kings and emperors had to have a large slaveholding. Such was the behavior of the Roman and other empires. After the industrial era and the use of carbon and oil, however, the energy needed for production is no longer obtained from slaves and animals. Today, the new emperors fight mainly for control of the supply of gas and oil. Few people know that Hitler and the Germans tried to conquer Russia in order to gain access to the oil fields of Central Asia: Iran, Turkmenistan, Azerbaijan and Kazakhstan. He nearly succeeded in this strategy, but was stopped by the winter and by the Russian Army: he ran out of fuel for his tanks and trucks before he was able to conquer the oil fields of Central Asia.

Today we have similar wars. If you look at the crisis zones of the world, you will always see the presence of oil and the effort to procure it or seize these oil fields by aggressor nations. The Hormuz strait provides such an instance: 33% of world oil has to transit the strait on big oil tankers. Iran, where a government not aligned with the USA politics is ruling, is on its northern side. In the past Iran was governed by the Shah, a despot aligned with the USA, but due to his mistakes—he and his ministers and government living too luxuriously—a rebellion, headed by a religious leader, the Ayatollah Khomeini, overthrew his government. Currently the USA no longer has full control of the strait and is always trying to destabilize Iran's political power in many ways, such as the killing of Iranian general, Qassem Soleimani, on January 3, 2020 that nearly led to the outbreak of war by the USA against Iran. The same kind of events are happening in Venezuela as had previously happened in IRAQ and in Libya. In all these instances, if the local oil fields are not owned by the USA or are not managed by states close to the USA, destabilization and wars take place. Since the common people of the western democracies are always looking for morally acceptable behavior when it comes to electing new generations of their political leaders, the leaders of USA and the allied NATO countries are forced to use deceptive wording—"Peace Keeping" and "Peace Enforcing"— to justify their military interventions. That said, nobody cares about what is happening in some central African states, where despotic dictators exploit their peoples without any respect for human life.

A different situation and perception of antagonisms is happening in China. Here we have a country that is not democratic, that is developing at a very fast rate, doubling the economic development parameters of whichever western country. This occurred after the previous leaders of the communist party officially declared that private property is allowed and is good for people. While this is a theory that is not compatible with old fashioned communism as it is studied in our schools, in China it is running perfectly and the plans to take the Chinese people out of poverty are running at the speed of light.

There is a political theory, called the Thucydides trap: This great historian attributed the outbreak of the war between Athens and Sparta in the fifth century BC to the growth of Athenian power, and to the fear that this growth generated in its rival, Sparta. Today, as in the time of Thucydides, international relations are mostly thought of as zero-sum games: if a dominant but declining power is faced with an emerging power, it will similarly be afraid and lead it to make war against its rival. It is easy to understand why this affects us. We live in a historical phase in which a long dominant power (the United States) has to face an emerging power (China). Will the Thucydides trap set in? Will a war between the United States and China break out, sooner or later?

Since a typical war with bombs, missiles, aircraft, destroyers, soldiers, etc., is very expensive and causes extensive damage to foe and friend alike, new types of wars have been studied. Starting from the theory that the intent of war is to damage the enemy, it is understood that many types of damage can be inflicted on the enemy—economic, political, cyber-attacks, social destabilization, and public health destruction—instead of firing and bombing. "Hybrid warfare" has been developed as a result. The CIA is the master and specialist of this new type of war. It is very skilled in conducting secret operations, paid for with black money gained through dealing in opium from Afghanistan. An instance of this type of operation likely took place in Hong Kong during the protest against China in the winter of 2019, when a CIA official was photographed in a Hong Kong hotel together with the chiefs of the riot. But the people rioting in Hong Kong had to be paid, making the operation expensive. Might one conclude that an easier way of conducting hybrid warfare is to spread an artificially generated virus? Is this probable or improbable? Why should we think that someone in the CIA might have conducted a bio-attack on China?

The best investigation process was outlined by Sir Arthur Conan Doyle, author of a series of novels describing the exploits of the super sleuth, Sherlock

Holmes. And what was Holmes's working thesis? Give me a motive, a reason, and I will find the culprit.

Here are some points and indicators that address the doubt that something similar has happened.

In November 2018, the Republican and Democrat parties bilaterally signed the paper, "Providing for the Common Defense,"[1] which clearly declared that China is the greater enemy of the USA and that the USA should prepare for a devastating war between 2018 and 2024. This paper also pinpoints some areas and possibilities whereby the war might be started. It is obvious that a very good way to avoid a military confrontation might be by weakening the enormous commercial and economic power of China by spreading a killer virus.

If a fire happens to a building, the first thing to do is to put out the fire. After this it is usual for everybody to investigate whether the fire occurred spontaneously, naturally, or was the result of a malicious act by somebody, whether to gain the insurance premium or to damage the owner of the building. Nobody questions that the authorities should conduct such an investigation.

Why is nobody starting an investigation to determine who, if anybody, is behind the spreading of the coronavirus in China, Iran, Italy and, by this time, all over the world? While there will never be 100% certainty that this has been planned, if the investigation is seriously undertaken, it seems highly likely information will be discovered which may point to potential culprits.

That an analysis of this type should be conducted, and how, had already been meticulously outlined by NATO; there are numerous documents demonstrating that.[2] It goes without saying that NATO officials undertook this study to counter a possible bio-attack by foes of the western alliance, but the same investigative principles can be easily applied to the opposite situation.

What does NATO declare? With absolute logic, they say that, if an animal or a human is killed by an unknown biologic agent, an investigation must be immediately started to determine if this occurrence was natural or caused by a potential enemy.

What are the main arguments, in NATO's view, to be taken into consideration? Here they are:

1. Is there a nation that is seeking the weakening of another country?

---

1 National Defense Strategy Commission, *Providing for the Common Defense,* November 13, 2018, United States Institute of Peace, https://www.usip.org/publications/2018/11/providing-common-defense.

2 Hunger et al., *Biopreparedness and Public Health: Exploring Synergies,* NATO Science for Peace and Security Series A: Chemistry and Biology (2013); Radosavljevic et al., *Defence Against Bioterrorism: Methods for Prevention and Control,* NATO Science for Peace and Security Series A: Chemistry and Biology (2018).

2. Does this nation have the capacity to bio-engineer an artificial bio agent?

3. Once the bio agent has been developed, has this nation the capability to use it against the other nation?

It appears evident that the answer to all the above questions, in the current instance, is: Yes!

If, in addition to this, if one were to apply the Grunow–Finke Assessment Tool to Improve Performance in Detecting Unnatural Epidemics[3]—a method to give a weight to every possible answer to the above questions—one surely will have a high degree of reliability, albeit not absolute certainty in determining who is the possible bio attacker.

Applying this method, it is possible to state the following.

In the past, bio-warfare has been used sparingly, due to the fact that, once you use it to attack your foe, nobody knows whether, due to today's globalization and the generalized air travel between the continents, this unnatural virus may come back to its creator like a boomerang.

The COVID-19 outbreak is an unusual epidemic event (UEE), since this type of coronavirus was an unknown virus.[4]

This unusual epidemic emerged at the same time as the trade war between the United States of America and the People's Republic of China, making the COVID-19 epidemic suspicious.[5]

When the source of an epidemic is suspect, methods of differentiation between natural and intentional epidemics[6] must be used, so that the degree of

---

3 Chen et al., "Recalibration of the Grunow-Finke Assessment Tool to Improve Performance in Detecting Unnatural Epidemics: Recalibration of the Grunow-Finke Assessment Tool," *Risk Analysis* 39/7 (2018).

4 *Biopreparedness and Public Health: Exploring Synergies* (2013), p. 18: "Basically, any unexpected occurrence of one or more patients or deaths in humans or animals which might have been caused by an intentional release of pathogens may be the first clue of an unusual epidemic event (UEE). Also, the occurrence of a single case or death caused by an unknown or already eradicated disease or agent may be considered as unusual."

5 *Biopreparedness and Public Health: Exploring Synergies* (2013), p. 19: "If political, military, ethnic, religious or other motives can be identified, this would lend credence to the assumption that an attack using pathogens or toxins as biological agents has taken place."

6 Springer, *Defence Against Bioterrorism: Methods for Prevention and Control,* NATO Science for Peace and Security Series A: Chemistry and Biology (2018), p. 76: "Early detection of a bioterrorist attack is crucial in order to engage security and law enforcement forces timely, because differing from natural epidemics, breaking an epidemiological chain is not sufficient against bioterrorism. Evil human mind might be willing to start another epidemic and perpetrators have to be neutralized as soon as possible. There are four available epidemiological methods in literature for differentiation between a biological attack and other epidemics."

likelihood of it being a biological attack can be assessed. Rejecting as far-fetched (or impossible) or accepting such a possibility as probable (or certain) without first applying a method of differentiation is uncritical, unreasonable and scientifically unfounded, even if you are the most authoritative virologist or the most respected epidemiologist in the world.

Therefore, it is incorrect procedure to simply write off the possibility of a U.S. biological attack at the origin of the COVID-19 epidemic as a conspiracy theory: Such a consideration is the normal procedure followed by the scientific community in cases like this.

The first in-concluding criterion of the Grunow-Finke method is the existence of a biological risk.[7]

Biological risk is defined as the presence of a political context from which a biological attack could result.[8]

Biological risk arises if political actors (1) have access to biological weapons, (2) have the ability to spread them at the epicenter of the epidemic, and (3) are willing to use it.[9]

1. Both the United States and China have access to biological weapons. The United States was known, in 2007, to have 15 maximum-security laboratories (BSL-4) dedicated to the study of biological weapons; in China there is 1. It should be recognized that in this area, distinguishing between scientific research and military development is extremely difficult.

2. Both the United States and China have the ability to spread bioweapons at the epicenter of the epidemic. COVID-19 appears to be transmitted by droplets, so it is sufficient, for example, for a nebulizer such as that of the fish market to start an epidemic. If, on the other hand, it was also transmitted by aerosols, which is doubtful,[10] a diffuser would be sufficient (such as a household or machine perfumer). So, in any case, there is nothing that the United States or China cannot

---

7 R. Grunow and E.-J. Finke, "A procedure for differentiating between the intentional release of biological warfare agents and natural outbreaks of disease: its use in analyzing the tularemia outbreak in Kosovo in 1999 and 2000," *Clinical Microbiology and Infection* 8/8, August 1, 2002, https://www.clinicalmicrobiologyandinfection.com/article/S1198-743X(14)62640-9/fulltext.

8 *Ibid.*: "A biological risk is considered to be the presence of a political or terrorist environment from which a biological attack could originate."

9 *Ibid.*: "A biological risk arises, for example, if states, groups or individual persons have access to biological warfare agents and the necessary means of distributing them and are willing to use them."

10 Stephanie Soucheray, "Unmasked: Experts explain necessary respiratory protection for COVID-19," Center for Infectious Disease Research and Policy, February 13, 2020, https://www.cidrap.umn.edu/news-perspective/2020/02/unmasked-experts-explain-necessary-respiratory-protection-covid-19.

employ, virtually anywhere, starting, for example in Chinese territory, without arousing the slightest suspicion (it may even be that the person that might have been used to do this was completely unaware of what he was doing).

3. There is no substantive reason why the United States would not use bio-weapons. We can assume that the United States, as a rational entity, would be willing to use it if the option of a biological attack is the best rational choice from their point of view; for example, when it has a formidable *raison d'etre* (stop Chinese economic growth, therefore the emergence of China as a global superpower, to escape the "Thucydides' Trap," that is, a world war within a few years) and when they run virtually no risk of being discovered—as in this case.

Taking into account these three factors we have to assign 3 points out of 3 [very likely/certain] to the biological risk criterion; we could also assign 2 [likely], but nothing less.

The second in-concluding criterion of the Grunow-Finke method is the existence of a biological threat.

A biological threat is defined as the presence, in a context of biological risk, of political actors who openly threaten to resort to biological weapons or if specific interests are recognized in their use.[11]

The first aspect, that of an open threat, is unrealistic in relation to the United States. It cannot openly threaten to resort to "dirty" weapons, insofar as they are particularly unacceptable to world public opinion.

We can recognize there exists in the United States a very strong interest, a deep national security interest, in the use of biological weapons against China. China is in fact perceived by U.S. strategists as the greatest long-term threat to the priority national objective of the United States, the "American Way of Life."[12,13]

There is probably no greater threat to a country than being considered the main threat to what the United States of America, the world's leading power,

---

11 Grunow and Finke, *op. cit.*: "A biological threat is to be assumed if, in the environment of a biological risk, individual states, groups or persons openly threaten to use biological warfare agents or if a specific interest in their use can be assumed."

12 George McGinn, "China Poses Largest Long-Term Threat to U.S., DOD Policy Chief Says," *The Daily Defense News,* September 23, 2019, https://dailydefensenews. wordpress.com/2019/09/23/china-poses-largest-long-term-threat-to-u-s-dod-policy-chief-says/: "It is not an exaggeration to say China is the greatest long-term threat to the U.S. way of life, but China also poses the greatest challenge to the Defense Department, DOD's policy chief said."

13 *National Security Strategy of the United States of America,* The White House, December, 2017, https://www.whitehouse.gov/wp-content/uploads/2017/12/NSS-Final-12-18-2017-0905.pdf: "First, our fundamental responsibility is to protect the American people, the homeland, and the American way of life."

considers most sacred: it is an incomparably greater threat than even that posed by the most dangerous terrorist group.

So, we have to assign 3 points out of 3 [very likely/certain] to the biological threat criterion; we could also assign 2 [likely], but nothing less.

The first criterion has as a multiplier of gravity 2, the second 3: if we add the products of the two criteria, we get 15 points (10, if we want to be sure not to exaggerate).

Since the total points of the Grunow-Finke method are 54 we have already exceeded the threshold of improbability, that is reaching 15%, taking into account only the first two criteria, a level of confidence of 27.8% (or 18.5%, if we want to be sure not to overdo it).

Therefore, according to the Grunow-Finke method, that is the most widespread used in the scientific community, it is false to consider the possibility of the U.S. biological attack as far-fetched: it is at least doubtful.

Let's consider other sly tactics:

1. Where did the coronavirus infection start?
2. When did the infection start?
3. Who gave the order for the bio-attack?

Answers:

1. It started in Wuhan, the city that has the only Chinese maximum safety bio-laboratory and, in addition, is in the center of China. Why not accuse the Chinese Government of responsibility for a leakage from the bio-lab? This would also lead to a political destabilization of China, since in that country it is common to give responsibility for every good or bad occurrence to the emperor.

2. It started in the period of the greatest holiday of China: the Chinese New Year, when everybody travels to meet their relatives!

3. The President of the United States is the chief commander of the Armed Forces and the use of military force can only be authorized by him. But, to start such an attack, it is absolutely not necessary to use a soldier. Only one person is necessary and, if presumably those who had the idea of doing this are smart enough, it may be that even the one who physically put the bio agent to work was not suspecting what he was doing. According to this scenario, it is quite likely that the President of the United States didn't even know anything about this bio-attack. So, that leads to alternative and high probabilities that the deep state could be involved in this conspiracy and mass destruction arm.

The above tactics demonstrate a very high level of intelligence, including the ploy to try to shift responsibility for what happened to the enemy—a Chinese BSL-4 leakage. Therefore it seems very probable that these eventualities are not casual, but have been carefully studied and planned.

But then, there's this. An article in the *Wall Street Journal* headlined as follows in 2019:

"Bridgewater Makes $1.5 Billion Options Bet on Falling Market"
World's largest hedge fund takes on a big bearish trade.

The question is this: How could Bridgewater in November 2019 bet on the fact that stock markets around the world would have fallen by March 2020?

Isn't there a possibility that a private special interest party, say, Bridgewater, has been conspiring with somebody at any one of the numerous global BSL-4 laboratories to use a new virus they have bio-engineered? This is only a doubt and not a certainty, but, since $U.S. 1.5 Billion is a big amount of money and the spreading of a virus is very easy and inexpensive, once the virus has been prepared, why not start an investigation on this possibility?

We must remember the following: The U.S. Centers for Disease Control owns a patent on a particular strain of Ebola known as "EboBun." It's patent No. CA2741523A1 and it was awarded in 2010. Perhaps the research to obtain the patent was undertaken to prepare the vaccine and to have a better knowledge of the virus, or, with a negative way of thinking, to preempt other pharmaceutical companies from preparing and selling the vaccine, which might prove very profitable if an outbreak were to occur—or useful for biowarfare purposes.

But the question is this: if a virus can be so deeply known as to obtain a patent for it, it is clear that a similarly devastating virus can be produced by a dedicated laboratory, for which the patent, due to the present outbreak of the virus all over the world causing thousands of death, has not yet been requested.

Now, let's pass to the way the economy has been impacted by this "pandemic."

It is evident that the first way in which China is impacting the American Empire is through Chinese products' permeation of the global economy.

It is also evident that a similar pandemic spreading all over the world, bringing a halt to nearly every economic activity and causing the closure of companies, is reflected in the falling of the world stock market.

And when this happens, there are a lot of people starving or reduced to poverty, but there are a few others too that will gain a lot from it.

When the value of their stocks fall, the value of big and important companies, the ones that create the real wealth of the world, fall, enabling these companies to be acquired for peanuts by the owners of great capital.

As an example, the day after the March 11 statement by Christine La Garde, the new president of the European Central Bank, that the ECB was not there to reduce the losses of the European countries, on March 12, in full coronavirus onslaught, the Stock Exchange of Milano, Italy, lost 16,92%, a total of 84,27 Billions of Euro, the worst loss since its foundation in 1998.

But Milan was not alone. It was also the worst day in their recent history for European stock exchanges in general. Overwhelmed by sales based on the COVID-19 emergency developments, the stock exchange in London ended with a slide of 10.9%, and in Paris and Frankfurt, both ended with a drop of 12.2%.

So, what happened? Is it possible that Christine La Garde, previously president of the International Monetary Fund is incompetent and made her declaration without thinking of its effects?

Maybe, but might it also be that she made this declaration, knowing the likely effects perfectly well, with a view to facilitating the efforts of some "friends" seeking to procure some good companies for peanuts? Or to grease the game of Bridgewater, which was betting on the falling of the stock markets in March 2020?

Looking at each sector of the economy, none of them has increased. When considering just China: production of every type of goods, from heavy industry to electronics, to food and fashion has fallen.

The best way to stop China's fast-growing economy—if bombing and destroying its cities and plants is left to the future or only a recourse to be undertaken by stupid dictators—is a pandemic, stopping every activity, every travel, every social contact. This result has been perfectly obtained with COVID-19, much better than by the spread of previous viruses such as SARS and bird-flu. If the previous incidences were also bio attacks, it seems that with this last coronavirus, many improvements have been obtained by the servants of death.

This argument might be criticized by saying that COVID-19 is now spreading very quickly in the USA as well. But maybe it was not the U.S. government that spread the new virus—or somebody miscalculated. If you look at present situation, July 29, the confirmed cases in the USA are 4,390,500, with 150,000 total deaths, in Italy there are 246,776 cases with 32,658 victims, in China there are 4,658 deaths with over 87,108 infected.

COVID-19 is certainly a danger, from which we must defend ourselves with the necessary precautions, which medical science is putting in place. But it presents a much lower danger than an infinitely older and more potent virus: that we can incidentally call the "Finanz-virus."

The Finanz-virus bears primary responsibility for the destruction of the real economy, the destruction of labor, the destruction of human rights, the destruction of the environment, and, most seriously, the destruction of the human psyche, that is, the natural solidarity of peoples, the ones who are mentally healthy.

Today the world is dominated by a small number of psychopathic bankers, who have no regard for human life, and who are leading humanity to complete ruin.

Let's try to understand how this Finanz-virus is destroying the economy and therefore the base of civilization. By destroying the economy, it is possible to acquire the real wealth created by labor of whatever kind: land, buildings, companies manufacturing cars, ships, aircraft etc. Since these human activities will be stopped, they will no longer be capable of surviving, so the stockholders will be obliged to sell their ownership shares in these activities for peanuts. We must remember that the two main banks of the world are privately owned: the FED and the European Central Bank (ECB), and are the only ones allowed to print Dollars and Euros. Now we have to remember that, after the Nixon Order that stopped the convertibility of dollars into gold during the summer of 1971, money is now printed freely, without requiring its convertibility to gold, and is therefore called "fiat money" (where fiat is the Latin term meaning "let's make"). So, from that date, money has been printed by central banks that are owned not by their respective countries but by private bankers, for just the cost of printing the paper. We all think of money as an absolute indicator of wealth. But we must remember that the value of the money is relative and is only the one that we, with our mind and psychology, give to it. So, just by printing money as they like, these private bankers have come to own the world, not just its material wealth but its political institutions, since these are usually corrupted and purchased by them, using their formidable power of being the only owners and creators of money.

In Europe the situation is the same of the USA, maybe worse: or maybe the final list of shareholders of the ECB is the same as that of the FED...

The European Union is not the Union of European Peoples, it does not concern solidarity between the European peoples and workers. The European Union is the Union of Private Banks that exploits both peoples and workers, acting against the real economy made by labor, and against the health and well-being of people.

The European Union is a financial dictatorship that concentrates wealth in the hands of a small group of capitalists, taking it away from the workers who produce it. This fuels poverty and war between the poor peoples.

Capitalists, by owning the mass media, prevent people from seeing this very simple truth.

However, this biologic attack, that started to damage mainly China, is now damaging Italy, Europe and the USA. China, being a dictatorship, has been capable of stopping the circulation of its people in one day and the diffusion of COVID-19 has been stopped in one month. But people in Europe are ruled by democracies and one of the main rights is the one of freedom of movement within each state and within Europe. So, the new provision of the governments, stopping the free circulation of citizens, is illegal and against European constitutions. Everybody understands this, but what will be the impact on European economies? At present nobody knows how much the damage will be, but surely, they will suffer great damage, similar to that of a real war.

All of this may have been obtained by just spreading a laboratory-made virus, unknown by everybody and for which, it may be, vaccines have already been prepared and are available. Considering this last hypothesis, why were 20,000 U.S. Army soldiers to be sent to Europe to run a big war game named "Defender 2020"? Defender 2020 in Europe was set to be the largest mobilization of NATO troops against Russia in 25 years, according to Lt. Gen. Chris Cavoli, the U.S. Army Europe commander. But now, because of COVID-19, it has been cancelled.

Though now, because of COVID-19, Defender 2020 has been cancelled, the question remains: why should the USA defend Europe? Where is the threat? How can we consider Russia a threat: they have the largest land surface of the world (7 time zones), the lower density of population in the world and, after the Berlin Wall fell, western Europe took over many former Soviet Union countries: East Germany, Poland, Romania, Bulgaria, Estonia, Latvia, Ukraine.

The NATO countries are the main risk for Russia, surely much more than the risk that it is for Europe. In addition to this, if a WW3 will be fought, it will surely not be with tanks and ground armies, it will surely be the most devastating war fought with ICBMs (Inter Continental Ballistic Missiles) and atomic bombs. So again, here is the question: why 20,000 U.S. soldiers sent to Europe, in the midst of the COVID 19 crisis, without biologic protections, in the first place? They arrived in Europe, hugging their brothers in arms already present in Europe without any precautions like those that European citizens have now been trained to take.

Maybe that their commander is unaware, or had they been vaccinated?

But the game is not ending here. After the first shock of the stock market, China is recovering with new and smart ideas.

As more central banks around the world are cutting interest rates to zero or even entering negative territory to release liquidity into the market amid the coronavirus (COVID-19) pandemic, China's central bank is one step closer to issuing its official digital currency. It seems the People's Bank of China (PBC), in collaboration with private companies, has completed development of the sovereign digital currency's basic function and is now drafting relevant laws to pave the way for its circulation, industry insiders said.

Alipay, the financial arm of the Chinese tech firm, Alibaba, reportedly publicized five patents related to China's official digital currency from January 21 to March 17.[14] The patents cover several areas of digital currency, including issuance,

14 CBN Editor, "Alipay Helps Chinese Central Bank Complete Initial Development of Statutory Digital Currency," *China Banking News,* March 27, 2020, http://www.

transaction recording, digital wallets, anonymous trading support and assistance in supervising and dealing with illegal accounts, industry media reported.

Cryptocurrency is seen as the most convenient tool to translate a central bank's zero and negative interest rate policy to commercial banks.

China's central bank will accelerate the launch of its digital currency in the face of the unprecedented COVID-19 pandemic. The global virus outbreak has prompted central banks like the European Central Bank and the Bank of Japan to cut their benchmark interest rates to near zero or moved into negative territory.

So, after the first big alarm, the world is now learning that there are not only negative economic impacts that can be achieved with a voluntary bio attack, but many other unforeseen positive economic possibilities may result.

Here are just some examples.

Online services are satisfying changing consumer needs:

Challenges	Solutions
A new forced consumer "lifestyle" to use grocery delivery and mobile apps. The surging demands and limited logistic utilities challenges grocery supply sides.	Yonghui to package vegetables as combo product to sell instead of letting customers pick. 4Paradigm's machine learning services to automate combo configurations according to needs and inventory.
Rapidly transmission of coronavirus brings intense worries for citizens. The huge pressure of inquiry volume for hospitals and government.	JD's medical chatbot services can answer common questions of medication and symptoms. Integration of support centers with outpatient departments in hospitals.

JD and Meituan's delivery and zero-touch logistics services (JD's autonomous vehicles deliver medical and essential supplies to hospitals in Wuhan), leading to:

- Autonomous delivery vehicles
- Reduction in contagion risks in hospitals and epidemic areas
- Increased in-region delivery efficiency

Yitu's medical imaging system:

- Can analyze CT scans for pneumonia infection
- Automatically highlights special regions
- Automatically computes quantitative indexes to accelerate diagnoses processes for radiologists

chinabankingnews.com/2020/03/27/alipay-helps-chinese-central-bank-complete-initial-development-of-statutory-digital-currency/.

Cloud-based IoT (Internet of Things) solutions for manufacturing leads to:
- Remote operations for unmanned factories
- Mobile apps for workforce mobility
- Cloud platforms with AI, big data, IIoT and AR capabilities to automate business operations

SaaS offerings for education:
- TalkWeb collaborated with WeLink based on Huawei Cloud, extended its services to public schools
- JD Cloud & AI provided online classrooms for school and educational institutions

Blockchains build distributed trust within digital ecosystem:

DAQSoft
- Nationwide scenic hotel ecosystem Supply chain financing for hardware equipment manufacturers and hotels

Alipay
- Anti-epidemic materials information service platform
- Reviews the information on the demand, supply, and transportation of materials (food, medical, infrastructure...)

Hyperchain
- Charity donation platform to Improve transparency

Many other improvements have already been obtained due to the compulsory directives to "stay at home" in this very reduced period of time:
- Collaboration platforms transform workforce cooperation models for "social distancing"
- RPA tools improve productivity and experiences
- Dynamic sourcing and motivation strategy maintains employee productivity

It is essential to note how things changed in just two weeks. At the beginning of the COVID-19 outbreak, China was the observed patient and the rest of the world was the "observer." Now the situation is the opposite: the world's sick nations are the observed ones and China is the observer.

How will the world be after this? Nobody was expecting a change like this: no economist, no scientist, no politician. The world seemed to run every day as usual, but in just two months everything is changed. No more work, no travels, no restaurants, no gymnasium, no movie, no theater. Will the situation recover as before?

I don't think so. Remember after 9/11? Nothing came back to the previous way of living: the security controls in the airports and in the cities have been increased, the funding of the government agencies related to the control of terrorism have been increased and the costs to maintain our governments increased to a very high level.

How will society deal with this pandemic? Will we continue to look at each other as possible infectors? How can we feel secure against the spread of whichever new virus, as we become increasingly aware of the many possibilities for such an occurrence? Shall our governments ask for new taxes to implement organizations, new systems to take care of new diseases, and new laws and means of enforcement to ensure our compliance?

Every way is open but, surely, the world will not be the same as before.

CHAPTER ELEVEN

BIOWARFARE AS GENOCIDE: THE DEVELOPMENT OF ETHNIC-SPECIFIC VIRUSES

Cynthia McKinney

"The United States has renounced these weapons, as have all civilized countries, by joining the Biological Weapons Convention of 1972."

—President of the United States George W. Bush, 1990

INTRODUCTION

On January 30, 2020, a research paper, entitled "Uncanny similarity of unique inserts in the 2019-nCoV spike protein to HIV-1 gp120 and Gag,"[1] written about the new, heretofore unknown coronavirus then just erupting in China, set the internet abuzz. The paper, published on *biorxiv.org,* a peer-reviewed journal of the Cold Spring Harbor Laboratory that fashions itself as "the preprint server for biology" concluded:

First, we identified 4 unique inserts in the 2019-nCoV spike glycoprotein that are not present in any other coronavirus reported till date. To our surprise, all the 4 inserts in the 2019-nCoV mapped to short segments of amino acids in the HIV-1 gp120 and Gag among all annotated virus proteins in the NCBI database. This uncanny similarity of novel inserts in the 2019- nCoV spike protein to HIV-1 gp120 and Gag is unlikely to be fortuitous.... Taken together, our findings suggest unconventional evolution of 2019-nCoV that warrants further investigation. Our work highlights novel evolutionary aspects of the

---

1 Prashant Pradhan et al., "Uncanny similarity of unique inserts in the 2019-nCoV spike protein to HIV-1 gp120 and Gag," *bioRxiv,* January 30, 2020 (accessed March 27, 2020), https://www.biorxiv.org/content/10.1101/2020.01.30.927871v1.full.pdf.

EXECUTIVE OFFICE OF THE PRESIDENT
OFFICE OF SCIENCE AND TECHNOLOGY POLICY
WASHINGTON, D.C. 20502

February 3, 2020

Dr. Marcia McNutt
President, National Academy of Sciences
2101 Constitution Ave, N.W.
Washington, D.C., U.S. 20418

SUBJECT: Rapid Response Assessment of 2019-nCoV Data Needs

In support of the Office of Science and Technology's (OSTP) National Science and Technology Committee (NSTC) rapid research response work for the 2019-nCoV response, and the Administration's efforts to characterize and provide evidence-based assessments for outbreak response efforts, I am writing to ask the National Academies of Sciences, Engineering, and Medicine (NASEM) to rapidly examine information and identify data requirements that would help determine the origins of 2019-nCoV, specifically from an evolutionary/structural biology standpoint. I also ask NASEM to consider whether this should include more temporally and geographically diverse clinical isolates, sequences, etc.

Although a widely-disputed paper, "Uncanny similarity of unique inserts in the 2019-nCoV spike protein to HIV-1 gp120 and Hag," posted on the pre-print server bioRxiv last week has been withdrawn, the response to that manuscript highlights the need to determine information and data requirements as quickly as possible to better perform and validate such analyses of origin. These questions are important not only for this current situation, but to inform future outbreak preparation and better understand animal/human and environmental transmission aspects of coronaviruses. As part of a broader deliberative process, this review will aid preparedness for future events by establishing a process that quickly assembles subject matter experts for evaluating other potentially threatening organisms.

OSTP requests NASEM convene a meeting of experts, particularly world class geneticists, coronavirus experts, and evolutionary biologists, to assess what data, information, and samples are needed to address the unknowns, in order to understand the evolutionary origins of 2019-nCoV and more effectively respond to both the outbreak and any resulting misinformation. I request a letter statement from the National Academies be prepared and provided in response to this solicitation. A more in-depth examination of the issues will be established as a follow up as needed.

Sincerely,

Kelvin K. Droegemeier
Director

[*screenshot*]

2019-nCoV and has implications on the pathogenesis and diagnosis of this virus."[2]

---

2 Ibid.

The paper drew from an article written by Chinese scientists published earlier on the same biorxiv.org website. That paper, entitled "Discovery of a novel coronavirus associated with the recent pneumonia outbreak in humans and its potential bat origin,"[3] had three important findings: 1) that the new virus was somewhat (79.5%) similar to SARS-CoV; 2) that the new virus was 96% similar to bat coronaviruses; and 3) that the new coronavirus "uses the same cell entry receptor, ACE2, as SARS-CoV." However, it also noted the presence of "three short *insertions.*"[4]

Thus began the rife speculation that the new coronavirus might actually be a bioweapon let loose among the general population, even prompting President Trump to instruct the National Academy of Sciences, Engineering, and Medicine (NASEM) to create a team to determine the origin of the new coronavirus, now officially known as SARS-CoV-2. Soon, China and the United States were locked in a war of words (and tweets) over the origin of SARS-CoV-2, with China accusing the U.S. of bringing the new coronavirus to China with its 300+ soldier delegation that traveled to Wuhan for the World Military Games held in 2019 in October.[5]

Iran's Supreme Leader Imam Khamenei soon tweeted that the new disease might be a "#BiologicalAttack." President Trump slapped back that the world knew where the new disease (COVID-19) started and characterized the new virus as the "Chinese Virus." With the jury still out on whether the release of SARS-CoV-2 was accidental or intentional, whether it is a biological weapon or not, whether its evolution is wholly natural or accompanied by a laboratory intervention, the questions have now been publicly raised at the highest political levels and this compels us to take a look at the historical use of biowarfare as a form of "Hybrid Warfare" in which genocide becomes "a politically useful tool." In this chapter, I will now discuss Hybrid Warfare, Biowarfare, and Genocide.

---

3 Peng Zhou, et al., "Discovery of a novel coronavirus associated with the recent pneumonia outbreak in humans and its potential bat origin," *bioRxiv,* January 22, 2020 (accessed March 27, 2020), https://www.biorxiv.org/content/10.1101/2020.01.22.914952v1.full. Please be sure to refer to Version One of this article.

4 Ibid. Emphasis added.

5 Read about U.S. participation in the World Military Games at https://www.defense.gov/Explore/Spotlight/CISM-Military-World-Games/ (accessed March 27, 2020).

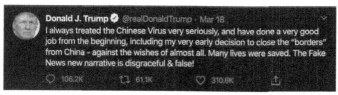

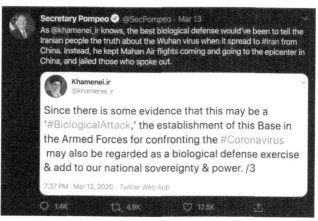

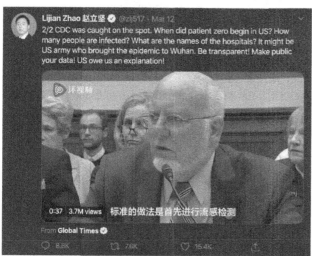

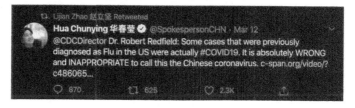

[*screenshots*]

*"To win one hundred victories in one hundred battles is not the acme of
skill. To subdue the enemy without fighting is the acme of skill."*

—Sun Tzu, *The Art of War*

HYBRID WARFARE

Sun Tzu wrote his time-tested volume over 2,500 years ago. And, while many
consider "Hybrid Warfare" to be a new phenomenon, actually, it is as old as is
war, itself—as the quote above attests. Because "Hybrid Warfare" is a form of
warfare, it involves the process of marshaling all available resources, including
psychological, in order to achieve certain political objectives short of the use
of "hot" tactics, that is, short of war using conventional or nuclear weapons.
Everything short of that *could* be considered hybrid warfare. The North Atlantic
Treaty Organization, NATO, considers Hybrid Warfare to be that part of an ac-
tor's military strategy that includes "propaganda, deception, sabotage, and other
non-military tactics."[6] In 1947, the United States embarked upon a strategy of
"Containment" of Communist expansionism and "Rollback" of governments that
refused to adhere to the Washington Consensus of that time. The geo-strategic
goal of these twin strategies was to make the world safe for U.S. hegemony.
When Containment and Rollback were to be achieved without resort to military
aggression or conflict, then hybrid warfare tactics were used. Hybrid warfare can
also be seen as a strategy that softens the target and makes it easier to defeat in a
direct military conflict: as in a strategy of tension. Of course, the target state or
government or set of non-state actors could be defeated as a result of such tactics
before the onset of hostilities, thus achieving Sun Tzu's maxim of winning the war
before a [hot] battle has been waged. U.S. prosecution of the Cold War against
the Soviet Union is an example of Hybrid Warfare. NATO's *Operation Gladio*[7]
was a Cold War era tactic of irregular war, fought against European socialists and
communists, whose political objective was to keep Western Europe, especially

---

6 North Atlantic Treaty Organization, "NATO's response to hybrid threats," https://
www.nato.int/cps/en/natohq/topics_156338.htm (accessed March 28, 2020).

7 *Operation Gladio* was a secret network, created by the Central Intelligence Agency
(CIA), of armed paramilitary forces in all NATO countries of 1959 whose stated purpose
was to protect Western Europe in the event of an invasion by the Soviet Union, but whose
real purpose was to keep a lid on Europe's politics and pro-socialist intellectuals. The
Operation escalated to bombings and kidnappings and resulted in the 1978 murder of
Italy's Prime Minister, Aldo Moro. The network was finally dismantled just prior to the
1990s.

Greece and Italy, two countries where socialism and communism had strong popular bases, within the U.S. orbit. *Operation Gladio* denied self-determination to the people of Western Europe.

As *Operation Gladio* shows us, contenders in Hybrid Warfare can be states or non-state actors while non-state actors can be proxies for states. And as technologies change and the world becomes more connected, the nature of hybrid wars will also change. As NATO notes, the "speed, scale, and intensity" of hybrid engagements is "facilitated by rapid technological change and global interconnectivity."[8]

Hybrid Warfare today includes "irregular tactics and formations, terrorist acts including indiscriminate violence and coercion, and criminal disorder."[9] Thus, NATO expanded its definition of Hybrid Warfare to include "a broad, complex and adaptive and often highly integrated combination of conventional and unconventional means, overt and covert activities, by military, paramilitary, irregular, and civilian actors, which are targeted to achieve (geo)political and strategic objectives."[10] Hybrid Warfare thus includes the use of insects (Entomological Warfare), chemicals (Chemical Warfare), Artificial Intelligence and Robotics (Electronic Warfare), the internet (Cyber Warfare), and more.[11] Regime Change can also be carried out with the use of Hybrid Warfare.[12]

One tactic of both regular and irregular warfare is "Germ Warfare," the use of biological toxins as part of a military effort to achieve strategic or political goals. Since the 20th century, what is now known as Biological Warfare, or Biowarfare—the strategic use of biological toxins to achieve political objectives—has become commonplace and with the enhanced sophistication of recent scientific discoveries, has been increasingly used *instead* of conventional war rather than as its mere complement.

---

8 "NATO's Response" op. cit.

9 Chiyuki Aoi, et al., "Introduction 'hybrid warfare in Asia: its meaning and shape,'" *The Pacific Review,* 31:6 (2018) accessed March 28, 2020, https://www.tandfonline.com/doi/full/10.1080/09512748.2018.1513548?src=recsys.

10 Ibid.

11 Please see Joan Nairuba, "modern means of warfare and the humanitarian issues involved," accessed March 28, 2020, https://www.academia.edu/7439736/modern_means_of_warfare_and_the_humanitarian_issues_involved.

12 For a deeper discussion of hybrid warfare inside the U.S., please see: Cynthia McKinney, "The 'Purple Revolution:' U.S. Hybrid Warfare Coming Home To Roost?" https://www.academia.edu/37864137/The_Purple_Revolution_U.S._Hybrid_Warfare_Coming_Home_To_Roost; and Cynthia McKinney, "Ruminations At the Margins: Brett Kavanaugh Confirmation Fight—Deep State Factions On Display?" https://www.academia.edu/37834159/_Ruminations_At_the_Margins_Brett_Kavanaugh_Confirmation_Fight_Deep_State_Factions_On_Display (both articles accessed March 28, 2020).

Table 1*	
Examples of biological and chemical warfare use during the past 2000 years	
600 BC	Solon uses the purgative herb hellebore during the siege of Krissa.
1155	Emperor Barbarossa poisons water wells with human bodies in Tortona, Italy.
1346	Tarar forces catapult bodies of plague victims over the city walls of Caffa, Crimean Peninsula (now Feodosia, Ukraine).
1495	Spanish mix wine with blood of leprosy patients to sell to their French foes in Naples, Italy.
1675	German and French forces agree to not use "poisones bullets."
1710	Russian troops catapult human bodies of plague victims into Swedish cities.
1763	British distribute blankets from smallpox patients to Native Americans.
1797	Napoleon floods the plains around Mantua, Italy, to enhace the spread of malaria.
1863	Confederates sell clothing from yellow fever and smallpox patients to Union troops during the U.S. Civil War.
World War I	German and French agents use glanders and anthrax.
World War II	Japan uses plague, antrax, and other diseases; several other countries experiment with and develop biological weapons programs.
1980–1988	Iraq uses mustard gas, sarin, and tabun against Iran and ethnic groups inside Iraq during the Persian Gulf War.
1995	Aum Shinrikyo uses sarin gas in the Tokyo subway system.
*Source: Stefan Riedel, Ph.D., M.D., "Biological warfare and bioterrorism: a historical review," Baylor University Medical Center Proceedings (October 2004), https://www.ncbi.nlm.nih.gov/pmc/articles/PMC1200679/ (accessed April 5, 2020).	

"When dumped into a water supply, one gram, one gram of typhoid culture has an impact roughly equivalent to 100 grams of the "V" chemical nerve agent, or almost 40 pounds of potassium cyanide. The point is that a minute tiny amount of biological toxins can have the same lethal effect of a larger amount of a chemical weapon."

—U.S. Senator David Pryor, 1990

BIOWARFARE

While we might think of biological warfare, or Biowarfare, as something completely modern and new, the fact is that Biowarfare is as old a phenomenon as is war. Ancient Africans in what is now Nigeria used bees in battle while ancient Iraqis used scorpions against their enemies, according to Jeffrey Lockwood.[13] Britain used biological agents against China in its Opium Wars in order to colonize and further steal resources from China. "In the 19th century, the British used blankets infected with smallpox in an attempt to wipe out whole tribes of North American Indians."[14] And in the 20th Century, the infamous Japanese General Shiro Ishii's Unit 731 "produced hundreds of millions of infected insects and dispersed them across China."[15] General Ishii's work caught the attention of the U.S. military which, after World War II, helped to cover up Japanese crimes and shielded Unit 731 scientists from prosecution.[16] Of this shameful episode in U.S. history—not its first and certainly not its last—Jeffrey Kaye writes: "The original promise of amnesty [for General Shiro Ishii and the scientists of Unit 731] for information was made after a discussion some months after the end of World War II between Ft. Detrick's Colonel Murray Sanders and General Douglas MacArthur."[17] This amnesty came despite the U.S. learning that even U.S. soldiers

---

13 Jeffrey A. Lockwood, *Six-Legged Soldiers: Using Insects as Weapons of War* (Oxford University Press, 2008), https://play.google.com/store/books/details?id=FN_QCwAAQBAJ&rdid=book-FN_QCwAAQBAJ&rdot=1&source=gbs_vpt_read&pcampaignid=books_booksearch_viewport (accessed March 28, 2020).

14 Lockwood, "Entomological Warfare: History of the Use of Insects as Weapons of War," *Bulletin of the Entomological Society of America*, 33, 2 (Summer 1987), https://academic.oup.com/ae/article-abstract/33/2/76/2841930 (accessed March 28, 2020).

15 Lockwood, *Six-Legged Soldiers*, op. cit.

16 Please see DoJ Letters explaining U.S. government treatment of Unit 731 scientists, shielding them from war crimes prosecution, and saving their research for itself.

17 Jeffrey Kaye, "Department of Justice Official Releases Letter Admitting U.S. Amnesty of Japan's Unit 731 War Criminals," *Medium*, May 2017 (accessed March 28,

that had been captured by the Japanese as Prisoners of War (POWs) in Manchuria had been experimented upon by the scientists in Unit 731. One Fort Detrick scientist wrote, "Such information could not be obtained in our own laboratories because of scruples attached to human experimentation."[18] Further, it was later learned that the U.S. government made payments in the form of "money, food, gifts, entertainment, and other kinds of rewards to the former Unit 731 members" in exchange for their data.[19] It is believed by historians that some 3,000 people died in the Japanese experiments carried out in China by Unit 731.[20]

Table 2*		
Biological warfare programs during World War II		
Nation	Numbers of workers (estimated)	Focus
Germany	100-200	Offense research forbidden
Canada	small	Animal and crop diseases, rinderpest, anthrax
United Kingdom	40-50	Animal and crop diseases, anthrax, foot and mouth disease
Japan	several thousand	Extensive; official information suppressed by a treaty with USA in which all charges for war crimes were dropped for exchange of information from experiments
Soviet Union	several thousand	Typhus, plague
*Source: Stefan Riedel, op. cit.		

The United States used biowarfare against China and North Korea during the Korean War and learned from its British brothers how to use drugs and the drug trade to further geopolitical goals. Journalist Gary Webb's exposé on the CIA's role in drug trafficking in general and in the creation of crack cocaine in particular

---

2020),   https://medium.com/@jeff_kaye/department-of-justice-official-releases-letter-admitting-u-s-amnesty-of-unit-731-war-criminals-9b7da41d8982.

18 Ibid.

19 "U.S. paid Unit 731 members for data," *Japan Times,* August 15, 2005 (accessed March 28, 2020), https://www.japantimes.co.jp/news/2005/08/15/national/u-s-paid-unit-731-members-for-data/#.Xn-sjtb450I.

20 Whatever scruples the U.S. government officials might have had about human experimentation must have been race specific, because at the same time as the U.S. was paying and rewarding Japanese scientists for their human experimentation on Chinese subjects, the Tuskegee Study was ongoing, being carried out by the U.S. Centers for Disease Control (CDC) and its precursor on Black U.S. citizens.

is an extremely painful read on many levels—from the lost generation of mostly Black crack addicts who victimized themselves and their families because of their addiction, to the mysterious death of Gary Webb, himself, who reportedly committed suicide with two shots to the head.[21] Sadly, Webb would not be the first or the last journalist who died mysteriously after exposing or while on the hunt to expose the sordid history of the U.S. government and its deadly trade in drugs. In short, whatever scruples the U.S. might have had regarding human suffering, nothing stopped the U.S. from making lethal drugs available to populations, including its own and using and testing biological weapons abroad and on its own citizens—of every race and color. Here is just a brief listing of some of the testing or use incidents carried out by the U.S. government on its own citizens:

- Ticks, Lyme Disease;
- Bacteria, Pentagon Air Conditioning System;
- Bacteria, Spraying Along the California Coast;
- Fungal Spores, Released Among Black Dock Workers;
- Zinc Cadmium Sulphide, Released Over St. Louis and Minneapolis To See Effect on Terrain;
- Operation Big Itch, To See If Fleas Could be Loaded Into Bombs;
- Bacteria, New York Subway.[22]

In 2008, the U.S. General Accounting Office published a study that found that these tests exposed thousands of U.S. military personnel and tens of thousands of U.S. civilians to U.S. bioweapons.[23] The Church Committee Reports and other documents pertaining to the assassination of President Kennedy show that individuals inside the U.S. government wanted to (and likely did) use biological weapons against Fidel Castro's Cuba to destroy the Revolution. (We also know that the United States wanted the ultimate in biological weapons to be used to

---

21 For more information on the involvement of the U.S. government in international drug trafficking, see the works of Dr. Peter Dale Scott at https://www.peterdalescott.net/q/ (accessed March 29, 2020).

22 Michelle Bentley, "The US has a history of testing biological weapons on the public—were infected ticks used too?" *The Conversation,* July 22, 2019, https://theconversation.com/the-us-has-a-history-of-testing-biological-weapons-on-the-public-were-infected-ticks-used-too-120638.

23 United States Government Accountability Office, "CHEMICAL AND BIOLOGICAL DEFENSE: DOD and VA Need to Improve Efforts to Identify and Notify Individuals Potentially Exposed during Chemical and Biological Tests," https://www.gao.gov/products/GAO-08-366 (accessed March 29, 2020).

kill Fidel Castro.[24]) Recently declassified documents expose the lengths that
the governors of policy in the U.S. were willing to go in order to achieve their
political objectives.

> The U.S. military tried to enter the covert action domain, too, against
> Castro during the early years of the Johnson Administration. In response
> to a Presidential request for new ideas on how to deal with the Cuban
> leader, the Pentagon proposed 'Operation SQUARE DANCE:' the
> destruction of the Cuban economy by dropping from the cargo hatches
> of aircraft late at night a parasite known as Bunga that would attack the
> island's sugar cane plants. 'The economic and political disturbances
> caused by this attack could be exacerbated and exploited,' claimed a
> DoD memo, 'by such measures as spreading hoof-and-mouth disease
> among draft animals, controlling rainfall by cloud seeding, mining
> cane fields,, burning cane, and directing other acts of conventional
> sabotage against the cane milling and transportation system.' The
> hoped-for end result, concluded the memo, would be 'the collapse
> of the Castro regime.' The military planners conceded that adoption
> of SQUARE DANCE 'would introduce a new dimension into Cold
> War methods and would require a major change in national policy.'
> But they were ready to carry out these measures anyway, if the White
> House so desired. . . . The DoD memo provides startling insight into
> America's capacity and, evidently at some levels of government, its
> willingness to engage in radical covert economic operations in order
> to achieve U.S. foreign policy goals.[25]

The Church Committee also uncovered the fact that toxic agents had been
illegally stored at Fort Detrick despite an order from President Nixon to destroy
them. "These toxins, stored at the Army's Fort Detrick in Maryland, included

---

24 Read the fascinating, but unfortunately true, account of the many ways in
which poisons were prepared by the U.S. government and its cooperation with crime
world figures to ensure the assassination of Fidel Castro in the official papers of the
COINTELPRO investigation led by Senator Frank Church: *The Senate Select Committee
to Study Governmental Operations with Respect to Intelligence Activities Interim Report
on Cuba* (accessed March 29, 2020), https://history-matters.com/archive/church/reports/ir/
pdf/ChurchIR_3B_Cuba.pdf.

25 Loch K. Johnson, *National Security Intelligence: Secret Operations in Defense
of the Democracies,* Second Edition (Cambridge: Polity Press, 2017), https://books.
google.com/books?id=GkO9DgAAQBAJ&printsec=frontcover&source=gbs_ge_
summary_r&cad=0#v=onepage&q=dance&f=false (accessed March 29, 2020).

anthrax and tuberculosis bacteria, the encephalitis virus, salmonella, shellfish toxin, the smallpox virus, and various other poisons and biological warfare agents."[26] Page 192 of this Report has a partial listing of the illegal toxins found to still be in U.S. government possession at both the CIA Headquarters and at Fort Detrick (see Appendix). In 2015, two Cuban scientists won the Grand Award in Cuba's annual Public Health Contest by tracing an unprecedented 1981 outbreak of dengue hemorrhagic fever in the Americas to a deliberate release by the United States. Modern automatic sequencing technology allowed the Cuban scientists to trace the source from samples that had been saved for more than thirty years in a refrigerator.[27]

In at least one instance the United States government admitted that its bio-weapon technology was turned against its own elected leaders: the 2001 anthrax attacks.

U.S. BIOWARFARE ATTACKS ON AMERICANS

Anthrax is a naturally-occurring substance that was clinically first described in the 1700s. By the early 1900s, anthrax was pretty well known in the U.S. and in Europe, but remained relatively unknown in Asia and Africa. However, in World War I, anthrax is acknowledged to have first been used as a weapon by the Germans. In World War II, Japan is acknowledged to have used anthrax as a weapon in China. During World War II, the United States greatly expanded its bioweapons program and even went so far as to fill more than 5,000 bombs with anthrax for use against Germany.[28] We now know that the U.S. has used biological or 30 chemical weapons against "Philippines, Puerto Rico, Vietnam, China, North Korea, Vietnam, Laos, Cambodia, Cuba, Haitian boat people, and Canada."[29] What is less known is that the U.S. actually used deadly anthrax against itself. Or rather, that some actors inside the U.S. military-industrial complex used a deadly strain of anthrax against U.S. elected officials and the media.

---

26 The Senate Select Committee to Study Governmental Operations with Respect to Intelligence Activities, Volume One, *Unauthorized Storage of Toxic Agents* (accessed March 29, 2020), https://www.aarclibrary.org/publib/contents/church/contents_church_ reports_vol1.htm.

27 "Study Confirms that US Introduced Dengue Fever in Cuba in 1981," *Cubadebate,* February 1, 2016 (accessed March 29, 2020), http://en.cubadebate.cu/news/2016/02/01/ study-confirms-that-us-introduced-dengue-fever-cuba-1981/.

28 Centers for Disease Control and Prevention, "The History of Anthrax," accessed March 29, 2020, https://www.cdc.gov/anthrax/resources/history/index.html.

29 Jeffrey St. Clair, "Germ War: the US Record," *Counterpunch,* September 3, 2013 (accessed March 30, 2020), https://www.counterpunch.org/2013/09/03/germ-war-the-us-record-2/.

Graeme MacQueen, the scholar who wrote what is widely acknowledged to be the definitive book on the anthrax attacks in the United States that were a part of the September 11, 2001 attack, wrote in a personal note to me specifically for this chapter:

> How many people know that in 2001 Congress was attacked with a weapon of mass destruction? Two countries were framed for this biological attack, Afghanistan (giving refuge to al-Qaeda) and Iraq. But neither country had anything to do with the attacks, as is now admitted by U.S. authorities. The perpetrators, still on the loose, came from within the U.S. military-industrial complex.
>
> The anthrax letter attacks of 2001 began in September, shortly after the events of 9/11. Victims of the disease were identified between October 3 and November 20. At least 22 people are thought to have become infected, 11 with cutaneous anthrax and 11 with inhalation anthrax. Five people died.
>
> As October, 2001 progressed, the view promoted was that the anthrax attacks were carried out by al-Qaeda, which supplied the foot soldiers, and Iraq, which supplied the anthrax spores. But this story held together only until the Patriot Act was passed, after which it fell apart quickly. Scientists who studied the anthrax spores concluded that the spores came from one of three highly secure facilities in the U.S. that serve the Pentagon and the CIA. The insiders who committed this crime were highly placed in the executive branch of the U.S. government and were linked to, or identical with, the perpetrators of the 9/11 attacks. There are numerous specific, corroborated connections between the 9/11 'hijackers' and the anthrax perpetrators.

At the time, former United Nations Weapons Inspector for Iraq (from 1991 to 1998), Scott Ritter, found that the cost of producing a powdered form of anthrax was too expensive and too complicated to be used as a weapon. Moreover, the "military grade" anthrax that had been sent in the mail to Congressional and media offices required large centrifuges and intensive heat for repeated washings and dryings. Scott Ritter said, "Terrorists do not have the facilities to weaponize anthrax, so if you have military grade anthrax being used, this would be the first solid evidence of state sponsorship."[30]

---

30 UCLA Department of Epidemiology School of Public Health, "Using Anthrax As A Weapon," *BBC News,* October 17, 2001 (accessed March 30, 2020), https://www.ph.ucla.edu/epi/bioter/anthraxasweapon.html.

With the cat out of the bag on the variety and strength of the anthrax used in the attacks, the hunt proceeded to find the culprit who would have had access to this weaponized version of the bacterium. Focus then turned to U.S. government scientists at the United States Army Medical Research Institute of Infectious Diseases (USAMRIID) at Fort Detrick just outside of Washington, D.C. in Maryland. Steven Hatfill, a Fort Detrick scientist, was named as a person of interest by the Department of Justice, but he fought back and sued the government for libel, winning almost $6 million in a settlement. However, when another scientist suspect who was never charged, Bruce Ivins, committed suicide, enabling the government to conclude its investigations and name Ivins as the culprit. However, as Barbara Honegger, a former senior Pentagon journalist, writes, "By insisting that Bruce Ivins, a biodefense scientist then with the Army's Fort Detrick laboratory, was behind the anthrax attacks, the Bush-Cheney Administration has officially acknowledged that those attacks were perpetrated by a U.S. Government insider—and not by bin Laden or by Iraq."[31]

Readers are encouraged to go directly to the MacQueen book, *The 2001 Anthrax Deception: The Case for a Domestic Conspiracy*[32]—that reads like a mystery thriller novel, but, unfortunately, is actually the reality show—of how a U.S. biowarfare laboratory was the source of the deadly anthrax attack on members of the U.S. Congress in 2001.

Unfortunately, those who create bioweapons cannot always control them. Sometimes there are accidental, but deadly, leaks from the facilities that create them and at other times there is deliberate use of these products for terrorism, as weapons intended to threaten or kill.

Mysteriously, in August 2019, Fort Detrick failed a Centers for Disease Control and Prevention (CDC) inspection and was shut down for two containment leaks. While not exposing exactly what the substances were that leaked from USAMRIID, documents reveal that among other failures, USAMRIID did not even keep an up-to-date log on hand of all of its toxins; the CDC also found that USAMRIID failed to "'implement and maintain containment procedures sufficient to contain select agents or toxins' that were made by operations in biosafety level 3 and 4 laboratories…. Biosafety level 3 and 4 are the highest levels of containment, requiring special protective equipment, air flow and standard

---

31 Barbara Honegger with Barry Kissin, "'Scarlet A:' Anthrax Links to The Day of 9/11 Itself," unpublished paper, September 25, 2008. Another version of the paper was published by Barbara Honegger alone, accessed March 29, 2020 at https://www.opednews.com/populum/page.php?f=Anthrax-Links-to-9-11-by-Barbara-Honegger-080925-678.html.

32 Graeme MacQueen, *The 2001 Anthrax Deception: The Case for a Domestic Conspiracy* (Atlanta: Clarity Press, 2014).

operating procedures."[33] These uncontrolled leaks constitute unintentional dangers—but dangers nonetheless—to the surrounding communities, and quite possibly to communities around the world. Today, Fort Detrick has quietly reopened and is back at work "manufacturing strains of the virus as it gears up to test a slate of potential vaccines"[34] for the coronavirus SARS-CoV-2 outbreak that has caused a pandemic of the COVID-19 disease. On March 30, 2020, Yahoo News broke the story that an unclassified FBI report revealed that a Chinese biologist who had traveled to the U.S. with vials of what was labeled "Antibodies" in his luggage, but when stopped by the U.S. Customs and Border Patrol Agency (CBP), at Detroit Metro Airport, was feared to be viable Severe Acute Respiratory Syndrome (SARS) and Middle East Respiratory Syndrome (MERS) samples. The biologist said that he was bringing samples "to a researcher at a U.S. institute."[35]

On the other end of the spectrum from the accidental breaches that caused the shutdown of Fort Detrick—or security risks in transporting dangerous materials as discovered by the CBP at Detroit Metro Airport—are acts of terrorism that are intentional, like the Anthrax attacks and another sordid episode in U.S. history that could have resulted in global repercussions: Operation Northwoods. Operation Northwoods demonstrated that some individuals at the highest levels of the U.S. government were willing to inflict terrorist acts on the American people in order to promote a policy change intended to lead to war on Cuba. In fact, the U.S. Joint Chiefs of Staff itself approved a plan to hijack planes, blow up ships, and cause a wave of terror to be blamed on Castro's Cuba. The Pentagon writes, "Casualty lists in U.S. newspapers would cause a helpful wave of national indignation." The hoped-for policy result was summed up in the name of the memorandum from the Chairman of the Joint Chiefs of Staff to the Secretary of Defense at the time, Robert McNamara: "Justification for U.S. Military Intervention in Cuba."[36] It was

33 Heather Mongilio, "CDC Inspection Findings Reveal More about Fort Detrick Research Suspension," *The Frederick News-Post,* Maryland, November 24, 2019 (accessed March 30, 2020), https://www.military.com/daily-news/2019/11/24/cdc-inspection-findings-reveal-more-about-fort-detrick-research-suspension.html.

34 Nancy Youssef, "A Onetime Germ-Warfare Site Is Army's Front Line in Coronavirus Battle," The Wall Street Journal, March 22, 2020 (accessed March 30, 2020), https://www.wsj.com/articles/a-onetime-germ-warfare-site-is-armys-front-line-in-coronavirus-battle-11584886591.

35 Sharon Weinberger, Jana Winter, and Martin de Bourmont, "Suspected SARS virus and flu samples found in luggage: FBI report describes China's 'biosecurity risk'" *Yahoo News,* March 30, 2020 (accessed March 30, 2020) located at https://news.yahoo.com/suspected-sars-virus-and-flu-found-in-luggage-fbi-report-describes-chinas-biosecurity-risk-144526820.html.

36 Memorandum for the Secretary of Defense: Justification for US Military Intervention in Cuba, March 13, 1962 (accessed March 30, 2020), https://nsarchive2.gwu.edu/news/20010430/northwoods.pdf.

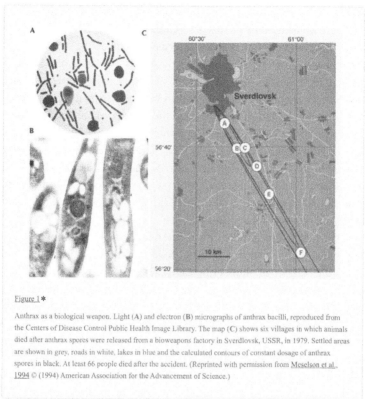

Figure 1 *

Anthrax as a biological weapon. Light (**A**) and electron (**B**) micrographs of anthrax bacilli, reproduced from the Centers of Disease Control Public Health Image Library. The map (**C**) shows six villages in which animals died after anthrax spores were released from a bioweapons factory in Sverdlovsk, USSR, in 1979. Settled areas are shown in grey, roads in white, lakes in blue and the calculated contours of constant dosage of anthrax spores in black. At least 66 people died after the accident. (Reprinted with permission from Meselson et al., 1994 © (1994) American Association for the Advancement of Science.)

* Figure 1 is a screenshot fromn Friedrich Frischknecht, "The History of Biological Warfare," *EMBO Reports,* June 2003 (accessed April 5, 2020), https://www.ncbi.nlm.nih.gov/pmc/articles/PMC1326439/.

only the moral convictions of President John F. Kennedy that led to his denial of the Pentagon's request and prevented it from undertaking the actions described in Operation Northwoods.

U.S. Biowarfare Attack on a Head of State

"The virus is in the safe." The President of the United States wanted the Head of Government representing the newly-independent state of Congo dead. Charismatic and articulate, Patrice Lumumba, the democratically elected leader of Congo was a thorn in the side of colonial powers. Lumumba advocated independence, freedom, sovereignty, and dignity: all the things that colonial masters had denied Africans on the Continent and their progeny around the world. Lumumba was inspiring other Africans to throw off their colonial yokes and with them, the capitalist ties that had brought slavery and colonialism to the Continent.

Lumumba's ideas, combined with his personal magic, threatened the global order that included colonization of Asians and Africans by U.S. allies. It was a bipolar world then, and former colonies had a choice of friends in the international arena between the United States and their former colonial masters or the Soviet Union that was helping countries attain independence from those masters. Congo was too wealthy and Lumumba was too smart to be "lost" from the U.S. orbit. Thus, President Eisenhower, himself, authorized the murder of Lumumba. The Office of the Historian of the United States Department of State writes, quoting a memo of and the recollection of participants in a National Security Council meeting held on August 18, 1960, "Eisenhower turning to CIA Director Allen Dulles 'in the full hearing of all those in attendance and saying something to the effect that Lumumba should be eliminated.' After that there was a stunned silence for about 15 seconds and the meeting continued."[37]

On August 26, 1960, head of the Central Intelligence Agency (CIA) sent a cable to the Leopoldville (now Kinshasa) Station Office authorizing $100,000 to be spent for the purpose of eliminating Lumumba. The memo read, "To the extent that the Ambassador may want to be consulted, you should seek his concurrence. If in any particular case, he does not wish to be consulted, you can act on your own authority where time does not permit referral here."[38] When Lumumba was finally overthrown, the United States was still not satisfied. The Leopold CIA Station met with "a high level Congolese politician" and reported to Washington, D.C.: "Lumumba in opposition is almost as dangerous as in office. [The Congolese politician] indicated understood and implied might physically eliminate Lumumba."[39] The CIA further concluded that Lumumba was so dangerous because every time he had the last word, "he can sway events" and decisions are made "to his advantage." Thus steps were taken to carry out the assassination that some have called one of the most consequential assassinations of the 20th Century.[40]

---

37 Office of the Historian, United States Department of State, *Foreign Relations of the United States, 1964–1968, Volume XXIII, Congo 1960–1968*, 11. Editorial Note, https://history.state.gov/historicaldocuments/frus1964-68v23/d11 (accessed March 31, 2020).

38 The Senate Select Committee to Study Governmental Operations with Respect to Intelligence Activities, *Interim Report on Congo* (accessed March 31), 2020, https://www.aarclibrary.org/publib/church/reports/ir/pdf/ChurchIR_3A_Congo.pdf.

39 *Interim Report on Congo,* Ibid., CIA Cable Leopoldville to Director (9/7/60).

40 Georges Nzongola-Ntalaja, "Patrice Lumumba: the most important assassination of the 20th century: The US-sponsored plot to kill Patrice Lumumba, the hero of Congolese independence, took place 50 years ago today," *The Guardian,* January 17, 2011 (March 31, 2020), https://www.theguardian.com/global-development/poverty-matters/2011/jan/17/patrice-lumumba-50th-anniversary-assassination accessed.

"The plot proceeded to the point that lethal substances and instruments specifically intended for use in an assassination were delivered by the CIA to the Congo Station."[41] One CIA agent explored injecting a toxic material into Lumumba's food or even into his toothpaste. Unfortunately from the point of view of the U.S. government, the CIA was not able to get to Lumumba before the expiration date of the poisons that had been prepared. As a result, the first "preparation" was disposed of in the Congo River, according to one version of events. Amid the comings and goings of different CIA agents and representatives, a message was communicated in various ways to various agents that the "gloves, mask, hypodermic syringe" and a lethal virus to carry out the assassination were all left in a CIA Station safe. There were four or five ways discussed to carry out the murder that all included the use of poisons and a virus.[42] Patrice Lumumba was eventually killed on January 17, 1961. With the help of the colonial master and U.S. ally, Belgium, Lumumba was shot and his body was dissolved in acid. The government of Belgium investigated its role in the sordid murder and in 2004 published its findings. The government of Belgium concluded that it "had a moral responsibility in the assassination of Lumumba and that it 'acted under pressure from the Belgian public, which had heard for days about violence against Belgian citizens in Congo.'"[43] No one in either Belgium or the United States has been held accountable for the murder of Patrice Lumumba. Moreover, it took 19 years for the truth to be told by the United States Department of State that the President of the United States at the time, General Dwight D. Eisenhower, personally approved the killing of his equal on the world stage. Patrice Lumumba stands today as the first time ever that a Head of Government was authorized by a President of the United States to be assassinated. And the CIA found that the use of a virus could work very well for this "project."

---

41 The Senate Select Committee to Study Governmental Operations with Respect to Intelligence Activities, *Assassination Planning and the Plots: Congo (*accessed March 30, 2020), https://www.aarclibrary.org/publib/church/reports/ir/pdf/ChurchIR_3A_Congo.pdf.

42 *Interim Report on Congo,* op cit.

43 Ismail Akwei, "The chilling details of Patrice Lumumba's assassination and how he was dissolved in acid," *Face2FaceAfrica.com,* January 17, 2019 (accessed March 31, 2020), https://face2faceafrica.com/article/the-chilling-details-of-patrice-lumumbas-assassination-and-how-he-was-dissolved-in-acid.

U.S. Biowarfare Attacks Against China and Korea

Both China and North Korea accused the U.S. of attacking them with biological weapons. At first, the U.S. denied the charges and forced retractions from the Chinese and Koreans. However, it was unknown at the time that there was an investigative Report produced by internationally eminent persons that corroborated the Chinese and Korean accusations. That Report was only recently made public, although it was written originally in 1952.[44]

Comprised of Europeans and South Americans, the International Scientific Commission landed in China in June 1952 and traveled to the affected areas in China and then proceeded to Korea. In each location, personal tests, interrogations, and examinations were made by the members of the Commission.

The Report begins by recognizing the role of the Japanese during World War II in the use of "Bacterial Warfare." It notes that the Japanese introduced bubonic plague in China by dissemination of infected fleas. And the members of the Commission wondered if the Americans merely took up where the Japanese left off in the use of these bacterial agents as weapons. The Commission documented never-seen-before-insects: mosquitoes (that carry yellow fever), flies, spiders, beetles (a source of anthrax), cholera, and more; Purple Spot Fungus that destroys soybean crops and other plant pathogens never seen before in Asia; Plague; what they called "Phytopathological Data" that included infected North American grains of corn dropped with the intention of destroying legumes. The Commission noted that insects were used as vectors for human and plant diseases.

Fort Detrick came under the scrutiny of the Commissioners who noted, "Researches from Camp Detrick published in 1946 and 1947 show that it has been possible to obtain new strains of anthrax bacilli cultured on synthetic media which not only possessed unusually high virulence, but which are especially adapted to the respiratory route of infection."[45] Captured Air Force officers and auxiliary (local) intelligence agents exposed the use of non-conventional containers and "bombs" like paper packets filled with infected insects as the preferred method of delivery. The U.S. even delivered freeze-dried bacteria to its China and Korea targets. The Commissioners noted that "technical and scientific advances extend the range of what may be done, and throw light, as here, on apparent contradictions." The Commissioners were specifically discussing what the Americans wrote as theoretical limitations versus what the Americans did in the field and so,

---

44 Report of the International Scientific Commissioner the Investigation of the Facts Concerning Bacterial Warfare in Korea and China (with Appendices) (1952), accessed April 4, 2020, https://www.documentcloud.org/documents/4334133-ISC-Full-Report-Pub-Copy.html.

45 Ibid.

chose to believe more in what they found in the field rather than to concentrate on or rule out actions based on what the Americans wrote. The Commissioners also found evidence of an unusual outbreak of encephalitis, but were not able to pin it on the U.S. They did conclude, however, that the people of the world need and have a right to know about what happened in China and Korea and the potentialities represented by "this kind of warfare, with its incalculable dangers."[46] The Commissioners wrote in conclusion:

> The peoples of Korea and China have indeed been the objective of bacteriological weapons. These have been employed by units of the U.S.A. armed forces, using a great variety of different methods for the purpose, some of which seem to be developments of those applied by the Japanese Army during the Second World War.
>
> The Commission reached these conclusions, passing from one logical step to another. It did so reluctantly because its members had not been disposed to believe that such an inhuman technique could have been put into execution in the face of universal condemnation by the peoples of the nations.
>
> It is now for all peoples to redouble their efforts to preserve the world from war and prevent the discoveries of science being used for the destruction of humanity.

So, What's the "Spanish" Flu Got to Do With it?

Early in the Trump Administration, the CDC held a one-day symposium on the 1918 Flu, also sometimes called the "Spanish Flu." What is less known about the "Spanish Flu" is that it actually started in Kansas, U.S. in the middle of World War I. In fact, several researchers into the origins of the 1918 Flu concluded that "the disease started in the United States and spread with 'the arrival of American troops in France.'"[47] Dr. Loring Miner, located in Haskell 49 County, Kansas, was so struck by this new influenza that he reported it to the U.S. Public Health Service. Barry writes of Miner:

> Miner considered this incarnation of the disease so dangerous that he warned national public health officials about it. Public Health Reports

---

46 Ibid.

47 John M. Barry, "The site of origin of the 1918 influenza pandemic and its public health implications," *Journal of Translational Medicine,* January 20, 2004, *U.S. National Library of Medicine, National Institutes of Health* (accessed April 3, 2020), https://www.ncbi.nlm.nih.gov/pmc/articles/PMC340389/.

(now Morbidity and Mortality Weekly Report), a weekly journal produced by the U.S. Public Health Service to alert health officials to outbreaks of communicable diseases throughout the world, published his warning. In the first six months of 1918, this would be the only reference in that journal to influenza anywhere in the world.[48]

The importance of the truth about the origin of the 1918 Flu cannot be understated. Barry writes, "The fact that the 1918 pandemic likely began in the United States matters because it tells investigators where to look for a new virus."

Finally, Kevin Barry raises a new issue surrounding the 1918 Flu, suggesting that it might not have been the flu at all, but instead was another disease. He asks whether the vaccination of U.S. troops might have had something to do with the origins of the 1918 Flu.[49] Dr. Frederick Gates writes about the 1918 soldier vaccinations at the Base Hospital at Fort Riley, Kansas, carried out with the cooperation of the New York-based Rockefeller Institute for Medical Research. These were anti-meningitis vaccinations. Gates cited "relative immunity" for the soldiers who were vaccinated.[50] Thus, Kevin Barry concludes that insofar as the Rockefeller Institute sent the antimeningococcic serum around the world to England, France, Belgium, Italy, and other countries, that the 1918 Flu might actually have been a bacterial meningitis epidemic.[51] Barry bolsters his conclusions on a study of the results of 167 autopsies performed in 1918 on fatalities from "flu," and found that 164 of 167 autopsies showed the presence of streptococci or pneumococci in the lung tissue of those dead from the flu. He writes, "Pneumococci or streptococci were found in 164 of (the) 167 lung tissue samples" autopsied. That is 98.2%. Bacteria was the killer."[52] Not a virus.

Brundage and Shanks go further and hypothesize that the influenza experienced by many in 1918 was compounded and complicated by the vaccinated

---

48 Ibid.

49 Kevin Barry, "Did a Vaccine Experiment on U.S. Soldiers Cause the 'Spanish Flu'? The 1918-19 bacterial vaccine experiment may have killed 50-100 million people," *Vaccine Impact* (accessed April 3, 2020) located at https://vaccineimpact.com/2018/did-military-experimental-vaccine-in-1918-kill-50-100-million-people-blamed-as-spanish-flu/.

50 Frederick L. Gates, M.D., First Lieutenant Medical Corps, U.S. Army, "A Report on Antimeningitis Vaccination and Observations on Agglutinins in the Blood of Chronic Meningococcus Carriers," July 20, 1918, *U.S. National Library of Medicine, National Institutes of Health* (accessed April 3, 2020), https://www.ncbi.nlm.nih.gov/pmc/articles/PMC2126288/pdf/449.pdf.

51 Kevin Barry, op. cit.

52 Ibid.

"antimeningitis bacteria carriers" who carried the bacteria in their noses. They write, "Persons with active infections were aerosolizing the bacteria that colonized their noses and throats, while others—often, in the same 'breathing spaces'—were profoundly susceptible to invasion of and rapid spread through their lungs by their own or others' colonizing bacteria."[53] Thus, Brundage and Shanks suggest that, from firsthand accounts from 1918–1919 army camps, first came the influenza which then decreased the body's ability to respond to the secondary bacterial pneumonia infection. It was this "One, Two" punch that increased the mortality of the 1918 Flu. Non-pharmaceutical interventions like "isolation, quarantine, and other social distancing measures," were recommended. Barry concludes that the 1918 Flu could have been the product of a pharmaceutical mistake. He writes,

> In 1918-19, there was no independent investigative follow up challenging the official story that "Spanish Flu" was some mystery illness which dropped from the sky.
>
> I suspect that many of those at the Rockefeller Institute knew what happened, and that many of the doctors who administered the vaccines to the troops knew what happened, but those people are long dead.
>
> In 2018, the Pharmaceutical industry is the largest campaign donor to politicians and the largest advertiser in all forms of media, so not much has changed over 100 years. This story will likely be ignored by mainstream media because their salaries are paid by pharmaceutical advertising.

So: is the United States research on vaccines and possible emergent pathogens more of a problem than anyone has thus far in officialdom been willing to admit? Do the people of the world and the U.S. need to be protected from the death scientists working in the BSL-3 and -4 labs of the United States, the production of whose noxious materials is at the behest of U.S. elected and non-elected leaders?

CURRENT U.S. BIODEFENSE POLICY

Despite its track record, the United States calls its efforts in this realm, "defense."

In 2018, President Trump produced his Administration's National Biodefense Strategy. It states:

---

53 John F. Brundage and G. Dennis Shanks, "Deaths from Bacterial Pneumonia during 1918–19 Influenza Pandemic," *Emerging Infectious Diseases,* 14(8), August 2008 (accessed April 3, 2020), https://wwwnc.cdc.gov/eid/article/14/8/07-1313_article.

Natural or accidental outbreaks, as well as deliberate attacks, can originate in one country and spread to many others, with potentially far-reaching international consequences. Advances in science promise better and faster cures, economic advances, a cleaner environment, and improved quality of life, but they also bring new security risks. In this rapidly changing landscape, the United States must be prepared to manage the risks posed by natural outbreaks of disease, accidents with high consequence pathogens, or adversaries who wish to do harm with biological agents. . . . This National Biodefense Strategy brings together and puts in place for the first time, a single coordinated effort to orchestrate the full range of activity that is carried out across the United States Government to protect the American people from biological threats.[54]

On September 18, 2018, President Trump issued National Security Presidential Memorandum 14 (NSPM–14)[55] which explained the Administration's biodefense strategy. It mandated an annual "Biodefense Assessment to identify any gaps, shortfalls, and redundancies; describe any challenges to the implementation and execution of the Strategy; and recommend any necessary updates or changes to the Strategy."[56] It created a biodefense steering committee headed by the U.S. Secretary of Health and Human Services and explained the "whole of government" approach that is seen today in the U.S. COVID-19 approach. Additionally, President Trump's approach includes a call to the private sector and federal responsiveness to all levels of government from the Federal Agencies to the States and Local Governments to be coordinated in the event of a biological event. In practice, we saw President Trump act on a 2015 bipartisan recommendation made by the Blue Ribbon Study Panel on Biodefense, co-chaired by Tom Ridge and Joe Lieberman, to have the Vice President "synchronize" U.S. national defense efforts.[57] NSPM–14 superseded previous biodefense directives issued by previous

---

54 National Biodefense Strategy, 2018 located at https://www.whitehouse.gov/wp-content/uploads/2018/09/National-Biodefense-Strategy.pdf accessed April 4, 2020.

55 National Security Presidential Memorandum–14: Presidential Memorandum on the Support for National Biodefense (September 18, 2018) located at https://www.whitehouse.gov/presidential-actions/presidential-memorandum-support-national-biodefense/ accessed April 4, 2020.

56 Ibid.

57 Daniel M. Gerstein, "Achieving the Trump Administration's National Biodefense Strategy," Rand Corporation, *The Rand Blog* (October 2, 2018) located at https://www.rand.org/blog/2018/10/achieving-the-trump-administrations-national-biodefense.html accessed April 4, 2020.

presidents. Interestingly, among all of the documents reviewed, only one mentioned the dangerous research, utilizing dangerous pathogens, that takes place inside the global network of U.S.-funded Levels 3 and 4 biolabs. Only the General Accounting Office (GAO) document, entitled, "The Nation Faces Long-Standing Challenges Related to Defending Against Biological Threats," mentioned the threats that come from biolabs:

> Since 2008, GAO has identified challenges and areas for improvement related to the safety, security, and oversight of high-containment laboratories, which, among other things, conduct research on hazardous pathogens—such as the Ebola virus. GAO recommended that agencies take actions to avoid safety and security lapses at laboratories, such as better assessing risks, coordinating inspections, and reporting inspection results. Many recommendations have been addressed, but others remain open, such as finalizing guidance on documenting the shipment of dangerous biological material.[58]

Two weeks before Donald J. Trump was sworn in, the then-short-lived Obama Administration left a document from the U.S. Northern Command (NorthCom) of the Pentagon entitled, "Pandemic Influenza and Infectious Disease Response" just lying around. It was a memo from the Northern Command to itself. This document reads like a science fiction B movie in that everything that is occurring now, is presaged in this document. Everything. The Obama Pentagon Northern Command describes the situation as, "The causative agents of biological incidents are microorganisms (or toxins produced or derived from them) which causes [sic] disease in humans, plants or animals."[59] It described the potential as "real" for a 61 "catastrophic biological incident" that threatens the national security of the United States. It describes that threat as being to the humans, animals, economy, plants, and the environment. It went on to describe the danger as follows:

> (b) Unique or novel pathogens are likely to defy conventional diagnostic and treatment tools which can result in rapid spread throughout the world, posing risk to national security;

---

58 General Accounting Office, "The Nation Faces Long-Standing Challenges Related to Defending Against Biological Threats," June 2019 (accessed April 4, 2020), https://www.gao.gov/assets/710/700014.pdf.

59 U.S. Northern Command, "Pandemic Influenza and Infectious Disease Response," passim, accessed April 3, 2020, https://www.scribd.com/document/454422848/Pentagon-Influenza-Response..

(c) Novel contagious pathogens capable of human-to-human transmission via aerosols with high virulence for which no MCM (medical countermeasures) exists may present the greatest challenge to response and recovery;

(e) Widespread and improper use of antibiotic, anti-viral, anti-malarial treatments or other medical countermeasures (MCM) are accelerating the emergence of drug-resistant pathogens that are unresponsive to available pharmaceutical interventions.

The document goes on to state the obvious in terms of U.S. history already cited, important for our purposes here: "(2) The deliberate employment of biologicals as a weapon does exist."[60] The plan it puts forward was developed after the outbreaks of "2009 H1N1 Pandemic Influenza, 2012 Middle Eastern Respiratory Syndrome Coronavirus (MERS-CoV), 2013 H7N9 Avian Influenza, 2014 Ebola Virus Disease (EVD) and 2015 Zika Virus outbreaks."[61] The document goes on to mention that both states and non-states harbor the desire to use biologicals as weapons and even points to the 2001 anthrax attacks in the U.S. as an example of a deliberate biological incident that reinforces the need for "seamless interagency planning in advance of any deliberate incident."[62] What the document fails to acknowledge is the fact that the U.S. anthrax attacks of 2001 were a self-inflicted wound. Finally, I'd like to turn to an important statute that remains on the books today in 2020: S.993—Biological Weapons Anti-Terrorism Act of 1989. This piece of legislation is designed to "implement the Biological Weapons Convention and to protect the United States from biological terrorism."[63] S. 993:

- Imposes "criminal penalties upon anyone who knowingly develops, produces, stockpiles, transfers, acquires, retains, or possesses any biological agent, toxin, or delivery system for use as a weapon or assists a foreign state or any organization to do so" and

- "Provides for extraterritorial Federal jurisdiction over an offense committed by or against a U.S. national."

---

60 Ibid.
61 Ibid.
62 Ibid.
63 S. 993 – Biological Weapons Anti-Terrorism Act of 1989 (accessed April 5, 2020), https://www.congress.gov/bill/101st-congress/senate-bill/993.

The U.S. Department of State characterizes the Biological Weapons Convention (BWC) as "critical to international efforts to address the threat posed by biological weapons—whether in the hands of governments or non-state actors. To remain effective, it must deal with all biological threats we face in the 21st century."[64] The BWC requires its Party States:

> Never to develop, produce, stockpile, or otherwise acquire or retain: 1) biological agents or toxins of types and in quantities that have no justification for peaceful uses; and 2) weapons, equipment, or means of delivery designed to use such agents or toxins for hostile purposes (Article I).
>
> To destroy or divert to peaceful purposes all agents, toxins, weapons, equipment, and means of delivery specified in Article I in their possession, or under their jurisdiction or control (Article II).
>
> Not to transfer or in any way to assist, encourage, or induce any entity to manufacture or otherwise acquire any of the agents, toxins, weapons, equipment or means of delivery specified in Article I (Article III).
>
> To take any necessary measures to prohibit and prevent the development, production, stockpiling, acquisition, or retention of any of the agents, toxins, weapons, equipment, and means of delivery specified in Article I under its jurisdiction or control (Article IV).[65]

The BWC was signed on April 10, 1972 in London, Moscow, and Washington, D.C. Thus, the Biological Weapons Anti-Terrorism Act criminalized violations of the BWC. Only a few states have failed to sign the BWC: The People's Republic of China did not sign the Convention, but acceded to it on November 15, 1984. In its accession statement, it wrote:

> 1. The basic spirit of the Convention on the Prohibition of Biological Weapons conforms to China's consistent position and is conducive to the efforts of the world's peace-loving countries and peoples in fighting against aggression and maintaining world peace. China once was one of the victims of biological (bacteriological) weapons. China has not produced or possessed such weapons and will never do so in future. However, the Chinese Government considers that the Convention has its defects. For instance, it fails to provide in explicit

---

64 United States Department of State, *Biological Weapons Convention*, accessed April 5, 2020, https://www.state.gov/biological-weapons-convention/.

65 Ibid.

terms for the "prohibition of the use of" biological weapons and the concrete and effective measures for supervision and verification; it lacks forceful measures of sanctions in the procedure of complaint against instances of violation of the Convention. It is the hope of the Chinese Government that these defects maybe made up or corrected at an appropriate time.

2. It is also the hope of the Chinese Government that a convention on complete prohibition and thorough destruction of chemical weapons will soon be concluded.

3. The signature and ratification of the Convention by the Taiwan authorities in the name of China on 10 April 1972 and 9 February 1973 are illegal and null and void.[66]

Israel neither signed nor acceded to the BWC in the name of keeping its capabilities "ambiguous." In fact, its Israel Institute for Biological Research (IIBR) is known to conduct "research on several select agents and toxins, including plague bacterium (Yersinia pestis), typhus bacterium (Rickettsia prowazekii), staphylococcal enterotoxin B (SEB), rabies, anthrax bacterium (Bacillus anthracis), botulinum bacterium (Clostridium botulinum), botulinum toxin, and Ebola virus."[67] Few were surprised when IIBR scientists announced that a vaccine for SARS-CoV-2 would be available in a matter of "weeks," a process that normally takes years. The Israeli newspaper, *Haaretz,* carried the news, thusly: "Scientists at Israel's Institute for Biological Research are expected to announce in the coming days that they have completed development of a vaccine for the new coronavirus COVID-19."[68] Moreover, scientists at Israel's Galilee Research Institute (MIGAL) stated that it was "pure luck" that they started studying coronaviruses four years ago in discussing their new technology that could also lead to an oral vaccine.[69]

---

66 United Nations Office for Disarmament Affairs (UNODA), "China: Accession to Biological Weapons Convention," accessed April 5, 2020, http://disarmament.un.org/treaties/a/bwc/china/acc/london.

67 Nuclear Threat Initiative (NTI) (accessed April 5, 2020), https://www.nti.org/learn/countries/israel/biological/.

68 Ido Efrati and Chaim Levinson, "Israeli Research Center to Announce It Developed Coronavirus Vaccine, Sources Say," *Haaretz,* March 18, 2020 (accessed April 5, 2020), https://www.haaretz.com/israel-news/.premium-coronavirus-vaccine-israel-biological-research-institute-develope-1.8665074.

69 Maayan Jaffe-Hoffman, "Israeli scientists: 'In a few weeks, we will have coronavirus vaccine,'" March 15, 2020 (accessed April 5, 2020), https://www.jpost.

The big loophole in both the BWC and the Act are that they both permit research and maintaining biological agents for peaceful purposes. The Act states, "Nothing in this Act is intended to restrain or restrict peaceful scientific research or development."[70] For the big and little states that were conducting research into biological pathogens, nothing changed, except the self-congratulating and hortatory language that they used to describe their efforts on the subject.

In fact, the Soviet Union had a massive BW program that employed 50,000 people at its height, even after it signed the BWC. Frischknecht writes, "Nevertheless, nobody really knows what the Russians are working on today and what happened to the weapons they produced. Western security experts now fear that some stocks of biological weapons might not have been destroyed and have instead fallen into other hands."[71] We now know that apartheid era South Africa and Israel[72] developed or are still developing race-specific biological weapons.

As we saw with the 1918 Flu, the Rockefeller Institute for Medical Research played a key role in the deaths attributed to the "Flu." Today, there is an explosion of private companies that work hand in glove with government agencies in the realm of biomedical research and that includes experimentation on human and ecological pathogens. This surge of actors also carries with it a multiplication of motives and varying means for intentional and unintentional actions that, as we will see in the next section, imperil global stability, increasing the possibility that these new agents and technologies could even be used, not against humanity en masse, as has largely been discussed thus far, but most horrifically against a specific slice of humanity for purposes of genocide—the elimination in whole or in part of an entire people.

---

com/HEALTH-SCIENCE/Israeli-scientists-In-three-weeks-we-will-have-coronavirus-vaccine-619101.

70 101st Congress (1989-1990), "S.993 - Biological Weapons Anti-Terrorism Act of 1989," *Congress.gov* (accessed April 5, 2020), https://www.congress.gov/bill/101st-congress/senate-bill/993/text.

71 Friedrich Frischknecht, "The History of Biological Warfare," *EMBO Reports,* June 2003 (accessed April 5, 2020), https://www.ncbi.nlm.nih.gov/pmc/articles/PMC1326439/.

72 Israel significantly complicates calculations because of its many hidden relationships with other countries, its sophisticated intelligence operations, and its commitment to what is known as "The Samson Option," which is Israel's threat to annihilate any county or countries that threaten what it views to be its existential state interests. See Seymour Hersh, *The Samson Option: Israel's Nuclear Arsenal and American Foreign Policy* (New York: Random House, 1991), https://archive.org/details/Sampson_Option/mode/2up (accessed April 7, 2020).

> *"[A]dvanced forms of biological warfare that can 'target'*
> *specific genotypes may transform biological warfare*
> *from the realm of terror to a politically useful tool."*

—Project for a New American Century, 2000

GENOCIDE

Genocide is the elimination, in whole or in part, of a people or nation—where nation is a body of people who believe themselves to be a nation. So, when I write the word "nation," I am not referring to either the state—the governing apparatus of a country or a nation— or the country—the geographic territory of either a state or a nation. Genocide can be cultural or physical or both. And recently, scholars have begun to address the issue of "Genetic Genocide" as it relates to health care and the disability communities in which the rights of the disabled are circumscribed, such as the right to reproduction. However, any compassionate consideration of those who are differently abled—or who are just plain different, period—is a far cry from what took place in the early history of the United States, including its current practices. In this section, I will cite the U.S. recent experiences with genocide, just so that we understand that this is not simply something buried in our past, and then move to a deeper consideration of recent experience and the impact that technology might have on the ability to carry out a genocide with very few people even realizing what is happening—including the intended genocide's targeted victims. While the world is aware of Nazi Germany's genocide against Jews, World War II was not the world's introduction to genocide nor was it the last genocide in our lifetime. But, for all that we know about Germany's Nazi-era genocide, we know very little about other genocides that have taken place around the world, including those whose occurrence we may have witnessed.

A short inventory of today's genocides, since World War II, would include:

- Khmer Rouge's Cambodia;
- Myanmar's Rohingya;
- Indonesia against East Timor;
- Rwandans against each other—Hutus versus Tutsis;
- Rwandan Tutsis against Congolese in Congo;
- Burundians against each other—Hutus versus Tutsis;
- West Pakistanis against East Pakistanis;
- Guatemalans against each other—Non-Indigenous versus Indigenous Guatemalans;

- Bangladeshis against each other—Non-Indigenous versus Indigenous Bangladeshis;
- Indians versus each other—Hindus versus Muslims in Gujarat and Hindus versus Sikhs in Punjab;
- Israelis versus Palestinians.

And this is not even an exhaustive list. But the diversity of examples should make it clear that genocide can be the result of ideological, religious, or political conflict—many of which are the result of earlier conflicts fanned by the colonial experience where one group was favored over another in order to make the colonial project successful and long-lived. Thus, a look at the colonial project in establishing the current world order is instructive. And therein lies the importance of the U.S. experience as it informs us of the nature of the current world order for which the U.S. serves as "global enforcer" for ongoing genocides of which most have no knowledge whatsoever.

WHENCE THE *TRAJECTORY* OF THE UNITED STATES OF AMERICA?

The foundations of the enumerated genocides are expressions of what Anibal Quijano called, "The Coloniality of Power."[73] That is, the current order of the world, which is built on European supremacy by way of imperialist conquest. This enabled Europeans to travel to any part of the non-European world and reap from it an excessive reward, which then further enabled them to construct the values, preferences, and historiography of the entire globe based on, and with a view to cementing, their control. The global result of this comprehensive exercise of power and control is Eurocentrism for all.[74] Eurocentrism is what former World Bank President James Wolfensohn is describing when he told a group of Stanford Masters of Business Administration (MBA) students that when he was growing up he had the "80–20 Rule"[75] tucked neatly into his hip pocket. What that meant is that he could travel anywhere in the world and have an advantage over the local people because of the way the world had been constructed by Eurocentrism to work in the favor of Europeans and their descendants all over the world. In

---

73 Anibal Quijano, "Coloniality of Power and Eurocentrism in Latin America," *International Sociology,* June 2000 (accessed April 6, 2020), https://journals.sagepub.com/doi/10.1177/0268580900015002005.

74 Eurocentrism is the belief that European culture and values and history ("Western Civilization") are superior to those of other nations or races.

75 Wolfensohn defined the "80–20 Rule" as the fact that approximately 1 billion of the world's population enjoyed 80% of global GDP and that the world's remaining population had to eke out a living on the remaining 20%. Please see an excerpt of Wolfensohn's speech (accessed April 6, 2020): https://www.youtube.com/watch?v=bpCKhJ9egvM&t=5s.

his speech to the Stanford students, Wolfensohn goes on to tell them that all of the organs that run the world were designed "to accommodate that fact." The so-called Washington Consensus, then, is the economic design for the world in which we currently live, enforced with the military might of the U.S., that ensures the continuation of this coloniality/neocoloniality of power—Eurocentrism—and Western European supremacy. Since its inception, sitting at the top of this design was the Anglo-American partnership. That, however, has morphed into a Zionist-Anglo partnership that has different membership criteria and different priorities.

Putin is so disdained in the West because he rejected Russia being consigned to subservience to the economic empowerment of "The West." The BRICS, the organization named for the acronym of its member states Brazil, Russia, India, China, and South Africa, was the opening shot of resistance, with many more to come, to the Washington Consensus by Russia, China, and Britain's former colonies of India and South Africa. The formation of the Shanghai Cooperation Organization (SCO), the Eurasian Economic Union (EAEU), the Asian Infrastructure Investment Bank (AIIB), UNASUR in Latin America, and the Africa South America Summit should all be seen in this light as challenges to the West's global coloniality of power. In 1998, the American Anthropological Association began the uphill task of trying to correct centuries of dogma and racist practice by issuing its statement on race:

> Today scholars in many fields argue that "race" as it is understood in the United States of America was a social mechanism invented during the 18th century to refer to those populations brought together in colonial America: the English and other European settlers, the conquered Indian peoples, and those peoples of Africa brought in to provide slave labor. . . . Thus "race" was a mode of classification linked specifically to peoples in the colonial situation. It subsumed a growing ideology of inequality devised to rationalize European attitudes and treatment of the conquered and enslaved peoples. Proponents of slavery in particular during the 19th century used 'race' to justify the retention of slavery. The ideology magnified the differences among Europeans, Africans, and Indians, established a rigid hierarchy of socially exclusive categories underscored and bolstered unequal rank and status differences, and provided the rationalization that the inequality was natural or God-given. The different physical traits of African-Americans and Indians became markers or symbols of their status differences. As they were constructing U.S. society, leaders among European-Americans fabricated the cultural/behavioral characteristics associated with each 'race,' linking superior traits with Europeans and

negative and inferior ones to blacks and Indians. Numerous arbitrary and fictitious beliefs about the different peoples were institutionalized and deeply embedded in American thought."[76]

Thus, once BRICS (and its New Development Bank) is seen as a response to the coloniality of Western power, the U.S. response to BRICS then becomes instructive and predictable: regime change for Brazil, divide and rule for the BRICS as a whole and for India in particular, and hybrid warfare against China and Russia. These strategies are replayed over and over again for the other resisting organizations mentioned above as the immense resources of the United States are used to subjugate, destroy, and destabilize the dreams of sovereignty, dignity, and freedom held by the rest of the non-Western world. Thus, before we tackle and try to save the world from the genocides of the future, it is important to understand this ongoing practice of genocide that we normally don't see. Thus, in order to answer the question of Whence the Trajectory of the United States of America, let us turn for a short while to the U.S. practice of Eugenics—the belief in and the practice of selectively breeding (and sterilizing) human beings for the purpose of creating a "Master Race." Even the assumptions underlying the founding of the United States of America must be seen to include the principles of Eugenics. Advances in biotechnology enable eugenics to be in even greater practice and a guiding principle in the U.S. and the rest of the Eurocentric world.

At least one scholar, Edwin Black, believes that the Nazi German "Master Race" quest was actually a U.S. export resulting from a very strong Eugenics movement in the U.S. I would venture further and posit that it is impossible to understand U.S. domestic and foreign policies today without an understanding of the drivers of those policies and that U.S. continued rootedness in the eugenics orientation and practices of its very founding lies at the bottom of them. As a precursor, let us turn to Stephen Jay Gould's *The Mismeasure of Man*. Here, Gould attacks an idea that animated U.S. policy throughout the 20th Century—that of being able to measure and rank human intelligence. (Before the IQ measure, of course, the issue was whether or not North America Natives had souls [before the westward expansion] and whether imported Africans were even humans, despite Africa being the cradle of homo sapiens. In 2015, the Catholic Church announced the elevation of Junipero Serra to sainthood despite the fact that he oversaw the brutalization of Native Americans who were "brutalized—beaten, pressed into

---

76 American Anthropological Association, "Statement on Race," May 17, 1998 (accessed April 6, 2020), https://www.americananthro.org/ConnectWithAAA/Content.aspx?ItemNumber=2583.

forced labour and infected with diseases to which they had no resistance,"[77] defeating them via diseases which decimated their populations.)

Of his book, Gould writes, *"The Mismeasure of Man* treats one particular form of quantified claim about the ranking of human groups: the argument that intelligence can be meaningfully abstracted as a single number capable of ranking all people on a linear scale of intrinsic and unalterable mental worth."[78] Thus, from the very inception of the U.S., based on biological determinism, there was a projection of the inferiority of the imported Africans and their progeny as well as of the Indigenous North Americans whose land was needed to complete the U.S. project. Cornel West drives the point home in his epic book, *Race Matters.* He writes:

> Yet the enslavement of Africans—over 20 percent of the population— served as the linchpin of American democracy; that is, the much- heralded stability and continuity of American democracy was predicated upon black oppression and degradation. Without the presence of black people in America, European-Americans would not be "white"—they would be only Irish, Italians, Poles, Welsh, and others engaged in class, ethnic, and gender struggles over resources and identity. What made America distinctly American for them was not simply the presence of unprecedented opportunities, but the struggle for seizing these opportunities in a new land in which black slavery and racial caste served as the floor upon which white class, ethnic, and gender struggles could be diffused and diverted. In other words, white poverty could be ignored and whites' paranoia of each other could be overlooked primarily owing to the distinctive American feature: the basic racial divide of black and white peoples. From 1776 to 1964... this racial divide would serve as a basic presupposition for the expansive functioning of American democracy, even as the concentration of wealth and power remained in the hands of a Few well-to-do white men.[79]

---

77 Andrew Gumbel, "Junípero Serra's brutal story in spotlight as pope prepares for canonisation," *The Guardian,* September 23, 2015 (accessed April 6, 2020), https://www. theguardian.com/world/2015/sep/23/pope-francis-junipero-serra-sainthood-washington- california.

78 Stephen Jay Gould, *The Mismeasure of Man,* Revised and Expanded (New York: W.W. Norton & Co., 1996) https://www.amazon.com/Mismeasure-Man-Revised- Expanded-ebook/dp/B007Q6XN2S/ref=sr_1_2 (accessed April 6, 2020).

79 Cornel West, *Race Matters,* (Beacon Press, 1993).

Thus, the United States was fertile ground on which the ideas and practices of biological determinism, racism, Eurocentrism, could prosper. Edwin Black argues that U.S. eugenicists were responsible for the spread of Eugenics around the world. Everything that happens in the U.S. and outside the U.S. and The West, must be viewed through this prism or analyses and interpretations of events involving the U.S. and The West will fall short. The application of this context to all of the sister Anglo-American settler-colonial states of Australia, New Zealand, Canada, is particularly apt. Hence, the "Five Eyes" exist to work with each other against the rest of the world that desires recognition, sovereignty, and freedom. Western policy has been explicitly to deny these values to the non-Western rest of the world. It is within this context that the virulent racism of U.S./Western wars must be seen: wars that destroyed the drinking water system in Iraq and the Great Manmade River piping water into the Sahara desert in Libya; sprayed Agent Orange on the Vietnam countryside and the Vietnamese people who are still suffering the ill health effects fifty years later. Even the dropping of atomic bombs and the use of depleted uranium weapons—another form of nuclear weapon attack—have mostly taken place against non-Western peoples. The Republic of South Africa used to be a part of the Anglo-American club until Blacks won the right to control the politics of their land—not the economy and not even the land, itself, yet. Bear in mind, European-descendant South Africans, before the handover of political power to the Indigenous Africans, created a covert BW-program that sought to find a "Black Bomb" biological agent that could be deployed, for example, in the water, that would kill only the Blacks and not the Whites. The Jewish State of Israel, controlled by Western-descendant and Western-oriented Jews, maintains a BW program, as has been discussed earlier, and some of its research, like that of apartheid-era South Africa, was based on the specific desire to kill Muslim Arabs. Now, let's turn to Edwin Black to see how pernicious this line of thinking is. Black writes that so-called "elite" White European-descended Americans came to believe in "Negative Eugenics" which is based on two points:

1. Minorities (Blacks, Native Americans, Mexicans) and poor whites are genetically inferior; and

2. They are by definition of unfit heredity only capable of reproducing genetically inferior offspring.[80]

---

80 Rodney J. Daniels, Review of Edwin Black, *War Against the Weak: Eugenics and America's Campaign to Create a Master Race* (New York: Four Walls Eight Windows, 2003), https://inside.nku.edu/content/dam/hisgeo/docs/archives/Vol20_2004-2005perspectives.pdf#page=79 (accessed April 6, 2020).

The magazine, *Catholic Stand,* wrote:

> [These] American eugenicists …were often political and social liberals—advocates of social reform, partisans of science, critics of stasis and reaction. [Quoting author Richard Conniff] "They weren't sinister characters …but environmentalists, peace activists, fitness buffs, healthy-living enthusiasts, inventors and family men…who saw the quest for a better gene pool as of a piece with their broader dream of human advancement."[81]

This Negative Eugenics was supported at the highest financial levels inside the U.S. in high schools, colleges, and universities; at private foundations like Rockefeller and Carnegie. Wealthy individuals financed scholars at universities who wrote journal articles that were read by the world's intelligentsia. Pro-eugenics candidates were elected to office flush with campaign cash and changed policies in the U.S. that resulted in the castration or sterilization of more than 80,000 people in the U.S. The Planned Parenthood organization was at the forefront of the U.S. movement. American and European eugenicists joined hands "across the pond" on their mission to improve mankind and sterilize the unfit. Even Bill Gates—one of the richest men on the planet today—admits that his father, who was an advocate for Planned Parenthood, impacted his views on population. The idea of eugenics is embedded in the DNA of the U.S.A.

Black writes:

> When we were done, we had assembled a mountain of documentation that clearly chronicled a century of eugenic crusading by America's finest universities, most reputable scientists, most trusted professional and charitable organizations, and most revered corporate foundations. They had collaborated with the Department of Agriculture and numerous state agencies in an attempt to breed a new race of Nordic humans, applying the same principles used to breed cattle and corn. The names define power and prestige in America: The Carnegie Institution, the Rockefeller Foundation, the Harriman railroad fortune, Harvard University, Princeton University, Yale University, Stanford University, the American Medical Association, Margaret Sanger, Oliver Wendell Holmes, Robert Yerkes, Woodrow Wilson, the American Museum of Natural History, the American Genetic Association and a sweeping

---

81 Mary Pesarchick, "Eugenics in America: The Legacy of Sanger and Gates," *Catholic Stand,* August 31, 2017 (accessed April 6, 2020), https://www.catholicstand.com/eugenics-in-america/.

array of government agencies from the obscure Virginia Bureau of Vital Statistics to the U.S. State Department."[82]

Thus, in an environment steeped in this kind of thinking, one should not be surprised that U.S. foreign and domestic policies—and those of its allied states—might turn a blind eye toward policies and behaviors that look a lot like genocide. This is the stuff of which The West is made. Non-Western actors, both state and non-state, and even individual actors, must understand the fullness and totality of this bottom line in order to adequately understand and engage the West. Technological advances can only worsen this situation unless there are fundamental values changes in the U.S. and The West, accompanied by a significant shift in power to the rest of the non-Western world.

What, then, are the interlinkages that exist between the government of the People's Republic of China and/or institutions located there and the organizations mentioned above, particularly in the biomedical or biotechnology fields? What does such collaboration mean for the Chinese people and for the rest of the non-Western world that looks to China for help in the balancing act that smaller states have to perform in their relations with The West? Or rather, in the absence of a multipolar world, will The West have no choice—in the face of dwindling population—to rely more and more on technologies for the few that control the many? (The population of Europeans has been stagnating and in some cases, actually declining for some time now—as the 2017 and 2020 population growth rate charts below demonstrate.)

Any shift away from a unipolar world to a more multipolar world will give breathing room to smaller countries and allow them to exercise a modicum of sovereignty otherwise non-existent in a unipolar world led by the U.S. and The West. Such a multipolar world will also usher in the end of Wolfensohn's "80-20 Rule"—as he indeed predicted in that same speech before the Stanford MBA students.

Are Chinese relationships with certain organizations from the West a cause for concern or alarm? Putin recently expelled George Soros organizations that were operating in Russia. I would love to be able to delve deeply into these questions in the search for more answers. That is not going to be possible here. However, I will try to provide an overview of a few of the concerns that I have seen expressed.

---

82 Edwin Black, *War Against the Weak: Eugenics and America's Campaign to Create a Master Race* (New York: Four Walls Eight Windows, 2003).

Which Way, China?

In an April, 2020 *Geopolitics and Empire* interview, Dr. Francis Boyle, who drafted the U.S. implementing legislation for the Biological Weapons Convention (the U.S. Biological Weapons Anti-Terrorism Act of 1989), alleged that China is attempting to develop "dual use"[83] (both defensive and offensive) biological weapons because now it too has a Level 4 bio lab of the type that the United States has and supports throughout the world to research and develop "defensive" biological weapons that the U.S. has then actually used offensively. Boyle believes that the Chinese either stole or bought access to U.S. or Western technology and he points to two studies to provide evidence for his point:

1. A 2010 study of SARS and HIV carried out by the Chinese, Americans and Australians; and

2. A 2015 study into how to make SARS more lethal carried out by the FDA, U.S. and Swiss-based scientists.

The purpose of the 2010 study entitled, "Angiotensin-converting enzyme 2 (ACE2) proteins of different bat species confer variable susceptibility to SARS-CoV entry," was to understand exactly which bats might be reservoirs for SARS-CoV. In order to answer this question, an HIV–SARS-CoV preparation was made. The 2003 epidemic caused by SARS-CoV killed mostly people from China, Hong Kong, Vietnam, Singapore, and Canada. The Chinese, in 2010, were still trying to understand where SARS-CoV had come from. According to the U.S. C.D.C, there have been no known cases of SARS-CoV reported since 2004. The 2010 study was carried out by scientists from the Wuhan Institute of Virology, the Australian Animal Health Laboratory, and University of Minnesota Medical School.

Dr. Boyle sees sinister roots in the 2015 study, too. The purpose of the study was to examine the disease potential in humans of a known bat virus then circulating in China and the possibility of effective use of vaccines against the virus. The result of the study showed increased pathogenesis both *in vitro* and in mice *in vivo* occurring, with the effort at a vaccine failing. Because the U.S. government had paused "gain-of-function" studies that sought increased lethality, the scientists wrote of this study: "On the basis of these findings, scientific review panels may deem similar studies building chimeric viruses based on circulating strains too risky to pursue, as increased pathogenicity in mammalian models cannot

---

83 "Transcript: Bioweapons Expert Dr. Francis Boyle on Coronavirus," *GreatGameIndia,* February 5, 2020 (accessed April 7, 2020), https://greatgameindia.com/transcript-bioweapons-expert-dr-francis-boyle-on-coronavirus/.

be excluded."[84] The 2015 study was carried out by scientists from the University of North Carolina at Chapel Hill, the U.S. Federal Drug Administration, the Wuhan Institute of Virology, Bellinzona Institute of Microbiology in Switzerland, and Harvard Medical School. Interestingly, the authors omitted acknowledging USAID as a funding source in their original submission for publication, only correcting that eleven days after publication.

The 2010 study sets off alarm bells for Boyle for many reasons. Because of the Indian study that found HIV-like similarities in SARS-CoV-2 that was then affirmed by a Chinese study. Moreover, early on, Chinese doctors were using HIV drugs on themselves to treat their own mild infections. Then, another study produced news reports that testes could be affected by the new disease, possibly affecting fertility. The *South China Morning Post* wrote, "Both Covid-19 and SARS invade cells by combining with an enzyme called ACE2, which exists in large amounts in the testicles, as well as in other organs like the kidneys and heart." Like the Indian study, this study, too, was soon deleted from government websites.[85]

The 2015 study is important because the scientists performed this study during the pause that the U.S. government had imposed on this kind of research, deeming it too risky. The reason for the pause was consideration of the high possibility that the enhanced virus could escape the laboratory and could cause risks to the public. In fact, according to *Business Insider*, the U.S. National Institutes of Health found repeated dangerous slip-ups with pathogens:

> In one case, the NIH discovered that vials of smallpox had just been sitting in a cold storage room of a Food and Drug Administration lab (there are only two labs in the world authorized to possess smallpox, one at the CDC in Atlanta and another in Russia). In another case, the CDC accidentally exposed more than 75 workers to anthrax.

Remarkably, in 2017, the U.S. then lifted the ban on "gain-of-function" research despite security risks and the most lethal research was again "business-as-usual." One Chinese scientist explained the difference between SARS and COVID-19 for the *Thailand Medical News*. He said, "This finding suggests that 2019-nCoV coronavirus [SARS-CoV-2] may be significantly different from the

---

84 Vineet D. Menachery, "A SARS-like cluster of circulating bat coronaviruses shows potential for human emergence," *Nature Medicine* 21:12, November 9, 2015 (accessed April 7, 2020), https://www.nature.com/articles/nm.3985.

85 Caibin Fan, et al. "ACE2 Expression in Kidney and Testis May Cause Kidney and Testis Damage After 2019-nCoV Infection," *MedRxiv*, February 13, 2020 (accessed April 8, 2020), https://www.medrxiv.org/content/10.1101/2020.02.12.20022418v1.

SARS coronavirus in the infection pathway and has the added potency of using the packing mechanisms of other viruses such as HIV." This is exactly the kind of research that could produce a bioweapon. Boyle fears that China's research might have this as a goal.

Boyle considers all of this research done by all parties to be in violation of the Bioweapons Convention. If this is what the U.S. is doing, who can stop the U.S.? And what are the consequences of trying? A bioweapons arms race? That's as insane as was the nuclear arms race. But we lived through those insane times after the U.S. actually used nuclear weapons.

Is China's replication of these Level 4 biolabs an effort to understand and defend against the intentions of The West (as I am inclined to believe)? Boyle seems to believe that China and Russia are preparing to respond to the U.S. in kind. Boyle continues in this interview, "Basically, this is offensive biological weapons raised by the United States government and with its assistance in Canada and Britain. And so other States, the world have responded accordingly including Russia and China. They were going to set up a whole series of BSL-4 facilities as well. And you know Wuhan was the first. It backfired on them."[86] Without providing further evidence than the existence of the Wuhan BSL1-4 lab and the prior joint research efforts cited above, Dr. Boyle asserts that Ground Zero for the outbreak of SARS-CoV-2 is the Huanan Seafood Market, and that it got there via an accidental leak from the Wuhan lab, presumably replicating the kind of negligence reflected in the many accidents at American BSL-4 labs that Dr. Boyle cites in his 2005 book, *Biowarfare and Terrorism.*

The Chinese government contests such a view. Rather, it has publicly accused the U.S. of bringing the disease—not necessarily maliciously—to China, to Wuhan, during the World Military Games, a kind of Olympics for soldiers. It was during these games that some U.S. soldiers presented themselves with a "mysterious disease" unseen before at the hospital in Wuhan. Then, the CDC Director admitted before Congress that some deaths in the U.S. had been labeled the flu, but were actually COVID-19 deaths. In fact, the CDC had shut down USAMRIID at Fort Detrick in August, just before the October 2020 World Military Games for breaches discussed earlier.

At this writing, we still have no Patient Zero and no Ground Zero, either.

When you combine that with the publicly stated desire on the part of the Chinese to study Ebola in their Level 4 biolab—as it is clear that they were also studying HIV—from a U.S. government point of view, and now let me break out my Southern, here: "There ain't no telling what kind of 'boogers and haints'[87]

---

86 Ibid.

87 "Boogers and haints" was a term used down at the Georgia Legislature when I was a State Representative to mean all that ugly stuff that no one wants anyone to know about,

the Chinese would find once they conducted authoritative investigations into the origins of these diseases."

No wonder President Donald Trump had his staff write a letter on February 3, 2020 demanding to know the origin of the SARS-CoV-2 virus in light of scientists finding HIV-like inserts. Interestingly, after that letter, all COVID-19 meetings were classified, meaning that the information about the meetings' contents are all restricted. Once again, it appears Donald Trump, oblivious to protocol (that is to say, to obfuscation) has shed unwitting light where powerful actors might prefer it not to shine.

In the meantime, U.S. lawyer Larry Kudlow of Freedom Watch filed a $20 trillion lawsuit against China for unleashing SARS-CoV-2 and COVID-19 on the world and waging biological warfare against the world. The lawsuit was filed against the People's Republic of China and the People's Liberation Army and the Wuhan Institute of Virology and Shi Zhengli, Director of the Wuhan Institute and Major General Chen Wei of the People's Liberation Army.[88] Kudlow alleges that China violated the BWC and the Justice Against Sponsors of Terrorism Act by creating and releasing a bioweapon.

It is clear where some want the blame to lie.

THE CURIOUS CASES OF SARS, MERS, AND COVID-19

At the beginning of the SARS outbreak, Asians felt besieged. One study found that Asians outside of Asia felt as if they had been unfairly singled out and targeted as "a dirty race" and that the disease was being "racialized," making them the sole target of society's distress."[89] In January 2004, the disease returned to China prompting a cull of wild animals in Guangdong Province that might have contributed to its spread. The case of the 32-year-old television producer who was diagnosed as having SARS was the last person to test positive for the disease that infected almost 8,100 people and killed 774 people, according to the World Health Organization. It took a lot of research for the Chinese to understand exactly how SARS could infect over 8,000 people around the world, killing over 700 of them. And despite spreading to 28 countries, its seeming Asian "selectivity"—not restricted to Asians in Asia. So, what was going on?

---

hidden inside pieces of legislation. According to radio personality Neal Bootz, the phrase was coined by State Representative Ted Hanson: http://freedomkeys.com/boortzisms.htm (accessed April 7, 2020).

88 China Bioweapon Lawsuit (accessed April 8, 2020), https://www.freedomwatchusa. org/pdf/200317-CoronavirusFILEDComplaint177113137478.pdf.

89 Kevin Lee, "SARS and Its Resonating Impact on the Asian Communities," *Lehigh Preserve,* Volume 21, 2013 (accessed April 7, 2020), https://preserve.lehigh.edu/cgi/ viewcontent.cgi?article=1015&context=cas-lehighreview-vol-21.

In 2003, the same year as the outbreak, Chinese scientists were able to isolate how the human body received the virus that caused the disease of SARS, that is, SARS-coronavirus or SARS-CoV. It turns out that SARS-CoV attaches to human cells by way of angiotensin-converting enzyme 2 (ACE2). The scientists wrote, "Together our data indicate that ACE2 is a functional receptor for SARS-CoV.... These data demonstrate that the ability of the SARS-CoV S protein to mediate cell–cell fusion is dependent on the presence of ACE2." Moreover, they found "that ACE2 contributes substantially to the efficiency of SARS-CoV replication." This was an important part of the puzzle, but it didn't complete the picture by a long shot. Their findings were published in *Nature,* a peer-reviewed science journal.[90] The first shoe had dropped. Moreover, the discovery of SARS-CoV led to a stampede toward the patent office.

The second shoe became unlaced with the outbreak of the A(H1N1) flu in 2009. This flu hardly affected the Chinese people at all. Another kind of "selectivity?" Despite starting in Mexico, it was the South America region that was hardest hit by this flu. And China was barely touched. Taking into account differing ethnic susceptibilities would be helpful in building accurate computer models of how virulent a flu outbreak might become, especially in a second wave, the Chinese scientists who authored the 2009 study concluded. Therefore, the study recommended including ethnic viral susceptibility to epidemiological models. (Below is a screenshot of a graph from this 2009 study titled "Mortality rates of selected countries including Mexico, the country of the A (H1N1) outbreak origin.")[91]

A following study in 2012 concluded that "epidemiologic evidence shows that a particular ethnic group may have selected susceptibilities to various pathogens."[92]

Then, in September 2012, the Middle East Respiratory Syndrome (MERS) outbreak emerged in Saudi Arabia. The CDC provides a list of countries that reported MERS cases "in or near the Arabian Peninsula:" Bahrain, Iran, Jordan, Kuwait, Lebanon, Oman, Qatar, Saudi Arabia, United Arab Emirates (UAE), and

---

90 Wenhui Li, et al. "Angiotensin-converting enzyme 2 is a functional receptor for the SARS coronavirus," *Nature,* 2003 (accessed April 8, 2020), https://www.ncbi.nlm.nih.gov/pmc/articles/PMC7095016/.

91 C.L. Chen, "Ethnic differences in susceptibilities to A(H1N1) flu: An epidemic parameter indicating a weak viral virulence," *African Journal of Biotechnology* 8:25, December 2009 (accessed April 8, 2020), located at https://www.ajol.info/index.php/ajb/article/view/77746.

92 Kunlong Dung, "Chinese Residents to SARS and H1N1 Flu: Their Potential Value in Viral Virulence Estimation," *Advanced Science Letters,* 16:1, September 2012 (accessed April 9, 2020), https://www.ingentaconnect.com/content/asp/asl/2012/00000016/00000001/art00026.

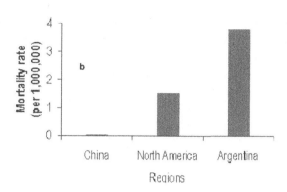

Yemen. Then travelers to and from the Arabian Peninsula carried MERS to other countries; for example, the U.S. experienced two cases from travel. The CDC goes on to report that more than 750 people tested negative in the U.S. MERS had been found in camels, believed to be the method of human transmission. Not much else is reported by the CDC on its MERS Factsheet. In 2014, Science Direct noted that "Bats are the major suspects in terms of zoonotic origin of both SARS and MERS-CoV."[93] Meanwhile, Rebecca Kreston, writing for Discover blog was preparing to make it easier for the other shoe to drop: she reported that "men have made up the majority of infected cases" and noted "the low rates of infection among women."[94] She also observes that Saudi Arabia is host to the Hajj, a religious pilgrimage that welcomes Muslims from all over the world. Less than one year out from the first case of MERS, she writes,

> The Hajj is a powerfully holy and social event for Muslims. But it's also unique from an epidemiological and public health standpoint: two to three million people from 70 countries meeting in one tiny place is the siren call for respiratory, water-borne and blood-borne microbial diseases. This year Saudi Arabian officials will have their hands full as they monitor and protect their pilgrims from a smorgasbord of pathogens that know no geographic borders, class or religion.[95]

93 Jaffar A. Al-Tawfiq and Ziad A. Memish, "Middle East Respiratory Syndrome-Coronavirus (MERS-CoV) Infection," *Emerging Infectious Diseases,* 2014 (accessed April 9, 2020), https://www.sciencedirect.com/topics/medicine-and-dentistry/middle-east-respiratory-syndrome-coronavirus.

94 Rebecca Kreston, "Purdah? I Hardly Know Ya!: Social Influences On Middle East Respiratory Syndrome," *Discover Blog,* June 30, 2013 (accessed April 9, 2020), https://www.discovermagazine.com/health/purdah-i-hardly-know-ya-social-influences-on-middle-east-respiratory-syndrome.

95 Kreston, "The Endless Public Health Challenges of the Hajj," *Discover Blog,* October 9, 2013 (accessed April 9, 2020), https://www.discovermagazine.com/health/the-

Al-Tawfiq and Memish write, "MERS-CoV appears to have a predilection for individuals with underlying medical comorbidities."[96] MERS-CoV was the first human coronavirus in the C lineage of BetaCoronaviruses.

And then, in 2020, came SARS-CoV-2 and COVID-19. According to the CDC, "Sometimes coronaviruses that infect animals can evolve and make people sick and become a new human coronavirus. Three recent examples of this are 2019-nCoV [SARS-CoV-2], SARS-CoV, and MERS-CoV."[97]

In January 2020, a group of Shanghai-based scientists wrote about a study performed on a small set of donors of differing races and genders:

> We further compared the characteristics of the donors and their ACE2 expressing patterns. No association was detected between the ACE2-expressing cell number and the age or smoking status of donors. Of note, the 2 male donors have a higher ACE2-expressing cell ratio than all other 6 female donors (1.66% vs. 0.41% of all cells, P value=0.07, Mann Whitney Test). In addition, the distribution of ACE2 is also more widespread in male donors than females: at least 5 different types of cells in male lung express this receptor, while only 2~4 types of cells in female lung express the receptor. This result is highly consistent with the epidemic investigation showing that most of the confirmed 2019-nCov [SARS-CoV-2] infected patients were men (30 vs. 11, by Jan 2, 2020).
>
> We also noticed that the only Asian donor (male) has a much higher ACE2-expressing cell ratio than white and African American donors (2.50% vs. 0.47% of all cells). This might explain the observation that the new Coronavirus pandemic and previous SARS-Cov pandemic are concentrated in the Asian area. [See Figure 2.][98]

This and other like studies caused Juergen Steinmetz, publisher of eTruboNews, a travel and tourism media outlet, to Headline the following on February 10, 2020: "Coronavirus risk for Asians, Africans, Caucasians revealed: Japanese and Chinese at highest risk for Coronavirus." He went on to write, "East Asians, Japanese, and Han Chinese are the most likely people to become severely sick by

---

endless-public-health-challenges-of-the-hajj.

96 Al-Tawfiq and Memish, op. cit.

97 CDC, "Human Coronavirus Types," https://www.cdc.gov/coronavirus/types.html (accessed April 9, 2020).

98 Yu Zhao, et al. "Single-cell RNA expression profiling of ACE2, the putative receptor of Wuhan 2019-nCov," *BioRxiv* (accessed April 9, 2020), https://www.biorxiv.org/content/10.1101/2020.01.26.919985v1.full.

	AGE	SEX	RACE	Smoking Status	Single Cell Number
Donor 1	63	F	African American	Never	5370
Donor 2	55	M	Asian	Former	3813
Donor 3	29	F	African American	Never	5150
Donor 4	57	F	African American	Never	5142
Donor 5	49	F	White	Active	5275
Donor 6	22	F	African American	Never	4208
Donor 7	47	F	White	Active	7446
Donor 8	21	M	African American	Never	6730

Figure 2.

the coronavirus with a chance of more than 90% when exposed. Europeans only rank in the 50%, Africans in the 60% range, and considered low to medium. It also makes a difference if one is a smoker or non-smoker." In plain English, he adds, "East Asians and men have more than say white Europeans and women. Being a white woman seems to be the way to have much lesser risk." Steinmetz goes on to delineate the danger:

> According to this preliminary study the risk of obtaining the virus:
> High risk 90%-99%
> Japanese in Tokyo, Japan
> Southern Han Chinese
> Kinh in Ho Chi Minh City, Vietnam
> Han Chinese in Bejing, China
> Chinese Dai in Xishuangbanna, China[99]

On February 24, the Chinese study entitled, "Comparative genetic analysis of the novel coronavirus (2019-nCoV/SARS-CoV-2) receptor ACE2 in different populations" would cause the other shoe to drop. It basically confirmed the findings of the January Shanghai study while also allowing for differing outcomes based on different methodologies. Lead scientist Yanan Cao and his group of eight other Shanghai-based scientists found that:

---

99 Juergen T. Steinmetz, "Coronavirus risk for Asians, Africans, Caucasians revealed," *ETurboNews,* February 10, 2020 (accessed April 9, 2020), https://www.eturbonews.com/542533/coronavirus-risk-for-asians-africans-caucasians-revealed/.

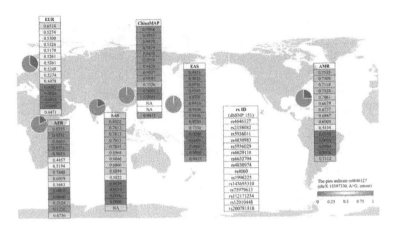

Figure 3.
[screenshot]

Recent reports of the ACE2 expression analysis in lung tissues from Asian and Caucasian populations are still controversial. The single-cell RNA-seq analysis reported that the Asian donor had much higher ACE2 expression cell ratio than white and African-American donors. In contrast, the ACE2 expression analysis using the RNA-seq and microarray datasets from control lung tissues indicated there were no significant differences between Asian and Caucasian, or male and female.[100]

Cao et al., however, produced the chart in Figure 3 above that seems to provide evidence for the conclusions drawn by Steinmetz in his article about who is most at risk of dying from SARS-CoV-2.

Finally, if these scientists are correct, then there is certainly, seemingly, some "selectivity" on the part of this new lineage of Betacoronaviruses represented by SARS-CoV, MERS-CoV, and SARS-CoV-2. What this all means is undeniably subject to the expertise of those who are better-trained in these matters than me.

---

100 Yanan Cao, et al., "Comparative genetic analysis of the novel coronavirus (2019-nCoV/SARS-CoV-2) receptor ACE2 in different populations," *Nature, Cell Discovery* 6:11, February 24, 2020 (accessed April 9, 2020), https://www.nature.com/articles/s41421-020-0147-1

PREVENTING BIOWARFARE

Will the new biowarfare-related sciences give different people the opportunity to take action based on their eugenicist convictions? Here are some still unresolved questions we might ponder, and some actions we might wish to prescribe:

1. Should the pharmaceuticals industries be nationalized to remove the profit incentive related to vaccine and antiviral production and to ensure their domestic availability?

2. How can all Level 3 and Level 4 biolabs, public and private, be monitored?

3. Should BSL-4 Labs be prohibited from developing "gain of function" viruses, pursuing the discovery of potentially threatening viruses and developing methods to support viral propagation, so that virus can be used for downstream studies?[101]

4. Should the global patents system related to vaccines and other antidotes to deadly viruses be abolished? Why is such research not in the public domain?

5. Why was the U.S. collecting DNA samples of Chinese[102] and Russians[103] surreptitiously?

6. What about the rights of small states when it comes to access to information about emergent diseases?

7. Why is research not in the public domain, with some privately owned peer-reviewed publishing companies—all owned by Western, mostly U.S. and U.K. companies, by the way, papers—charging as much as $100 for a single paper?

8. Why are education, knowledge, and health profitable pursuits for private individuals and companies?

9. What are Chinese geneticists' views of eugenics, even within their own group?

10. What role did MK Naomi (see Appendix) play in the creation of HIV?

11. Do pandemics demonstrate that healthcare for all is a necessity in order to protect the health of all?

---

101 See the chapter by Whitney Webb, "Bats, Gene Editing, DARPA and Bioweapons," herein.

102 Alliance for Human Resource Protection, "Article," May 21, 2002 (accessed April 6, 2020), https://ahrp.org/article-30/.

103 "Russian biological samples 'collected for research' – US Air Force," *RT*, November 1, 2017 (accessed April 6, 2020), https://www.rt.com/news/408416-russians-biological-samples-research/.

12. Did the COVID-19 pandemic originate in China or in the U.S.?

13. Was the virus human-originated rather than natural?

14. Was its release intentional—an act of biowarfare?

15. Is there a relationship between 5G technology and coronaviruses (that occur naturally in the human body), especially since the emergence of COVID-19?[104]

16. Has Frances Cress Welsing been vindicated?

I would love to have been able to apply the Peter Dale Scott Deep State/Deep Event template to my findings with respect to COVID-19, but I suspect that is an entirely new Chapter or maybe even a new book![105]

CONCLUSION

Just as the powers that be never let a good crisis go to waste, neither should we. As they are weakened and flailing, and we are jolted out of our complacency and forced to realize our medical common interests and endangerment, this is our opportunity to forge a new social reality in which science serves to illuminate, educate and better the wellbeing of humanity. Unfortunately, so many countries in the West seem to be saddled with leadership that alienates, misappropriates, and contaminates everything and everyone with its misleadership. We need a new way of living and a new way of being. Dr. Martin Luther King, Jr. said that we need a revolution in values. And then action. Let's get to it. Let truth, justice, peace, and dignity reign.

---

104 For more on this topic, please see "5G 'Mobile' Communications," *Physicians for Safe Technology,* updated June 23, 2020 (accessed July 22, 2020), https://mdsafetech.org/problems/5g/; and M. Fioranelli et al., "5G Technology and induction of coronavirus in skin cells," *Journal of Biological Regulators and Homeostatic Agents,* July 16, 2020 (accessed July 22, 2020), https://pubmed.ncbi.nlm.nih.gov/32668870/.

105 For an example of how the Peter Dale Scott Deep State/Deep Event analysis tool could work, please see "Je ne sais pas qui je suis," in Kevin Barrett, ed., *We are Not Charlie Hebdo! Free Thinkers Question the French 9/11* (Lone Rock, Wisconsin: Sifting and Winnowing Books, 2015), where I use the Scott template to analyze whether or not there could have been Deep State involvement in the "Je Suis Charlie!" movement in France.

POSTSCRIPT

This book was written between April and July. Information is being unveiled and events are unfolding rapidly. Literally, as chapters were being written, the need for updates became evident; and some chapters were updated as many as three times! I suspect that updates to the updated material presented here will be required because, in some instances, what we know is being overwritten by what those who are now controlling events want us to know through their media. On the last day before submitting the final version of this text to the publishers for type-setting, I spoke on a teleconference with Dr. Stella Immanuel, a much-maligned Christian doctor, who gave a speech on the steps of the U.S. Supreme Court in Washington, D.C., and was immediately censored by Facebook and Twitter due to her remarks in support of the 75+ year-old anti-malaria drug, Hydroxychloroquine. On the call with her were other pastors and doctors outraged by what they consider to be needless deaths occurring now, due to the denial of Hydroxychloroquine as a potential cure for COVID-19. They believe that politics and powerful pecuniary interests have prioritized profits and social control to the detriment of the interests of the people. The July 30, 2020 death of African-American politician and businessman, Herman Cain, only punctuated their outrage. Following is a message directly from the participants on this conference call, who are physicians and pastors, both Black and White, and who feel targeted by COVID-19:

> We The People of the United States of America believe that the people of the U.S. might be under attack by way of the use of a financial bioterror weapon designed to force long-tem control over the masses via indoctrination and subjugation to the Military Medical Congressional (Judiciary) Media Industrial Complex, marking all for mandatory vaccines—that may not be needed and might be detrimental. COVID-19 preferentially kills Black, Brown, Native, Diabetic, and Elderly Americans, and this vaccine may preferentially harm as well. Why so anti hydroxychloroquine (HCQ) and zinc and vitamins D3&C? Answer: if Zinc + HCQ is taken early, prior to Covid infection, the spike protein cannot bind to cells and virus cannot be taken intracellular and hide while replicating. With HCQ the virus remains outside the lung and heart cells so that T cells can see the Covid and make Interferon and create primal T cell immunity. Zinc blocks intracellular RNA polymerase but is a charged ion and cannot enter cells without an ionophore to open a channel and allow Zinc entry. Elderberry and Quercetin are zinc ionophores, although HCQ

is one of the best Zinc ionophores because of the long half life of at least 22 days. Zinc and HCQ early will stop Covid replication. So those who take zinc + HCQ may not have to isolate, contact trace, and may not need a vaccine. Those with lung symptoms may also need azithromycin (ZPac). HCQ breaks the plan of "Darkest Winter" 2020. That is why Governors and pharmacy boards must stop HCQ use at all costs. Darkest Winter mandates our U.S. military vaccinate the masses, Black and Brown people first.

APPENDICES

U. S. Department of Justice

Criminal Division

FAX SENT

Washington, D.C. 20530

Via Telefax   NOV – 3 1998

Rabbi Abraham Cooper
Associate Dean
Simon Wiesenthal Center
9760 West Pico Boulevard
Los Angeles, CA 90035-4792

Dear Abe:

Thank you for your letter of September 8, 1998, and
congratulations once again on the Center's successful and
historic August 16 international videoconference on World War II-
era Japanese atrocities. By holding this conference and by
preserving it on the Internet, the Center has made a significant
contribution to the historical record regarding an important
aspect of World War II that is still too little known.

In response to your specific questions about Unit 731, I can
confirm that all former members of Unit 731 of the Japanese
Imperial Army, as well as all Japanese military and civilian
personnel who were involved in Axis-sponsored acts of persecution
on the basis of race, religion, national origin or political
opinion during the period of Japan's alliance with Nazi Germany,
are ineligible to enter the United States under the provisions of
the Holtzman Amendment, 8 U.S.C. 1182(a)(3)(E). These provisions
also apply to individuals who participated in the atrocities at
Nanjing (which occurred after Japan signed the Anti-Comintern
Pact with Germany) and in the operation or utilization of so-
called "comfort stations" where women and girls were routinely
raped, brutalized, and sometimes murdered by Japanese military
personnel.

As you know, in addition to investigating suspected Axis
persecutors who have obtained U.S. citizenship or are residing in
the United States, OSI is charged with responsibility for
preventing the entry of such persons into the United States.
OSI's intensive efforts to identify suspected Axis persecutors
and have their names added to the U.S. Government's so-called
"watchlist" of excludable aliens have resulted in the exclusion
of nearly 150 such individuals at airports and other U.S. ports
of entry since 1989 (when we began compiling statistics on this

[screenshot]

- 2 -

aspect of our work). Last year alone, 23 suspected Axis
persecutors (all of them European suspects) were blocked from
entering. This year, as you will recall, we succeeded for the
first time in stopping a Japanese perpetrator and preventing his
entry into the United States.

OSI's addition of tens of thousands of names to the
interagency border control watchlist is an outgrowth of this
Office's unprecedented investigative effort, spanning nearly two
decades, to identify and obtain birthdate information on
suspected Axis persecutors. We have systematically checked the
names of such individuals against U.S. immigration records. The
names of those suspects who were not found to have immigrated to
the United States (i.e., the overwhelming majority of these
individuals) and who might still be alive have been added to the
watchlist for exclusion from this country. In all, the names of
more than 60,000 suspects have been added to the watchlist at
OSI's behest.

Unfortunately, despite years of work by this Office, we have
been able to identify fewer than a hundred suspected Japanese
participants in World War II-era crimes against humanity
(primarily individuals implicated in the "Unit 731" medical
atrocities and in the so-called "Comfort Women" mass rapes).
There are two reasons for this unfortunate situation. First,
whereas most documents captured by American forces in Europe
during and after the war were microfilmed prior to being returned
to Germany and other countries in Europe, the Department of
Defense decided in the 1960's to return to Japan, *without*
microfilming, nearly all of the vast documentation captured from
Imperial Japan. Second, despite U.S. Government entreaties over
the years, the Government of Japan has failed, to date, to grant
OSI meaningful access to these and related records. Access to
European archives has been crucial to this office's success in
identifying suspected Nazi persecutors who should be barred from
the United States. In addition, the Japanese Government has not
responded to this Office's longstanding request for birthdate
information on individual Japanese suspects whom OSI has
identified without assistance from Tokyo; the first such request
was made in December 1996. Lacking this data, we remain unable
to add these individuals' names to the watchlist and thus cannot
prevent their entry into this country.

Members of my staff are currently preparing a detailed
response to the historical questions posed in your letter of
September 8. That response will be sent to you shortly under
separate cover. Please do not hesitate to contact me should you
have additional questions about this or any other aspect of the

---

- 3 -

Justice Department's efforts to identify persons implicated in
the perpetration of Axis crimes and to remove and/or bar them
from the United States.

Sincerely yours,

Eli M. Rosenbaum
Director
Office of Special Investigations
1001 G. Street, N.W., Suite 1000
Washington, D.C. 20530
Telephone: (202) 616-2492
Fax: (202) 616-2491

[screenshots]

FAX SENT

U.S. Department of Justice

Criminal Division

Washington, D.C. 20530-0001

DEC 17 1998

VIA TELEFAX: 310/553-8007

Rabbi Abraham Cooper
Associate Dean
Simon Wiesenthal Center
9760 West Pico Boulevard
Los Angeles, CA 90035-4792

        Re: U.S. Non-Prosecution of Japanese War Criminals

Dear Abe:

        In my letter of November 3, 1998, I wrote that my staff was
preparing a detailed response to the historical question posed in
your letter of September 8, i.e., did the United States give
blanket immunity to Class A Japanese war criminals in return for
the results of their research and experimentation? Set forth
below is the analysis that I promised in that letter.

        As we have discussed, this issue was raised at the video-
conference arranged by the Wiesenthal Center and broadcast via
satellite and the Internet on August 16, 1998. A participant in
that conference reportedly stated that personnel of Unit 731 of
the Japanese Imperial Army who, "under any definition," were
"Class A" war criminals, were never tried by the International
Military Tribunal - Far East [IMTFE] because the United States
Government granted them immunity in return for their human
experimentation research data. This participant further charged
that the United States, by failing to prosecute Unit 731's
members and by classifying records pertaining to it, had
essentially assisted Japan in covering up the atrocities
perpetrated by the unit.

        This office has confirmed that the allegation regarding the

[screenshot]

-2-

United States' treatment of Unit 731 personnel is accurate, with
one exception: the term "Class A" war criminal was actually
applied only to twenty-eight key leaders and policymakers who
planned and executed Japan's war of aggression.   These
individuals were prosecuted before the IMTFE, nearly all were
convicted, and several were executed.   The members of Unit 731
did not qualify as Class A war criminals, and this office is
unaware of any evidence that immunity was ever conferred on
individuals who were given that designation.

In addition to Class A war criminals, however, the United
States, Australia, China, France, the United Kingdom, the
Netherlands and the Philippines tried 5,416 Japanese military and
government personnel for war crimes and crimes against humanity,
but no member of Unit 731 was ever included in such prosecutions,
to our knowledge.   Although allegations arose soon after the war
that U.S. occupation authorities under General Douglas MacArthur
had granted Unit 731 personnel immunity from prosecution in
return for access to the results of their criminal biological and
chemical warfare experiments, it was for many years impossible to
ascertain the truth about those allegations because the United
States classified its records pertaining to the unit.   In 1981,
after most of those records had been declassified, the Department
of the Army initiated a records review to determine whether the
allegations were true.   Norman M. Covert, the former Chief of
Public Affairs and current Command Historian for the Medical
Research and Materiel Command at Fort Detrick, Maryland (the
former site of the United States' early biological warfare
research programs), reviewed the voluminous records at Fort
Detrick as well as related Supreme Commander Allied Powers [SCAP]
records at the National Records Center at Suitland, Maryland. He
uncovered several documents, all now declassified and in the
public domain, which describe in some detail the biological
warfare data collected by the Japanese and the arrangement made
between the United States and Lieutenant General Shiro Ishii, the
commander of Unit 731.   Covert's findings are outlined in several
Army reports and information papers which, along with the
underlying documentation, have been reviewed by this office.   Two
of these reports, dated November 17, 1981 and May 5, 1982,
confirm that Ishii and his colleagues received immunity from
prosecution and that, in exchange, they provided a great deal of
information to U.S. authorities.

The section of the May 5, 1982 report pertaining to the
grant of immunity from prosecution (which is quoted here with the
permission of the Department of the Army) states as follows:

> 7. *The Joint Chiefs of Staff decided to keep Top Secret
> any information about the Japanese Biological Warfare
> Program.   The Joint State, War, Navy Coordinating
> Committee expressed its desire that the information be
> retained in US hands exclusively and certainly it*

- 3 -

*should be kept from the Soviet Union. The second
driving force in the protection of LTG [Lieutenant
General] Ishii and his associates was the precondition
established by the War Crimes Tribunal in Japan that no
prosecutions would be pursued unless a specific
incident could be identified and a single person
established as the responsible party. This could not
be done in LTG Ishii's case. It could not be said that
LTG Ishii personally ordered the death of prisoners
through experimentation on a particular date using
particular agents. This was the result of the US
withdrawal from Manchuria and the lack of incriminating
evidence from the wealth of material supplied on
testing at the Unit. Immunity from prosecution was
therefore granted to LTG Ishii and his associates and
they in turn provided much information.*

*8. In the memorandum written by Dr. Edward Wetter and
Mr. H.I. Stubblefield for the State, War, Navy
Coordinating Committee for the Far East, the decision
not to prosecute LTG Ishii was discussed. "An
agreement with Ishii and his associates that
information given by them on the Japanese BW
program will be retained in intelligence channels is
equivalent to an agreement that this government will
not prosecute any of those involved in BW activities in
which war crimes were committed."*

*9. Scientists in the US program said the information
was not of significant value, but it was the first data
in which human subjects were described. It indicated
the Japanese program reached a level of expertise in
1939 that was never advanced because of lack of
resources. Any prosecution of LTG Ishii and his
associates would have exposed the Japanese capability
in addition to US expertise. It would have been
difficult to retain such information in US-only hands
in such a case. LTG Ishii was thus able to escape
prosecution. The Joint Chiefs of Staff and SCAP
agreed there would be little gained by such prosecution
and deferred, offering LTG Ishii immunity in exchange
for detailed information.*

In a file memorandum dated June 27, 1995, Mr. Covert states
that since 1982, "the Army and DoD [Department of Defense],

[screenshot]

primarily through this office, have released all information
known in [their] possession on the subject.... All of the
material has previously been released to private citizens, news
media representatives (U.S., Japanese, British and Canadian),
authors, [and] other interested persons." Mr. Covert's research
and the documentation he uncovered at both Fort Detrick and the
National Records Center at Suitland are cited in Sheldon Harris'
1994 book, <u>Factories of Death: Japanese Biological Warfare 1932-
1945 and the American Cover-Up</u>. Professor Harris visited Fort
Detrick while conducting research for his book. He also cites
Covert's May 5, 1982 report several times and quotes, at page
222, the first sentence in Paragraph #9 of that report.

I hope that this information satisfactorily responds to your
question. Please do not hesitate to contact me should you have
additional questions or require further clarification. You may
also wish to contact Mr. Covert directly, as his office has been
designated by the Department of the Army to handle public
inquiries concerning U.S. knowledge of Japanese biological
warfare programs, including questions dealing with the U.S.
decision to decline prosecution. He can be reached at (301) 619-
3326 (voice) or by telefax at (301) 619-3131.

Sincerely yours,

Eli M. Rosenbaum
Director
Office of Special Investigations
United States Department of Justice
Criminal Division
1001 G Street, N.W., Suite 1000
Washington, D.C. 20530
(202) 616-2492; Fax (202) 616-2491

[screenshot]

Inventory of Lethal and Incapacitating Agents Found at a CIA Building
[*screenshot*]

EXHIBIT 2
INVENTORY OF LETHAL AND INCAPACITATING AGENTS
FOUND AT A CIA BUILDING (excerpted
from CIA Inventory)

Material	Class	Quantity	Characteristics	Dose
LETHAL AGENTS:				
Saxitoxin (shellfish toxin)	Lethal	11.405 gr.*	Highly lethal nerve toxin. Attacks cardio-vascular, respiratory, nervous, and muscle systems. Death in seconds.	
Cobra venom	Lethal	8 mg.	Lethal nerve toxin; attacks nervous system.	7 mg.
French compound	Lethal	1.83 gr.	Highly lethal	less than .1 mg.
Aconitum Ferox extract	Lethal	2 gr.	Lethal in overdose	20-40 ml.
Aconitine Nitrate	Lethal	.5 oz.	Lethal	
T-270	Lethal	1 cc		
Colchicine	Lethal	8 gr.	Lethal in overdose; death via muscular paralysis and respiratory failure.	7 mg.
Strychnine	Lethal	5 gr.	Lethal; attacks neuro-muscular system.	

*10.927 gr. of the total were transferred from Ft. Detrick to a CIA Building sometime in February 1970. the remainder (approximately .5 gr. had previously been delivered to the a CIA Building in the mid-1960's.

192

that no damage was done to individuals who volunteer for the experiments."[1] Overseas interrogations utilizing a combination of sodium pentothal and hypnosis after physical and psychiatric examinations of the subjects were also part of ARTICHOKE.

The Office of Scientific Intelligence (OSI), which studied scientific advances by hostile powers, initially led BLUEBIRD/ARTICHOKE efforts. In 1952, overall responsibility for ARTICHOKE was transferred from OSI to the Inspection and Security Office (I&SO), predecessor to the present Office of Security. The CIA's Technical Services and Medical Staffs were to be called upon as needed; OSI would retain liaison function with other government agencies.[2] The change in leadership from an intelligence unit to an operating unit apparently reflected a change in emphasis; from the study of actions by hostile powers to the use, both for offensive and defensive purposes, of special interrogation techniques—primarily hypnosis and truth serums.

Representatives from each Agency unit involved in ARTICHOKE met almost monthly to discuss their progress. These discussions included the planning of overseas interrogations[3] as well as further experimentation in the U.S.

Information about project ARTICHOKE after the fall of 1953 is scarce. The CIA maintains that the project ended in 1956, but evidence suggests that Office of Security and Office of Medical Services use of "special interrogation" techniques continued for several years thereafter.

3. MKNAOMI

MKNAOMI was another major CIA program in this area. In 1967, the CIA summarized the purposes of MKNAOMI:

(a) To provide for a covert support base to meet clandestine operational requirements.

(b) To stockpile severely incapacitating and lethal materials for the specific use of TSD [Technical Services Division].

(c) To maintain in operational readiness special and unique items for the dissemination of biological and chemical materials.

(d) To provide for the required surveillance, testing, upgrading, and evaluation of materials and items in order to assure absence of defects and complete predictability of results to be expected under operational conditions.[4]

Under an agreement reached with the Army in 1952, the Special Operations Division (SOD) at Fort Detrick was to assist CIA in developing, testing, and maintaining biological agents and delivery

---

[1] Memorandum from Robert Taylor, O/DD/P to the Assistant Deputy (Inspection and Security) and Chief of the Medical Staff, 3/22/52.
[2] Memorandum from H. Marshall Chadwell, Assistant Director, Scientific Intelligence, to the Deputy Director/Plans (DDP) "Project ARTICHOKE," 8/29/52.
[3] "Progress Report, Project ARTICHOKE." 1/12/53.
[4] Memorandum from Chief, TSD/Biological Branch to Chief, TSD "MKNAOMI: Funding, Objectives, and Accomplishments," 10/18/67. p. 1. For a fuller description of MKNAOMI and the relationship between CIA and SOD. see p. 360 ff.

[*screenshot*]

systems. By this agreement, CIA acquired the knowledge, skill, and facilities of the Army to develop biological weapons suited for CIA use.

SOD developed darts coated with biological agents and pills containing several different biological agents which could remain potent for weeks or months. SOD also developed a special gun for firing darts coated with a chemical which could allow CIA agents to incapacitate a guard dog, enter an installation secretly, and return the dog to consciousness when leaving. SOD scientists were unable to develop a similar incapacitant for humans. SOD also physically transferred to CIA personnel biological agents in "bulk" form, and delivery devices, including some containing biological agents.

In addition to the CIA's interest in biological weapons for use against humans, it also asked SOD to study use of biological agents against crops and animals. In its 1967 memorandum, the CIA stated:

> Three methods and systems for carrying out a covert attack against crops and causing severe crop loss have been developed and evaluated under field conditions. This was accomplished in anticipation of a requirement which was later developed but was subsequently scrubbed just prior to putting into action.[*]

MKNAOMI was terminated in 1970. On November 25, 1969, President Nixon renounced the use of any form of biological weapons that kill or incapacitate and ordered the disposal of existing stocks of bacteriological weapons. On February 14, 1970, the President clarified the extent of his earlier order and indicated that toxins—chemicals that are not living organisms but are produced by living organisms—were considered biological weapons subject to his previous directive and were to be destroyed. Although instructed to relinquish control of material held for the CIA by SOD, a CIA scientist acquired approximately 11 grams of shellfish toxin from SOD personnel at Fort Detrick which were stored in a little-used CIA laboratory where it went undetected for five years.[10]

4. MKULTRA

MKULTRA was the principal CIA program involving the research and development of chemical and biological agents. It was "concerned with the research and development of chemical, biological, and radiological materials capable of employment in clandestine operations to control human behavior."[11]

In January 1973, MKULTRA records were destroyed by Technical Services Division personnel acting on the verbal orders of Dr. Sidney Gottlieb, Chief of TSD. Dr. Gottlieb has testified, and former Director Helms has confirmed, that in ordering the records destroyed, Dr. Gottlieb was carrying out the verbal order of then DCI Helms.

MKULTRA began with a proposal from the Assistant Deputy Director for Plans, Richard Helms, to the DCI, outlining a special

---

[*] *Ibid*, p. 2.
[*] Senate Select Committee, 9/16/75, Hearings, Vo. 1.
[11] Memorandum from the CIA Inspector General to the Director, 7/26/63.

[screenshot]

References

Brundage, J. F., and Shanks, G. (2008). "Deaths from Bacterial Pneumonia during 1918–19 Influenza Pandemic." *Emerging Infectious Diseases,* 14(8), 1193–1199. https://dx.doi.org/10.3201/eid1408.071313.

Centers for Disease Control and Prevention (May 7, 2018). "1918 Pandemic Flu Symposium Agenda: 100 years of Influenza Pandemics and Practice: 1918–2018." https://www.cdc.gov/flu/pandemic-resources/1918-commemoration/agenda.htm (accessed April 3, 2020).

Chiyuki Aoi, Madoka Futamura & Alessio Patalano (2018). "Introduction 'hybrid warfare in Asia: its meaning and shape.'" *The Pacific Review,* 31:6, 693–713, DOI: 10.1080/09512748.2018.1513548.

Lockwood, Jeffrey A. "Entomological Warfare: History of the Use of Insects as Weapons of War," Bulletin of the Entomological Society of America, 33:2, Summer 1987, 76–82. https://doi.org/10.1093/besa/33.2.76

Nairuba, Joan. "Modern means of warfare and the humanitarian issues involved." https://www.academia.edu/7439736/modern_means_of_warfare_and_the_humanitarian_issues_involved (accessed March 28, 2020).

Pradhan, Pashant (January 30, 2020). "Uncanny similarity of unique inserts in the 2019-nCoV spike protein to HIV-1 gp120 and Gag." https://www.biorxiv.org/content/10.1101/2020.01.30.927871v1.full.pdf (accessed March 27, 2020); https://doi.org/10.1101/2020.01.30.927871 .

Riedel, Stefan, Ph.D., M.D. (October 2004). "Biological warfare and bioterrorism: a historical review." Table 1: Examples of biological and chemical warfare use during the past 2000 years and Table 2: Biological warfare programs during World War II. https://www.ncbi.nlm.nih.gov/pmc/articles/PMC1200679/ (accessed April 5, 2016).

World Health Organization Bulletin (February 2004) https://www.who.int/bulletin/volumes/82/2/News.pdf (accessed April 7, 2020).

Zhou, Peng (January 22, 2020). "Discovery of a novel coronavirus associated with the recent pneumonia outbreak in humans and its potential bat origin." https://www.biorxiv.org/content/10.1101/2020.01.22.914952v1.full (accessed March 27, 2020). https://doi.org/10.1101/2020.01.22.914952.

PART V
Biowarfare:
Dysfunctional, Inconceivable?

CHAPTER TWELVE

BIOWARFARE PAST AS PROLOGUE? THE IMMORAL AND CRIMINAL USE AND PURSUIT OF BIOWEAPONRY

Gary D. Barnett

Those that prevent disease and expose human intervention in virus genomes to create new viruses are heroic, but those that create these new "gain of function" viruses with a view to purposely spreading disease are inhuman. The history of the United States government and its military industrial complex's use of biological and germ warfare against large populations demonstrates their readiness to be compassionless purveyors of death to the innocent. Manmade viruses designed for warfare, whether with a view to causing economic destruction, starvation, or mass death, are the workings of the truly evil among us. Predation at this level could have been and can only be exercised by those in power.

Who would ever have believed that modern warfare could be more brutal, more torturous, more painful, and more harmful to innocents, especially children, than past atrocities committed in war? Human history is haunted by memories of millions sent to their deaths fighting in trenches, of cities obliterated by atomic bombs, entire countries destroyed, and millions purposely left to starve in order advance some leader or nation's interests. Where once nuclear war seemed most likely to signal the end of life as we know it, now uncontrolled and deadly viruses seem the most likely to obliterate the world's population, as one toxin after another is released in acts of hidden war. The madness amplifies with the prospect of retaliation in kind, leading to the further spread worldwide of disease.

As we look at the world today, the actual unleashing of biowarfare is not inconceivable, given the history of the U.S. government and its military industrial complex. In fact, as far as the ruling class is concerned, it has not been inconceivable for some time. The U.S. has had a massive biological warfare program[1] since at least the early 1940s and has used toxic agents against its own population and

---

1 James Corbett, *Corbett Report,* May 1, 2009 (accessed April 18, 2020), https://www.corbettreport.com/articles/20090501_biowarfare_history.htm.

others going back to the 1860s. By 1999, the U.S. government had deployed its chemical and biological weapons arsenal against the Philippines, Puerto Rico, Vietnam, China, North Korea, Laos, Cambodia, Cuba, the Haitian boat people, and even our neighbor, Canada. U.S. citizens have been used as guinea pigs many times as well, and exposed to toxic germ agents and deadly chemicals by government. Keep in mind that this is a short list, as the U.S. is well known for also using proxies to spread its toxic chemicals and germ agents, such as has happened in Iraq and Syria in recent decades.

Since 1999 there have been continued incidences of several different viruses, most of which are presumed to be manmade, including the current SARS-CoV-2 coronavirus variation that is afflicting us today. There is also much evidence of the research and development of race-specific biowarfare agents.[2] This is very troubling. One would think, given the race arguments currently being advanced by post-modern Marxists, that this would consume the mainstream news, and that any activities seeking to advance these atrocious race-specific poisons would be exposed at every level. That is not happening.

While the U.S. is not the only country that is developing and producing bio-warfare agents and viruses—many developed countries around the globe do so as well—the United States, as is the case in every other area of war and killing, is by far the world leader in its inhuman desire to be able to kill entire populations through biological and chemical warfare means. Because these agents are extremely dangerous and uncontrollable, and can spread wildly, the risk not only to isolated targeted populations, but also to the entire world is evident. What if it were discovered and verified that a deadly virus created by the U.S. had been used against another country and in retaliation, that country or others decided to retaliate with other toxic agents against America? Where would this end, and over time, how many billions could be affected in such a scenario?

All indications point to the fact that the most toxic, poisonous, and deadly viruses ever known are being created in labs around the world. In the U.S. think of Fort Detrick, Maryland, Pine Bluff Arsenal, Arkansas, Horn Island, Mississippi, Dugway Proving Ground, Utah, Vigo Ordinance Plant, Indiana, and many others. Think of the fascist partnerships between this government and the pharmaceutical industry. Think of the U.S. military installations positioned all around the globe. Nothing good can come from this, as such biological experimentation is not about finding cures for disease, or about discovering vaccines, but is fundamentally being done for this primary reason: for the purpose of biowarfare, for mass killing and economic destruction.

---

2 Tom Burghardt, "Biological Warfare and the National Security State: A Chronology," *Global Research,* August 9, 2009 (accessed April 21, 2020), https://www.globalresearch. ca/biological-warfare-and-the-national-security-state/14708.

How can such insanity at this level be allowed to continue?

While most everything concerning the creation of poisonous gases, new and more resistant virus strains, and other deadly toxins is mostly kept hidden from the public, U.S. development and use is no secret, and has been known for decades. As George Orwell so presciently stated in his book, *1984*: "In vast laboratories in the Ministry of Peace, and in experimental stations, teams of experts are indefatigably at work searching for new and deadlier gases; or for soluble poisons capable of being produced in such quantities as to destroy the vegetation of whole continents; or for breeds of disease germs immunized against all possible antibodies."[3]

In order to understand the scope of this subject, one must delve into the past so that the root of corruption can be known, and the patterns of U.S. bio-weapon history can be exposed for all to see. It is a sordid past, to be sure, and one that is often overlooked because the truth is not a pleasant sight. While combatants' use of the infected as biological weapons began a few thousand years ago, the modern age of bio-weapon use had its first major impact during WWI. Germany, Britain, France and others used chemical gases during the war, as did the United States after 1917.[4] Initially, Germany was by far the leader in science and chemistry, but that would change after the U.S. entry into the war. By 1918, the U.S. was using large quantities of mustard gas—a gas created by the Germans—and America was becoming more proficient in chemical weapon development and warfare.

> As the American war effort intensified, research expanded to include offensive weapons, resulting in numerous discoveries, including the creation of one of the conflict's only new chemical weapons, an arsenic-based agent similar to mustard gas called lewisite (β-chlorovinyldichloroarsine). Synthesized in his laboratory by Wilfred Lee Lewis, this deadly substance was soon mass-produced by the military under the direction of chemist and future Harvard president James. B. Conant. By July 1918, research and development on agents such as lewisite passed from civilian to military control as the entire chemical weapons program moved from the Bureau of Mines to the Army's newly organized Chemical Warfare Service.[5]

---

3 George Orwell, *1984* (Secker & Warburg, June 8, 1949).

4 Biological warfare and chemical warfare overlap to an extent, as the use of toxins produced by some living organisms is considered under the provisions of both the Biological Weapons Convention and the Chemical Weapons Convention.

5 Gerald J. Fitzgerald, "Chemical Warfare and Medical Response During World War I," *American Journal of Public Health,* 98(4), April 2008, 611–625 (accessed April 14, 2020), https://www.ncbi.nlm.nih.gov/pmc/articles/PMC2376985/.

At that time, chemical warfare research in the United States involved more than 1900 scientists and technicians, making it at that time the largest government research program in American history. By the time the war ended, historians estimated that more than 5500 university-trained scientists and technicians and tens of thousands of industrial workers on both sides of the battle lines worked on chemical weapons. Both the military use and industrial production of chemical weapons presented a number of health risks.[6]

Chemical agents developed during WWI and used by the U.S. included Chlorine, Phosgene, Carbonyl Chloride, Mustard Gas, and Lewisite. The U.S. had begun its programs in earnest, and never looked back. American research, development, and use of bioweapons are long-standing policies, and today the U.S. is by far the world leader in bio-weapon research, development, and production. The U.S. agencies concerned rarely do this for defensive or medical reasons, and if so, usually as a cover for offensive objectives.

There is nothing new about the U.S. using poisonous gasses, chemical weapons, radioactive weapons, nuclear weapons, and bioweapons against other countries, as well as experimenting with many of these types of weapons inside and outside the U.S. on civilians. Forty-five years ago, the Church Committee in the Senate stated that bioweapons were stored at Fort Detrick, Maryland that included anthrax, encephalitis, tuberculosis, shellfish toxins, and other poisons. This was confirmed due to a CIA memo, and exposed during the Church hearings. But the U.S. has been caught time and time again using these horrible weapons against people and countries going back to the middle of the 19th century when American Indians were purposely infected by smallpox-infected blankets.

USING AMERICAN CITIZENS AS GUINEA PIGS

The U.S. government has never been shy about using its own citizens as unwitting test subjects for its bio-weapon experiments. While there are many well-known cases, this has actually happened hundreds of times in U.S. history, demonstrating the utter contempt that those in power have had and have now for the general population of this country.

Some of the more famous incidents include the Tuskegee Syphilis Study[7] in 1932, when two hundred black men with Syphilis were lied to, and purposely not given treatment as an experiment. They all died horrible deaths without their families knowing that they could have been treated.

---

6 Ibid.

7 Ibid

There was the San Francisco biological attack scenario called "Operation Sea Spray"[8] in 1950 when the United States Navy sprayed pneumonia causing bacteria over the city so they could monitor the infections in the residents there. The coast of San Francisco in California was sprayed with two types of bacteria that cause food poisoning and can hurt anyone with a weak immune system.

A year later in 1951, the Norfolk Naval supply Center in Virginia carried out a test by dispersing fungal spores to purposely infect mostly African American workers at the center. This test was meant to find out if these spores would infect African Americans more than Caucasians. It seems that race specific bio-weapon use began earlier than once thought.[9]

In 1955, the U.S. military released Yellow Fever infected mosquitoes over Savannah, Georgia in an event called "Operation Big Buzz," so they could monitor the horrible effects on the people there. This was a planned experiment, but not the only one. From a report in 1981 called "An Evaluation of Entomological Warfare," by William H. Rose, a full report on cost to launch a bio-warfare attack on a city was done, including cost per death estimates. The report stated that these attacks should kill 40% to 50% of all infected. These tests concerning mosquito and other infected insect drops went on for decades.[10]

In 1962, huge increases in bio-weapon testing began when Project 112 was authorized by then U.S. Secretary of Defense, Robert McNamara. This led to massive testing with increased budgets for research. Because of this, one of the tests done took place in the New York subway system. Scientists filled light bulbs with deadly bacteria, and they were shattered on the tracks. The bacteria were spread broadly throughout the system, and exposed tens of thousands of American citizens to those biological agents.[11]

Later, in 1965, prisoners in Philadelphia were used as guinea pigs and subjected to dioxin, the horrible cancer-causing chemical toxin used in Agent Orange. They were studied to verify the resulting cancer.[12] During Vietnam, Agent

---

8 Jim Carlton, "Of Microbes and Mock Attacks: Years Ago, The Military Sprayed Germs on U.S. Cities," *The Wall Street Journal,* October 22, 2001 (accessed April 14, 2020), https://www.wsj.com/articles/SB1003703226697496080.

9 Tom Burghardt, op. cit.

10 William H. Rose, An Evaluation of Entomological Warfare as a Potential Danger to the United States and European NATO Nations, March 1981, in "Attack of the Killer Mosquitos," *The Smoking Gun,* September 28, 1998 (accessed April 21, 2020), http://www.thesmokinggun.com/file/attack-killer-mosquitoes-0.

11 "Project 112," *Wikipedia,* (accessed April 3, 2020), https://en.wikipedia.org/wiki/Project_112.

12 William Robbins, "Dioxin Tests Conducted in 60's on 70 Philadelphia Inmates, Now Unknown," *New York Times,* July 17, 1983 (accessed April 2020), https://www.

Orange was used as a way to destroy and defoliate all of Vietnam from 1961 to 1971. This was meant to starve all the people there, as farmlands and forests were decimated, but that was not all that was destined to be destroyed. The effects on the Vietnamese people were devastating, exposing 4 million innocent people to severe illness, birth defects, and many other health problems. Horrible cancers resulted not just in the Vietnamese, but in American soldiers as well. The extent of environmental and crop damage, and the loss of many animal species was horrendous.[13]

These are but a handful of abhorrent examples of the American government using American citizens as fodder for biological experimentation, experimentation seeking to prepare bioweapons to be used against claimed enemies in the future. How can one describe the mindset necessary to do such heinous things to innocent and unsuspecting people as other than pure evil? Any use of bioweapons against any country or people is immoral, and does not discriminate between men, women, and children. Some agents target every living thing, including animals and plants. This is the nature of biological poisons: to sicken, to sterilize, to maim, to torture, to destroy food supply to induce starvation, and to kill. There is no place for such horror in any civilized society.

COVID-19 SOCIETAL DYSFUNCTION FORESHADOWS THE DANGERS OF BIOWARFARE

The only possible good that could come out of this year's manufactured COVID-19 disaster is the possibility that the unbridled fear awakened in most of the earth's people, and the controlling and maniacal response by governments around the world, will alert a heretofore apathetic humanity to the risk of biological warfare at home. That risk is immense, and to date has not been fully understood by the American public—insofar as they know next to nothing about it.

So long as that risk seemed distant, fearful anxiety over biowarfare was not a factor for the common man. But now things have changed dramatically. This virus, whether or not it is an act of actual biowarfare, has been let loose on the world, forcing Americans to come to grips with what the effects of such a war might be like, should bioweapons be used against them at home. So long as all the risk was outside the country, Americans continued to stand and salute, to sing their nationalistic anthems, and to wave their flags of war. But biowarfare knows no boundaries and is a very unpredictable force that can get out of control quickly,

---

nytimes.com/1983/07/17/us/dioxin-tests-conducted-in-60-s-on-70-philadelphia-inmates-now-unknown.html?&pagewanted=all.

13 "Agent Orange," *Wikipedia* (accessed April 2020), https://en.wikipedia.org/wiki/Agent_Orange.

regardless of the intent of any of the players. Indeed, Americans need to come to understand this truth, because the research and development of these toxins is universal. While the United States government, its military, and its fascist partners in academia and the pharmaceutical industry are certainly the world leaders in the manufacture of bioweapons, many other countries now have bioweapons labs. Given the nature of these lab-created weapons, no one is exempt from the reach of infection or disease that is inherent in these contaminants.

A real risk that has not been given enough attention is that biological weapons can be easily distributed and dispersed among populations. Should the U.S. or any other country purposely use these weapons to infect those in another country, what is to stop any in-kind retaliation? Guns and bombs cannot stop the intentional spread of toxic bioweapons, because they can be carried anywhere, released anywhere, and without detection in most cases. Bioweapons put the entire world at risk and without any real defense against any enemy intent on infecting such a horrific harm.

This may be the most crucial aspect of this argument, because continued research and development leads to the possibility—even likelihood—of the use of bioweapons by any government or group against others. Is it unlikely, even unthinkable, that there would be no retaliation in kind in the future? Once initiated, that retaliation cannot be stopped or controlled.

Americans must bear this in mind: bioweapon development by any country, especially by the U.S., could lead to a biological war. The U.S. is hated by much of the world, and since almost any country can get their hands on bio-weapons, the U.S. has a great risk of being infected, if found to have purposely used viral weapons against any country claimed as an enemy. And there will be no defense against it. No possibility of vaccine development keeping up with the permutations and possible combinations of the virus. Should any country be proved to have manufactured this virus and purposely released it—indeed, should the propaganda organs of any country so argue, irrespective of proof—it would open the door for reprisal, and that reprisal could come from anywhere, just as, in point of fact, the original attack might have. It would be a war based on the spread of highly infectious germs. There would be no winners in such a conflict. All would lose. Retail bioterrorism too carries with it a risk to all mankind, even if initially isolated in scope. The resulting consequences are indeterminable, and brutal beyond sanity.

Many speak of "the alleged use" of bioweapons. This obfuscates the truth that all bioweapons are intentionally manufactured for offensive purposes. Whether they are released by design, or leaked accidentally matters not, for the very act of producing such heinous agents negates the non-charge of "alleged." They all know that these types of weapons that are biologically deadly and created in labs are meant to be a silent killer of masses of people, and intended, while so doing, to keep the guilty party hidden from view. This anonymity quickly becomes irrelevant once suspicions arise, whether accurate or not, and the prospect of revenge rears its ugly head.

Regardless of the type of agent used, whether chemical, biological, or radiological, and regardless of its origin, only one goal is sought. That is to make an organism, whether human, animal, or plant, or all three, completely dysfunctional. The problem now has expanded in scope, this due to the fact that technological advances are changing the landscape of research, development, and deployment of these modern weapons. The science and tools now available allow for such advanced research that any number of new strains of toxins with the ability to spread wildly throughout populations without resistance can be creatively manipulated and produced. The technology is not just available to a few countries, but to very many around the world. Because of this, any tension between countries today could lead to a perilous outcome where an unknown entity could release unknown biological agents in retaliation to an attack. This adds new meaning to false flag attacks, as one could easily play one party against another without ever divulging the true intent, and fatal harm would be widespread. The human race cannot afford to delve into biological weaponry and war. Any use of any harmful biological agent against any population through any means, including war, is pure terrorism against all.

The Origin of SARS-CoV-19 Is Unknown

The new Coronavirus, one in a line of many that were not just likely but most certainly produced by man in laboratories, initially affected almost exclusively the Chinese. This has seemingly opened the floodgates to speculation as to its exact origin. This virus has unique characteristics that have occurred before with SARS and MERS, but it also has genetic material that has never been identified and is not tied to any known animal or human virus. This should be troubling to all, because if this is manmade, it was manufactured as a weapon of war. So, who is responsible for its release? It is possible that this virus was created in China and was "accidentally" released into the population. But insofar as the strain of the virus in Wuhan appears to be especially destructive for people of Chinese descent, does it make sense to think that Chinese scientists or the Chinese government would create or accept to participate in the creation of a Chinese-race specific virus? The mere mention of that raises red flags.

Interestingly, in the past, U.S. universities and NGOs in league with government went to China specifically to do joint research, and at one point, were caught doing illegal biological experimentation, and covertly taking hundreds of thousands of Chinese DNA samples.[14] This was so egregious, in the view of Chinese officials, that forcible removal of these people was the result. Harvard University, one of the major players in this scandal, was accused of stealing the DNA samples, left China with those samples, and continued its illegal bioresearch in the U.S. It is thought that the U.S. military, which puts a completely different spin on the conversation, had commissioned the research in China at the time, and this is more than suspicious. The collection of Chinese DNA could be used to do race-specific bio-weapon research in order to develop race-specific virus strains. Collaboration between these countries has continued, and the biological lab in Wuhan received funding from the U.S. until as late as September 30, 2019. Close-working ties between the two countries remained in place until this supposed new outbreak.

Given that the U.S. had sent 300 military personnel to Wuhan for the world military games taking place there from October 18th to 27th, 2019, just two weeks before the new outbreak allegedly began there, also raises many questions. The U.S. team had always done well in these games, and had bragged about their performance, but on this trip, the U.S. team finished 35th, and little or nothing was mentioned about this failure. Why did they do so badly? Is it just coincidence that the U.S. military was in Wuhan right before the outbreak? Was this group of sol-diers a different group than normal for these games? Could there have been plants to make sure the virus was released? These questions have not been answered, but once again, too many coincidences should lead one to question the narrative, and in this case, questioning the narrative is imperative.[15]

To date, no one knows exactly where this coronavirus outbreak began. Speculation from the U.S. government and its mainstream media always fo-cuses on China, but there is no solid evidence to support that claim. The U.S. in any part of the world, including China, could easily have produced it, but at this time no solid proof is yet available to clarify exactly how or where this virus came from, and how it spread around the world with such speed. One thing that does seem certain is that this virus is not natural or organic in any way, and if in fact it is what is claimed, it was most likely produced in a lab, and then released accidentally or intentionally.

---

14 Yandong Zhao and Wenxia Zhang, "An International Collaborative Genetic Research Project Conducted in China," in Schroeder D., Cook J., Hirsch F., Fenet S., Muthuswamy V. (eds.), *Ethics Dumping* (Springer, Cham), *Springer Link,* December 5, 2017 (accessed April 10, 2020), https://link.springer.com/chapter/10.1007/978-3-319-64731-9_9.

15 "United States at the 2019 Military World Games," *Wikipedia* (accessed April 2020), https://en.wikipedia.org/wiki/United_States_at_the_2019_Military_World_Games.

Finding the origin of this virus, a virus that has allowed governments around the world to take full control of entire populations, is of vital importance. If it were produced in a lab, then finding the source would answer a lot of questions. If it were produced in the U.S. and intentionally released in China, that would be very damning information, and could lead to a similarly covert retaliation. But since this information is not now known and is likely to be suppressed by both sides if known, it is impossible to find the party responsible for such a release. What is clear is that governments, most all governments, have been able to use this pandemic to assert and extend their control over their respective populations and economies. In addition, monetary expansion has exploded, buying governments time, to say nothing of buying favors and enriching those controlling this situation. Governments and their elite controllers, especially the banking magnates, are all taking advantage of this forced response with a view to advancing globalist agendas at a rapid pace. So long as the truth remains hidden, resistance forces flounder, while the people continue to suffer and their dominant groups continue to gain wealth and power.

It cannot be forgotten that the U.S. narrative points to China as blameworthy. But which country's objectives seemed to have been furthered at the outset? The two biggest enemies of the U.S. have for some time been China and Iran. The U.S. had stated desires to destroy the economies of both, and was actively using brutal sanctions, tariffs, and many other protectionist measures to do just that. Once this virus erupted in China, its economy, an economy that was about to surpass that of the U.S., suffered severe shocks. The very next victim country was Iran, and Iran's already shaky economy that had been brutalized by the U.S. also suffered great harm—and they were the first two harmed by this virus outbreak. Once again, are these mere coincidences? The U.S. has had a definite biological lab research presence in China for years, and due to heavy sanctions, economic interference, and a desire to destroy economically both China and Iran, it is telling that these two countries were the first harmed due to coronavirus. These outbreaks have severely impacted two of the primary countries standing in the way of U.S. global control.

THE LONG ARMS OF BIOWARFARE DYSFUNCTION

The dysfunction of biowarfare impacts all aspects of life and the economy. What begins as research to discover deadly and toxic poisons turns into development of those toxins. Once a weaponized version is ready, and the delivery system is in place, it can be released virtually anywhere, and depending on the objective, that deployment can cause sickness and death over large areas. Once this stage is reached, and the diseased victims are aware of an unknown bacterial or viral agent, panic begins to consume the people affected. The more widespread the release and infection, the wider and greater the panic. What allegedly began in China caused panic there, but as this new coronavirus spread, or was said to have spread, the panic increased until it consumed the entire world. This is in essence, the all-encompassing nature of these kinds of evil creations. They have the potential to infect an isolated population but can be made to easily infect many others by mass contagion. Those producing bioweapons fully understand the potential for great harm and panic, but unlike traditional means of war, whose various impacts might be foreseen, predicting all outcomes in biowarfare, once these agents escape, is not possible.

It is staggeringly obvious that people all over the world have now been willing to allow the force of government to dictate their thought and behavior. This is due to the mentality of the herd, for without that dynamic, government fear mongering would be ignored. But the panic that is present today is astounding, and for what? The flu? While panic is a tool that has long been used by government to gain control over the general public, it appears to have been easier to generate more recently, as Americans appear to have become more indoctrinated, and to have learned to trust the most untrustworthy source possible—their government—failing to grasp that they have now lost control over their lives.

Something is amiss here, and corruption in high places seems evident. The CDC has been one of the main drivers of this inflated risk narrative, but CDC is not only in the vaccine business, but also is deeply in bed with the pharmaceutical companies.[16] In other words, the worse the panic, the more money to be made by the CDC and its partners. This should be very troubling to anyone paying attention, but other than in the alternative media, this issue is mostly ignored. (Links at this level should be thoroughly scrutinized.)

So what has changed due to the panic-stricken political authorities' mandates around the globe? Highly increased surveillance, monitoring, and the population control conversation have all been brought to center stage. The large pharmaceutical companies, the WHO, and all its donors and partners, and politicians (of course) are in line to receive huge amounts of money from the World Bank and governments to develop vaccines. Medical and economic martial law has been implemented around the world, and restrictive measures abound. Internet censorship is much more evident, police powers have expanded, economic instability has reached every corner of the planet, and talk of forced vaccination is

---

16 See "CDC Pressed to Acknowledge Industry Funding," *ASH Clinical News,* November 18, 2019 (accessed April 2020), https://www.ashclinicalnews.org/online-exclusives/cdc-pressed-acknowledge-industry-funding/ and "Patents Assigned to Centers For Disease Control and Prevention," *Justia Patents* (accessed April 2020), https://patents.justia.com/assignee/centers-for-disease-control-and-prevention?page=2

widespread. In other words, control over people everywhere has vastly increased, and even if this so-called pandemic were to end suddenly, these tyrannical control measures and the assault on economic activity will remain in place. The adverse effects of this paranoia will not go away quietly. The global elites have already gained much ground over the public due to this viral panic. Control is the name of the game, and this government created panic has allowed for that control to expand greatly. This is a globalist's dream, as this is being presented as a global catastrophe not just now but into the future, leaving the door wide open for more far-reaching global control overall.

The real risk of this so-called pandemic is the prospect of worldwide tyranny that could result, both in individual states and globally. This is much bigger than the impact of an unchecked virus. It could be not just an impetus to such an end, but an initial paradigm, a trial run demonstrating how to achieve much more world government and global control in the future.

When government-created panic becomes evident due to any bio-weapons release, a snowball effect of invasive government action results. Everything works together, as addressing each aspect of biowarfare leads to more totalitarian measures, all stated as intended to protect the safety of the public, but much deceit is evident in this approach. When this began, state governments referred to their purported legal authority in order to take control during the undue panic caused by a virus scare.

To provide medical context to this authority asserted by governments, the Center for Disease Control and Prevention drafted the Model State Emergency Health Powers Act (MSEHPA), designed to authorize "state health officials and their designees to take control of people, property, health care, communications and more in a public health emergency." This horrendous document has been adopted in one form or another by at least 40 states. Anyone with an interest in what is going on should read over this emergency health powers document. It is very scary to say the least. Here is how the controllers see things:[17]

- Articles I and II are for funding and planning for a health emergency.
- Article III covers detection, tracking, identifying and interviewing individuals, information sharing, and enforcement.
- Article IV concerns declaring a state health emergency, emergency powers, executive orders, and enforcement.

---

17 The Center for Law and the Public's Health at Georgetown and Johns Hopkins Universities, *The Model State Emergency Health Powers Act,* December 21, 2001 (accessed March 2020), https://www.aapsonline.org/legis/msehpa2.pdf.

- Article V concerns special powers and management of property. It spells out asserting access to and control of properties, of health care facilities, of all roads and public areas, disposal of human remains, control of all health care supplies, rationing, and destruction of property.

- Article VI concerns additional special powers to "protect society." Some of these include forced vaccination, treatment, isolation and quarantine—with or without warning, forced collection of samples and testing, criminal investigation, and access to all protected health information about individuals.

- Article VII concerns disseminating all information.

- Article VIII concerns what is labeled miscellaneous, but includes the transfer of funds, private liability, and federal supremacy in cases of conflicting law. This is important.

If total control over a population is the intended goal of this type of health emergency plan, there is no doubt that with these powers, there is little restriction to impede the implementation of medical martial law by the self-proclaiming state authorities. Allowing any takeover by government of this magnitude would be tantamount to a population submitting to the self-interested discretion of a ruling class.

The globalist agenda could not have a better excuse for establishing greater world governance and massive economic change than this new disease called COVID--19. Crisis creates opportunity for the ruling elites, as popular dependence on the authoritative ruling class vastly increases in times of fear and stress. Panic and uncertainty lead to a weak and compliant society, one easy to control, and that is exactly what the ruling powers desire. Any bioweapon attack, or mass viral outbreak, regardless of whether it was intentional or not, can only lead to tyrannical measures. The release of this agent creates a perfect storm of attendant ills of all kinds, setting the stage for radical global economic change. Even if the outbreak was unintentional, rather than initiated with any such extensive goal in mind, these changes are already set to take place, awaiting a catalyst.

One of the most important impacts on society of COVID-19 concerns the extent of economic destruction wreaked and to come, and the expansion of aggressive monetary policy in order to facilitate mass wealth transfers to deal with that. Many have been talking about the markets and economic risks apparent in this country and around the world for a long time. I began sounding alarms before 2008, and since that time the markets and the economy have become much worse, and more suspect. After all the manipulation, the Quantitative Easing (QE), and the continued debt growth, it seemed apparent to many knowledgeable people that a massive economic failure was likely in the future. That future is now, and that failure is about to come to fruition. Do the controlling powers that created the likelihood of this economic disaster understand this, and seek to place blame on this new coronavirus outbreak as the cause of all financial ills to come? Was this new coronavirus purposely created and released so that central bankers, investment bankers, corporate heads, and government puppets could use it as cover for an imminent economic collapse that has become impossible to contain?

The Federal Reserve and the Treasury now have been given an unlimited ability to print fake money out of thin air. A trillion dollars a day is being used to buy stocks, and to run the market up and down daily. With this amount of money flowing, trading profits in this high volatility are extreme, and this fraud also serves to falsely hold up a market that should be failing. It gives the appearance of some sort of stability where none exists. It also enriches those who are every day cheating American investors, which includes all those with retirement plans, by manipulating the market in their favor. The most wealthy and powerful will get most all this bailout money, and due to this transfer, they will be able to consolidate even more wealth.

With any financial collapse occurring in the wake of a pandemic, real or not, control over world populations is much easier to implement. Once martial law or medical martial law is in place due to panic, all of society is crippled in the sense that individual liberty and power is lost, economic freedom is restricted, and societal controls such as quarantine become reality. All monetary policy rules will be non-existent, as scrutiny for these measures will be lacking during times of extreme strife. But was that the plan all along?

These measures being forced on the public by the governing bodies stopped much if not most normal economic activity. This spread to all aspects of American society. All gatherings of people were suspended or eliminated. Events nationwide have been stopped, venues were closed down, and the precious right of movement was quickly curtailed. Normal functions required for survival have since become much more difficult or impossible to achieve. Businesses have been shut down, and those dependent on paychecks are facing dire consequences. There has been no thought or compassion evident when political decisions that affect the lives of so many have been arbitrarily mandated under the questionable auspices of safety and protection.

There are multiple agendas being achieved due to COVID-19.

The growing government takeover of all economic affairs is still expanding and has the potential to become all-consuming in nature. The massive economic chaos created out of this structured pandemic will linger for many years. It could change the entire world's economic outlook, and due to measures implemented without thought or caring, could destroy many families and businesses, and bring much more poverty, famine, and death than any virus ever could have achieved.

The economic reality that is America today is one of debt and consumption, and this extends well into the current middle class. By some studies, 70% of Americans have less than $1000 in savings. What will happen when government stipends of whatever kind cease or are never received? What will happen when people have no jobs, no food, and no staples required to live? How will they heat their homes, buy groceries, pay their bills, and handle medical costs for themselves and their families? How will the elderly fare when they are locked up in their homes and isolated without the ability to be with their families? How will the unemployed pay the rent? How will small landlords survive with no rental income? With restrictive laws prohibiting large gatherings and the ability to shop and to travel how will small businesses recover? Even if the coronavirus disappeared today, the devastating economic fallout would remain prevalent in this country for years to come. Already, many are on the edge of poverty, with prices in this country at unheard levels, and increasing constantly. The inflationary aspect of the coronavirus response alone will cause prices to continue to skyrocket at a time when the average American is unable to work, has no savings, and is completely unsure of the future. This is a recipe for economic disaster.

Besides the lockdowns and isolation, a surveillance state has been created the extent of which even science fiction writers would find difficult to imagine. There are a myriad of extremely invasive monitoring techniques already in place around the world, and these will increase as time goes by, as government "predicted" new stages erupt. This is not only heightened surveillance, but draconian measures are being implemented.

Many new terms have been initiated that indicate the level of insanity housed in the halls of government and its pawns in corporate and social media. Some of these are social distancing, self-isolation, phone data tracking, hot spots, shaming, contact tracing, social scoring, essential items, the new normal, obedience signaling, and more to come. The idea is to come up with a totalitarian agenda that sounds benign. The underlying implications of these terms are much more sinister than the terms themselves. That is how propaganda works.

Depending on what part of the world one lives in, many forms of government surveillance are fully in place. Facial recognition is rolling out worldwide, as is phone data tracking. Cell phone monitoring for all movement, including personal contact information, is now becoming rampant, and with that comes new apps that record every movement of any individual. Websites have been set up in order to identify those infected, so that contact can be tracked and avoided. Some airlines actually require blood tests taken on site to see if one is able to fly, and mandatory temperature checks are becoming more widespread in order for many to go to work. Monitoring apps are coming out constantly, and wristbands that sound an alarm if any come within 6 feet of a co-worker or friend are more prevalent. Hand stamps that can be tracked by mobile phones are being used in some parts of the world,[18] and some have been required to take a personal photo every hour and send it in for verification of quarantine.[19] Phone location data in some areas is being used to contact police if a quarantined person moves too far from their address. Tracking all credit card transactions for the purpose of monitoring location of people is being considered, although monitoring credit card transactions has been going on for a long time. The use of drones and robots to monitor citizens is becoming increasingly widespread—to name only some of the surveillance measures; in the future much more invasive surveillance will be forthcoming. These are not temporary measures. They will become the new normal.

Mass Psychological Damage That Leads to Disaster

Fear and panic have driven this monstrous response, and although government and the mainstream media knowingly fed this fear from all angles, the people at large accepted the fraud hook, line, and sinker. The death toll from the state response of shutting down the country, isolating people and families, forcing those most at risk into seclusion, and destroying the economic activity that sustains the lives of all will certainly be responsible for many more deaths than the so-called threat of any virus. From a health perspective, the psychological toll on Americans from this madness perpetrated by government is the real danger. This is the truth that is shunned, as isolation, economic collapse, financial ruin, poverty, bankruptcy, unemployment, and extreme fear will have enormous and deadly ramifications for a long time in the future. The psychological damage alone will be devastating, and sickness, immune system damage, suicide, abuse, and violence will escalate beyond anything imagined. When economic systems across all sectors do not magically go back to normal when things reopen, the fallout from these factors will cause further extensive harm to individuals, families, and businesses.

While the extreme stress caused by massive mainstream media coverage, including expansion of symptoms and morbidity statistics, has been devastating, many more sicknesses, disease, and deaths are occurring simply due to government

---

18 Roli Srivastava and Anuradha Nagaraj, "Privacy fears as India hand stamps suspected coronavirus cases," *Reuters,* March 20, 2020, https://www.reuters.com/article/us-health-coronavirus-privacy-idUSKBN21716U.

19 Pranav Dixit, "This Indian State Wants People In Coronavirus Quarantine To Send Them Selfies Every Hour," *Buzzfeed News,* March 30, 2020, https://www.buzzfeednews.com/article/pranavdixit/karnataka-coronavirus-quarantine-selfies

action. While suicide has been increasing every year, with the onslaught of government interventions due to coronavirus, many risk factors that cause suicide have been greatly enhanced, and this will most likely lead to ongoing higher suicide rates. How many more will kill themselves in the future due to measures initiated by government during this so-called crisis?

The bottom line is this; sickness and death due to the government response to this manufactured pandemic will be multiple times greater than the death toll due to this coronavirus. This fact is certainly known by those implementing these mind-destroying mandates. But it is much worse than that, because the deaths due to this response will continue to rise for years to come, as people struggle to stay afloat in a country whose economy has been destroyed. Early and unnecessary death, suicide, family abuse, violence, despair, starvation, and loneliness will continue to wreak havoc on Americans, causing any number of continuing health problems and death.

THE REAL THREAT TO HUMANITY TODAY IS NOT THE PANDEMIC

While biowarfare risks massive human sickness, suffering, and death, an actual biowarfare attack cannot be proved to have been behind this particular coronavirus event. Rather, it is simply being used to further particular agendas that will increase state power and control over their populations, monetary policy, economies, public and private behavior, and "healthcare." Some have even referred to it as a "plandemic."[20] The global elite desires this for multiple reasons: cover for private economic destruction, massive wealth transfers, the seizure of value-debased assets, the issuance of new digital money, the consolidation of power and control over the 99%, and strengthening the hold on all medical systems with a view to facilitating population control through eugenics and forced

---

20 Dr. Judy Mikovits, *Plandemic,* a film about the global plan to take control of our lives, liberty, health & freedom, May 5, 2020 (accessed May 6, 2020), https://www.youtube.com/watch?v=FnktXOXLhSw.

Additional references: Stephen Lendman, "Is COVID-19 a US Bioweapon?" *David icke,* March 24, 2020, https://www.davidicke.com/article/566369/covid-19-us-bioweapon; Larry Romanoff, "COVID-19: The Truth Has Three Stages," *Critical Studies,* March 24, 2020, https://criticalstudies.org/covid-19-all-truth-has-three-stages/; https://www.corbettreport.com; http://www.lewrockwell.com; and Margaret Sleeboom-Faulkner, "The Harvard case of Xu Xiping: Exploitation of the people, scientific advance, or genetic theft?" *New Genetics and Society* 24(1):57-78, May 2005, *ResearchGate,* https://www.researchgate.net/publication/7225984_The_Harvard_case_of_Xu_Xiping_Exploitation_of_the_people_scientific_advance_or_genetic_theft.

vaccination, among other nefarious agendas. At this time, this is the real threat, and much more dangerous than any virus whether organic or manmade.

The people of the world have now become a collective group of like-acting and like-thinking players in a game fully controlled by deep forces. Few have the desire or capability or knowledge basis to grapple with the issue. Because of this, the acquisition of knowledge that would normally lead to an understanding of conflicts and the contradictions in fraudulent narratives is no longer likely by the people at large. Americans are the worst in this light. In fact, whether with or because of the untold advantages they have enjoyed in this country's history, U.S. citizens are some of the weakest and most indifferent on this planet. To the extent that the world follows the U.S., failure by Americans to grasp and accept the truth will certainly lead to global governance and societal control. Most of the populations on this earth are now relegated to ignorance and are easily manipulated and frightened. If this does not dramatically change, the entire underclass, which now is most all populations, will be subdued.

Much of the reason for the fear can be attributed to the many strategies of deception being propagated by the WHO, the CDC, and by the government and the controlled mainstream media, in order to falsely present huge numbers of coronavirus deaths where few exist. False narratives abound, but due to a very dumbed-down populace, a phenomenon created by design over the past few decades, the task of fooling the public has been relatively easy to achieve.

THE UNITED STATES AS A BIOWARFARE ENEMY OF THE WORLD

The United States government is not to be trusted under any circumstances, given the sordid history of U.S. research, development, and use of deadly chemicals, gas, and toxic biological agents. The U.S. is by far the most prolific and devoted country on earth in its efforts to research, develop, and use biological agents as a means of warfare and geopolitical control. Considering the number of labs in the U.S., is it any wonder that the United States is the world leader in bio-warfare?

There are four laboratory bio-safety levels with levels 3 and 4 handling the most lethal disease-causing agents and organisms. BSL-3 labs work with microbes that are either indigenous or exotic, that can cause serious or potentially lethal disease through inhalation. Some examples include yellow fever, West Nile virus, and the bacteria that causes tuberculosis. Microbes at this level are so serious that the work is often strictly controlled and registered with the appropriate government agencies with personnel under medical surveillance who can receive immunizations for microbes present. The U.S., as of 2007, had a total of 1,356 CDC/USDA registered BSL-3 facilities.

BSL-4 labs, the highest and most dangerous level, work with very highly dangerous and exotic microbes. These microbes are often fatal and have as yet no treatment or vaccines. Some examples of such microbes include Ebola, Marburg, Nipah and Crimean-Congo hemorrhagic fever viruses. These facilities would of course handle the supposed new SARS-CoV-19 strain.[21]

The U.S. has 15 identified BSL-4 facilities inside U.S. borders, including nine federal labs. In addition, there are others around the world in which the U.S. has a presence,[22] but since they are located in other countries, and as information as to exact U.S. involvement is sketchy at best, it is difficult to know the actual extent of American involvement in all bio-weapon research and development. But counting only the 15 known BSL-4 labs, the U.S. has almost 30% of all BSL-4 labs in the world, with the joint ventures overseas not listed or secret making that number higher.[23]

To put this into perspective considering the hype about China during this coronavirus controversy. China has one BSL-4 lab in a country with well over four times the population of the U.S.. That is the lab in Wuhan. The U.S. has had a presence in Wuhan for many years, and actually funded that lab until September 30, 2019.

This massive U.S. commitment to dangerous and deadly biological research and development puts a new spin on where new agents of bio-warfare might originate. If one considers the U.S. preponderant position in military expenditures, nuclear weapons, arms production, and wars of aggression, its extreme level of bioweapon research, development, and use should come as no surprise. Viewed in this light, one might reasonably contend that the U.S. government and those that control it, are engaged in this research for the primary purpose of producing bioweapons for conquest and control. The fact that the United States is producing millions upon millions of liters of poisonous biological pathogens, indicates this can only be for biological warfare. But that warfare is not just against so-called enemies in stated wars but is being used against civilian populations around the world for sinister reasons that are geopolitical in nature. Regardless of who is targeted with these poisons, it is always for evil intent. While most claims by governments and militaries allude to this being research and development for defensive purposes, that is an outright lie perpetrated to fool the masses. Producing in large volumes

21 Arthur Trapolsis, "Do You Know The Difference in Laboratory Biosafety Levels 1, 2, 3 & 4?," *Consolidated Sterilizer Systems,* March 31, 2020 (accessed April 2020).

22 See map, Jeff Brown chapter herein.

23 "Biosafety Level - List of BSL-4 Facilities" *Liquisearch* [Source: Wikipedia Facilities (Creative Commons)] (accessed April 20, 2020), https://www.liquisearch.com/biosafety_level/list_of_bsl-4_facilities.

any agent in a lab that can sicken or kill large numbers of people, plants, and animals is never defensive; it is always offensive.

The global governmental response to COVID-19, the current virus scare, is a manufactured and purposeful conspiracy.

We are at a time of great importance and without recognition of the deeper implications of these current operations by governments and those pulling their strings, we will face an Armageddon where evil will become the controlling force in this country and around the world.

The insanity of bioweapon research, development, and use largely driven by the U.S., threatens not only every American, but puts everyone on earth at risk of sickness, suffering, and death. Due to these risks all of us are also subject to the prospect of abject slavery. The ongoing agenda of the ruling class is power and control of the entire planet, and bio-warfare against humanity is the tool envisaged to accomplish it. Foreign invasion or foreign wars are no longer necessary in order for the U.S. government to control the world's people, both at home and abroad. Once ignorance and apathy have become the defining characteristics of a population, fear will cause them to voluntarily surrender to their own servitude. That is the point we have reached in this country today.

CHAPTER THIRTEEN

THE POST–COVID-19 WORLD: A PERMANENT DYSTOPIA?

Helen Buyniski[1]

Whatever the nature of the novel coronavirus that hit the world in 2019, global reactions to the pandemic will change—indeed already have changed—life on this planet dramatically. It's difficult to deny that this was the goal of the national responses by the U.S., UK, and other powerful governments. Coronavirus has been pressed into service on countless levels as a means to an end, a vehicle for cementing control—of global trade and finance, of society, and ultimately of the individual—by powerful interests who have long been working behind the scenes to effect just such results.

However it began, the "planned chaos" of the greater epidemic is geared toward birthing the same new world order old John D. Rockefeller notoriously spoke about—the new globalist society which figures so prominently in what are pejoratively called "conspiracy theories" by people who believe in a benevolent ruling class. The fingerprints of the recently-deceased plutocrat, David Rockefeller, are all over the events of the last few months, dating all the way back to a publication titled "Scenarios for the Future of Technology and International Development,"[2] a quartet of simulations with a deceptively bland title that the Rockefeller Foundation funded in 2010 in conjunction with the Global Business Network.

The first of the four scenarios included in that publication, called "Lock Step," lays out a near-future in which a global pandemic has driven the world police-state crazy, in which sheer panic caused by a killer virus (like 2019's COVID-19, but deadlier) leads even so-called liberal democracies to look to China's authoritarian

---

1 Research for this article was contributed by Spiro Skouras.

2 *Scenarios for the Future of Technology and International Development,* The Rockefeller Foundation and Global Business Network, May 2010, https://www.nommeraadio.ee/meedia/pdf/RRS/Rockefeller%20Foundation.pdf (accessed April 17, 2020).

response for guidance—and one by one discard their liberal western freedoms in favor of a sanitized, technologically-enhanced Panopticon:

> During the pandemic, national leaders around the world flexed their authority and imposed airtight rules and restrictions, from the mandatory wearing of face masks to body-temperature checks at the entries to communal spaces like train stations and supermarkets. Even after the pandemic faded, this more authoritarian control and oversight of citizens and their activities stuck and even intensified.[3]

If *Lock Step* was the screen treatment for the film that the 2019 coronavirus outbreak has become, Event 201 was the screenplay. A simulation organized by vaccine enthusiast and Microsoft billionaire Bill Gates' Bill & Melinda Gates Foundation with the World Economic Forum, Event 201 was held at Johns Hopkins University's Bloomberg School of Medicine in October 2019. Prominent figures in business and government came together to participate in a "tabletop exercise," war-gaming a pandemic in which a novel coronavirus transmitted from bats to pigs to humans wreaked havoc on the global economy and killed 65 million people. As the real-world events of 2020 began to unfold, the event's host, the Center for Health and Security,[4] posted a disclaimer on its website warning that projections—that scary 65 million death toll—shouldn't be taken as a certainty, but did not take down several hours of video highlights from the exercise, which provide a fascinating window on the movers and shakers of Big Business and Big Government discussing how best to "triage" businesses and human beings with limited resources as a virus very much like Covid-19 lays waste to society.

It's difficult to watch the Event 201 videos[5] without developing a sinking feeling in the pit of the stomach, and this may be the point of leaving the videos up on normally-censorious YouTube. The U.S. Centers for Disease Control has admitted in internal powerpoint presentations that one way to maximize uptake of a new, untested vaccine, especially in the face of public opposition, is to create a sense of urgency and fear in the populace surrounding the disease it is

---

3 "Lock Step Scenario Narrative," *Scenarios for the Future of Technology and International Development,* The Rockefeller Foundation and Global Business Network, May 2010, https://www.nommeraadio.ee/meedia/pdf/RRS/Rockefeller%20Foundation.pdf (accessed April 17, 2020).

4 "The Event 201 Scenario," Event 201: *A Global Pandemic Exercise,* Center for Health Security, accessed April 17, 2020, http://www.centerforhealthsecurity.org/event201/scenario.html.

5 "Event 201 Videos," Event 201: *A Global Pandemic Exercise,* Center for Health Security, accessed April 17, 2020, http://www.centerforhealthsecurity.org/event201/videos.html.

supposed to prevent. As scientists supposedly scramble to develop a cure-all shot for Covid-19, the notion that tens of millions will die if the vaccine is not widely adopted will no doubt encourage not only individuals to rush to their local clinics, but governments to mandate the inoculation for their citizens. No one wants 65 million deaths on their conscience.

The presence of such "predictive programming" has become all but expected to those who study international crises. American media have leapt to draw comparisons between the coronavirus epidemic and the terror attacks of September 11, 2001, perhaps hoping to set the nation on the desired "war footing" that encourages populations to abandon concern for their civil liberties and embrace a jingoistic, unthinking form of patriotism. CNN's Chris Cuomo—himself an alleged coronavirus case—ordered his audience to "surrender the 'me' to 'we'" because "we're in a war"—insisting that complying with an increasingly draconian lockdown was just "doing our part" for the "war effort."[6] Certainly the government response from the U.S. and its allies has powerful echoes of the Patriot Act and other post-9/11 legislation, even as the "enemy" this time around is supposedly a microscopic virus.

However, drawing the obvious parallels between the two crises should invite other, more troubling similarities. By some counts, as many as 46 "drills" by various government agencies echoing certain elements of the 9/11 attacks were underway in the days and weeks before (and even during!) the real-life attacks. Indeed, Johns Hopkins was behind one of those drills—a scenario called "Dark Winter" which simulated a "covert smallpox attack on U.S. citizens," closely resembled the anthrax attacks that followed 9/11 right down to its claims that Saddam Hussein was building secret bioweapons labs and the involvement of an "al-Qaida operative" linked to "Usama bin Laden," and included in its participants notorious WMD propagandist Judith Miller of the *New York Times*.[7]

While pandemic "preparedness" exercises are not inherently sinister and indeed should be regarded as legitimate preparedness called for by government, the echoes with reality in something like Event 201 or Lock Step are too strong and too numerous to write off as coincidence.

As with 9/11, powerful interests shifted into action as soon as the novel coronavirus epidemic was declared, proposing "solutions" that had clearly been devised in advance. They were able to take advantage of the reigning confusion, smoothly assuming control even as many in their own governments were thrown

---

6 *CNN*, "Chris Cuomo: Coronavirus scares me as a parent," video, 5:42, March 17, 2020, https://edition.cnn.com/videos/us/2020/03/17/closing-argument-war-against-coronavirus-cpt-vpx.cnn.

7 "Dark Winter," Center for Health Security, accessed April 17, 2020, http://www.centerforhealthsecurity.org/our-work/events-archive/2001_dark-winter/index.html.

off balance by the crisis. "Simulations" like Lock Step and Event 201 allow powerful factions within the ruling class government-corporate nexus to ensure their interests are put first in any response to a crisis, laying out roadmaps for action while their adversaries are still scratching their heads trying to figure out what happened. By the time some rogue congress(wo)man has gotten around to demanding answers on how suspending habeas corpus or bailing out bloated corporations addicted to their own stock buybacks helps those dying of an unfamiliar plague, the measure has been rushed through and popular consent manufactured in the media.

It is thus impossible to go along with the prevailing narrative that the U.S. somehow "botched" its official response to coronavirus. Having run the simulation (along with representatives from China's Center for Disease Control and several international corporations) just months before at Event 201, Washington's point-people on disease response clearly knew what they were doing when they refused the WHO tests, ordered Dr. Helen Chu of Washington to stop testing her flu patients for coronavirus, and dragged their feet declaring a national emergency. Responding competently would not have created the same atmosphere of panic that ultimately developed, a frenzy that saw even prominent members of the typically anti-government "alternative media" demand lockdowns and mouth the propaganda phrases—"flatten the curve," "social distancing"—that became the scenario's calling card.

Such a crisis state, after all, is necessary to effect massive societal change—a phenomenon Naomi Klein describes in *Shock Doctrine,* and which has been used time and time again with resounding success by an international ruling class with its roots in the U.S., UK, and Israel. The coronavirus epidemic set the stage for a rollout of a nightmarish "new normal" in which everyone is perfectly alienated from their own humanity, outfitted with a biometric ID housing their social credit score and financial data, and wholly dependent on the benevolence of the corporate-state nexus for their next meal.

EMERGENCE OF A POLICE STATE?

Former U.S. President Barack Obama's chief of staff Rahm Emanuel once infamously recommended, "never let a serious crisis go to waste." It would be difficult to imagine an epidemic response better suited to the development of an authoritarian police state than the U.S.' reaction to coronavirus. Just as Lock Step predicted, the U.S.—like Italy, France, and other European "democracies"—took its cue from China and immediately began claiming authoritarian powers under the guise of a medical emergency. The U.S.' constellation of federal- and state-level responses to the epidemic has ripped huge chunks out of the First, Second, Fourth, Fifth, Sixth, Seventh, and arguably Third and Eighth Amendments, a shocking impingement not seen since the Patriot Act trampled the "land of the free" into the ground in the name of fighting terrorism. Given the precedents—emergency after emergency has been declared since 2001, never to be officially concluded—it is highly unlikely these rights will be returned to Americans when the epidemic is officially declared over—*if* the epidemic is officially declared over. And where the U.S. goes, so goes the rest of the world—until they've had enough...

Governments—especially those that style themselves as liberal democracies—have pounced on the coronavirus outbreak as a vehicle to accelerate their enactment of levels of authoritarian control with unprecedented speed. The only comparable example of such a grand-scale "problem-reaction-solution" in the last half century for Americans is 9/11, though the tradition dates back at least to World War 1, when the unconstitutional Espionage & Sedition Acts were used to squelch a rising socialist movement by making it illegal to criticize the war. And just as the Patriot Act, written years before 9/11 and placed in a drawer awaiting a "New Pearl Harbor," was triumphantly passed in the days immediately after the planes hit the towers, so an astonishing array of police state measures have been pulled out of cold storage and introduced—some quietly, and some with much fanfare—in the wake of the coronavirus.

The American government wasn't alone in whipping out its police-state wish-list as it watched China seal off 40 million people behind a giant cordon sanitaire in Hubei province in January. The UK, France, Italy, Australia, Israel, and many other countries seized various opportunities to ram through unpopular "emergency" legislation of their own. Just as predicted in the Lock Step scenario, much of this took the form of emulating China, which in addition to shutting down entire cities, had adopted unprecedented restrictions on internal movement of citizens, tightened controls on information, and deployed the military, constructing massive new hospitals in a matter of days to tackle the epidemic.

But the Chinese Communist Party did not have to nullify any constitution or otherwise violate its own laws in order to obtain the authority for its actions. A strong current of jealousy crackled through western media's hostile coverage of the Chinese coronavirus crackdown, even as pundits like Richard Haass of the Council on Foreign Relations gloated that China's heavy-handed response to the outbreak meant the government was surely on its last legs.[8]

As western governments scrambled to follow in China's footsteps, they had to sell the outbreak as a legitimate reason to suspend the rights of their people. Fortunately, weeks of shocking videos coming out of China—showing people dropping dead in the street, convulsing on gurneys, and other horrors—had

---

8 Richard Haass, "Why the coronavirus should change the way we think about China," *The Washington Post,* February 11, 2020, https://www.washingtonpost.com/opinions/2020/02/11/how-coronavirus-could-change-china.

convinced many that the coronavirus was not something to mess with, and fear-primed populations willingly gave up their rights. States of emergency were declared in some areas with just a handful of cases, and the military was soon rolling through the streets of "democratic" cities from Paris to San Diego.

Just as none of the many emergency measures declared in the U.S. since September 11 have been repealed, these "emergency" measures adopted to "fight" the "war" on coronavirus will not vanish when the virus does. A UK law allowing the indefinite detention of individuals on mere suspicion of having the virus remains in effect for *two years*, meaning not only police but also "public health officers" will—under the bill's vague wording—have the authority to pull people off the street, break up events, and otherwise behave like a military junta long after the epidemic is over.[9] The legislation was supposedly made necessary when a patient tried to "break out" of a quarantine hospital patrolled by armed guards.[10] Trials by jury were suspended across the UK.[11]

Things looked even worse on the other side of the Atlantic, where the Justice Department's requested suspension of habeas corpus, the statute of limitations, and the suspension of other legal protections once included in the Fifth and Sixth Amendment to the Constitution would conclude only upon the "termination of the COVID-19 national emergency or the Chief Justice's finding that the emergency conditions no longer materially affect the functioning of the federal courts." Unless the president were to declare the emergency over (something vanishingly rare in recent U.S. history), these rights could be gone for good.[12] When news the Justice Department was considering such an appalling power grab reached the public, the resulting outcry forced a spokeswoman to clarify that it would be the judicial branch, not the executive—unelected, appointed-for-life judges, rather than an elected president—who would exercise the expanded powers. It's not

---

9 *Coronavirus Bill: Explanatory Notes related to the Coronavirus Bill as introduced in the UK House of Commons,* March 19, 2020 (Bill 122), accessed April 17, 2020, https://publications.parliament.uk/pa/bills/cbill/58-01/0122/en/20122en.pdf.

10 James Tozer and Sophie Borland, "UK police can arrest anyone suspected of being infected with coronavirus," *IOL,* February 11, 2020, https://www.iol.co.za/news/world/uk-police-can-arrest-anyone-suspected-of-being-infected-with-coronavirus-42532401.

11 Chiara Giordano, "Coronavirus: All jury trials suspended in UK and Wales," *Independent,* March 23, 2020, https://www.independent.co.uk/news/uk/crime/coronavirus-trials-suspended-cancelled-jury-england-wales-a9417436.html.

12 Betsy Woodruff Swan, "DOJ seeks new emergency powers amid coronavirus pandemic," *Politico,* March 21, 2020, https://www.politico.com/news/2020/03/21/doj-coronavirus-emergency-powers-140023; Kerri Kupec, DOJ, (@KerriKupecDOJ), "Here's the full thread," Twitter, March 22, 2020, https://twitter.com/KerriKupecDOJ/status/1241938116757381121/photo/1 (accessed April 17, 2020).

clear how that was supposed to help Americans sleep easier at night—perhaps the somber black-robed judge is considered a more responsible steward of absolute power than the orange-skinned Commander in Chief.

The Justice Department even invoked the threat of coronavirus-related terrorism, essentially throwing everything it had at the "problem" of resistance to the shredding of the Constitution. Noting that the virus "appears to meet the statutory definition of a 'biological agent,'" deputy AG Jeffrey Rosen urged law enforcement agencies in a March memo to use "the nation's terrorism-related statutes" to punish "threats or attempts to use COVID-19 as a weapon against Americans."[13] Equating coughing on others—or even threatening to cough—to a deliberate act of terrorism wasn't the limit of the absurdity: the FBI put out a bulletin warning that "white supremacist groups" were urging their members to cough on police and Jews.[14]

People have already been charged under these respiratory-terrorism laws. A New Jersey man faced anywhere from 3 to 7 years in prison for coughing on a supermarket worker, laughing, and telling her he had coronavirus (and that her co-workers were lucky to have jobs); the stupid prank saw him charged with terroristic threats in the third degree, harassment, and obstructing administration of law in the fourth degree.[15] The UK, too, has charged multiple people under stepped-up penalties for malicious display of symptoms, warning anyone who coughs or spits at emergency workers or even threatens to do so that they could be charged with common assault and spend as much as 2 years in jail.[16]

Projecting into the future, it is clear that consent is being manufactured for the permanent suspension of basic judicial rights based on an invisible menace. This opens up a bonanza of opportunities for a police state determined to cleanse its territory of troublesome political dissidents, enabling it to—detain people indefinitely merely on suspicion of having a virus or charging them with terrorism

---

13 Paul LeBlanc, "People intentionally spreading coronavirus could be charged with terrorism, DOJ says," *CNN,* updated March 25, 2020, https://www.cnn.com/2020/03/25/politics/coronavirus-terrorism-justice-department/index.html.

14 Josh Margolin, "White supremacists encouraging their members to spread coronavirus to cops, Jews, FBI says," *ABC News,* March 23, 2020, https://abcnews.go.com/US/white-supremacists-encouraging-members-spread-coronavirus-cops-jews/story?id=69737522.

15 "Man Charged with Terroristic Threats for Allegedly Coughing on Food Store Employee and Telling Her He Has Coronavirus," State of New Jersey, Office of the Attorney General, March 24, 2020, https://www.nj.gov/oag/newsreleases20/pr20200324b.html.

16 Dominic Casciani, "Coronavirus cough attacks a crime, says prosecution chief," *BBC News,* March 26, 2020, https://www.bbc.com/news/uk-52052880.

for coughing. Quarantine facilities could soon fill up with political activists, detained on the basis of dubious and inaccurate tests like those devised by the WHO and CDC[17]—constantly-shifting lists of symptoms further expand the net until literally anyone on the street can be considered a possible coronavirus patient and dealt with accordingly.

The Trump administration's decision to frame the fight against the epidemic as a "war" should unsettle any American concerned with what few rights they retain. Wars have historically been cause for imprisoning massive numbers of people—from Japanese-Americans during World War II to black men during the War on Drugs—and in the last half century, the U.S. has failed to win a single one. The War on Poverty, the War on Cancer, the War on Terror—all have exacerbated the problems they claimed to seek to defeat and dragged on for decades, burning up billions (if not trillions) of dollars even as the government insisted there was no money in the budget for healthcare, housing, or education. Wars are cause for shutting down the press, imposing rationing of goods and services, even drafting segments of the population to help in the "war effort." UK utilities have already warned of potential blackouts, while both U.S. and UK governments have issued calls for retired medical professionals to return to work—essentially a medicalized version of the draft. Putting the country on a war footing also raises the risk that an excuse will be manufactured to swap out the virus-enemy with a real one—Iran, or even China, after both have been softened up by an epidemic that had a curiously voracious appetite for America's enemies.

LOCKED UP

The coronavirus has ushered in unprecedented restrictions on freedom of movement—both within countries and across national borders. While some level of border closure is reasonable under the epidemiological logic of quarantine—and, as Lock Step reminds us, "China did it and it worked" with their unprecedented lockdown of some 50 million people in 17 cities in Hubei province[18]—many countries reacted tardily to news of the pandemic's spread, alternating between foot-dragging and frenzied action, guaranteeing poor decisions would be made too late to achieve anything beyond instilling fear in their citizens. Indeed, one is forced to ask if that was the intent of such haphazard responses in the U.S., given

---

17 Bruce Y. Lee, "For COVID-19 Coronavirus, How Well Do Thermometer Guns Even Work?" *Forbes,* Feb. 16, 2020, https://www.forbes.com/sites/brucelee/2020/02/16/for-covad-19-coronavirus-how-well-do-thermometer-guns-even-work/#2f173deb2af9.

18 Joe McDonald, "China locked down 50 million people and has to keep them fed," *AP News,* January 31, 2020, https://apnews.com/ae3b771d965a635e438cfdeeedb62b71.

the almost yearly "pandemic preparedness exercises" which promised something better.

The EU's refusal to close its borders until mid-March, even as epidemics raging in Italy and Spain, forced hard-hit member countries to institute their own makeshift lockdowns, some riddled with giant loopholes like Spain's crowded commuter rail, which seemed to defeat the purpose utterly.[19] But internal restrictions on movement reached a pathological extreme on the east coast of the U.S. toward the end of March. Densely-populated New York City predictably became a national "hot spot," sending residents scattering into surrounding states, where they were briefly declared criminals. Rhode Island Governor Gina Raimondo issued an order barring New York refugees from her state, warning moneyed Manhattanites that attempting to flee to their homes in the Ocean State would result in having their cars pulled over and ultimately having their homes searched, door to door, by the National Guard. Violators would be forcefully quarantined for two weeks, and those found to be harboring fugitives from the Empire State would be punished with fines and jail time. These disturbingly gestapo-like tactics were only derailed at the last minute by New York's own governor, Andrew Cuomo, who threatened a lawsuit. Rather than repeal the order entirely, Raimondo merely expanded it to cover all out-of-state visitors. Florida and Texas also set up checkpoints for out-of-state drivers from "hotspot" states along major highways,[20] and other states eagerly seized the right to pull over out-of-state plates as the epidemic dragged on.

Lest anyone get the idea that the quarantine restrictions were optional, Cuomo set the militaristic tone of the official response with the epidemic barely arrived in the U.S., sending in the National Guard to police a "containment area" within the city of New Rochelle, 20 miles north of Manhattan. The "containment" wasn't rigid—residents could still come and go—and the Patient Zero of the cluster had already exposed countless people commuting back and forth from his job in midtown before his diagnosis. At first there appeared to be little epidemiological purpose to the military presence. But as Trump mulled cordoning off the city entirely, then backed off building his wall around the city that never sleeps, local government stepped in where federal will fell short. Nearby New Jersey cities of Newark, East Orange, Orange, and Irvington locked themselves

---

19 Al Goodman, Laura Perez Maestro, Sheena McKenzie and Tara John, "European Union will close its borders to all non-essential travel to fight coronavirus," *CNN World,* March 16, 2020, https://www.cnn.com/2020/03/16/europe/spain-coronavirus-lockdown-intl/index.html.

20 Roberto Baldwin, "Rhode Island, Texas, Florida Cops Target Out-of-State Plates to Curb Virus Spread," *Yahoo! News,* April 1, 2020, https://news.yahoo.com/rhode-island-texas-florida-cops-181700389.html.

down. Residents, forbidden to so much as sit on their stoops, were also banned from traveling between the municipalities. "It's dangerous to come out," Newark mayor Res Baraka told reporters.[21]

Some of the newly-defined "crimes" within the pandemic police state seemed designed with the idea of quashing protest against the first round of draconian measures. "Social distancing"—alienation by another name—required individuals to keep more than six feet away from one another and forbid more than a handful of people from deliberately gathering. Mandated by most governments (with a few outliers like Sweden and Belarus), fines for violations could be steep. A British man who failed to "self-quarantine" upon arrival on the Isle of Man was threatened with a £10,000 fine and three months' prison.[22] Australia warned citizens caught out without one of 16 pre-determined "excuses" for leaving their homes could be fined as much as $11,000 or jailed for six months in New South Wales, fines that could go as high as $19,800 in Victoria.[23] The government banned gatherings of more than two people even as infection numbers there declined by half.[24]

Enforcement of such measures—not only in Australia but in nearly every country where fines have been rolled out—has been uneven. Individuals complained of being cited for nonexistent violations, and even in the most heavily-policed cities, there were not enough police to arrest or fine everyone who violated "social distancing." The arbitrary nature of enforcement encouraged the development of a resigned awareness that even following the rules to the letter was not enough to "save" a person from fines they certainly cannot afford.

The stay-at-home orders didn't just stop people from partying or protesting. Most countries and municipalities restricted workers involved in "non-essential" industries or occupations to working from home, permitting only travel to supermarkets, pharmacies, medical facilities, and exercise. Which industries were

---

21 FOX 5 NY Staff, "3 municipalities join Newark lockdown; cops issuing summonses," *FOX 5 New York,* March 31, 2020, https://www.fox5ny.com/news/3-municipalities-join-newark-lockdown-cops-issuing-summonses.

22 Jamie Johnson, "First British arrest for failing to comply with coronavirus isolation measures made on Isle of Man," *The Telegraph,* March 20, 2020, https://www.telegraph.co.uk/news/2020/03/20/first-uk-arrest-failing-comply-coronavirus-isolation-measures/.

23 Michael McGowan and Ben Smee, "Man eating kebab on bench among 50 people fined in NSW and Victoria for violating coronavirus laws," *The Guardian,* updated April 9, 2020, https://www.theguardian.com/law/2020/apr/03/man-eating-kebab-on-bench-among-50-people-fined-in-nsw-and-victoria-for-violating-coronavirus-laws.

24 Robert Gearty, "Australia bans gatherings of more than 2 even as coronavirus daily infection rate declines by half," *MSN,* March 29, 2020, https://www.msn.com/en-us/news/world/australia-bans-gatherings-of-more-than-2-even-as-coronavirus-daily-infection-rate-declines-by-half/ar-BB11S6nE.

deemed "essential" varied by country—U.S. states closed their few remaining bookstores but kept marijuana dispensaries open. Some countries even required citizens to carry documents verifying their "right" to be out of their home—even if, as in France, they could print or hand-write the documents themselves. The idea seems to have been merely to get populations accustomed to producing papers on demand—to ask permission to exist in public space.

In Tunisia, the government deployed tank-like surveillance robots to patrol the streets of the capital,[25] and video posted to social media appeared to show one of the dystopian enforcers scanning a woman's "papers."[26] It's a chilling window on learned helplessness—the 'bot appears to be equipped with facial recognition, so she knows that even though she can outrun it there's no use, she's been spotted. She rummages around, produces her papers, and even thanks the inanimate object as it goes on its way, satisfied she is allowed to be outside.

Quarantine-enforcing robots were not confined to the streets, either—contagion proved a golden opportunity to step up the rollout of robotic patrols of land and sky. Since the epidemic exploded in Wuhan, drones were used to scold quarantine-breakers, and while the concept was sneered at as Orwellian when it debuted in China, parts of the U.S. and Europe quickly embraced the airborne proximity police. Less than two years after buying its first drones and promising citizens they wouldn't be used for routine police patrols or warrantless surveillance,[27] the New York Police Department was doing just that, proudly flying them over Central Park, looking for social-distance violators and bragging about the "nearly 100% compliance" it was seeing.[28] Residents of Western Australia posted video to social media of a hefty black drone outfitted with red and blue lights and a mechanical voice reminding locals to maintain "social distancing" at all

25 Christian Fernsby, "Tunisia using unmanned robots to enforce lockdown during coronavirus," *Post Online Media,* March 27, 2020, https://www.poandpo.com/news/tunisia-using-unmanned-robots-to-enforce-lockdown-during-coronavirus-2732020506/.

26 Beach Milk (@BeachMilk), "In Tunisia you must show your "papers" to patrolling robots if you are on the streets during their #COVID_19 lockdown! Get used to it people(or not!)" Twitter, March 29, 2020, https://twitter.com/BeachMilk/status/1244208975576535045 (accessed April 17, 2020).

27 Ashley Southall and Ali Winston, "New York Police Say They Will Deploy 14 Drones," *The New York Times,* December 4, 2018, https://www.nytimes.com/2018/12/04/nyregion/nypd-drones.html.

28 Matt Agorist, "NYPD Releases Orwellian Video of Drones Spying on Citizens to Enforce Social Distancing," *Activist Post,* March 27, 2020, https://www.activistpost.com/2020/03/nypd-releases-orwellian-video-of-drones-spying-on-citizens-to-enforce-social-distancing.html.

times.[29] Another line of drones, made by the U.S. company Draganfly, was rolled out by the University of Southern Australia with the ability to detect fever, cough, respiratory and heart rates, and blood pressure from a distance.[30] While nothing currently on the market couples these capabilities with the ability to "neutralize" the infected, the U.S., through IARPA (the intelligence equivalent of DARPA), had been working on technology to identify targets via facial recognition since before the pandemic began. The Office of the Director of National Intelligence put out a call in September 2019 for solutions to facial recognition and other biometric recognition technologies' weaknesses at distance—currently an obstacle on the path toward AI-enabled drones that will eventually be able to identify a target from the air and decide, without human input, whether or not to destroy it.[31]

Even in those countries whose lockdowns didn't require citizens to carry and display "papers," the conditioning still pointed toward a submissive, permission-oriented model of domestic movement. Australians were forced to choose from 16 authorized "excuses" to be outdoors. The UK warned as March turned into April that being caught out "without a reasonable excuse" would trigger a fine that doubled with every offense. In a disturbingly vague order, police were given the authority to "ensure parents are doing all they can to stop their children breaking the rules" or face quarantine—presumably without their children. When the hashtag #FilmYourHospital was trending on social media, with many convinced the whole epidemic was a hoax after comparing news reports showing packed hospitals and busy ambulance bays with the tumbleweeds blowing through the empty ERs and parking lots they saw at their own local facilities, a British man was shamed in the media and supposedly jailed for "bragging" about filming an empty hospital in Aylesbury.[32]

---

29 Lee Adam Wilshier (@LeeAdamWilshier), "What kind of hell is this... Pinch me. This is in Western Australia," Twitter, April 1, 2020, https://twitter.com/LeeAdamWilshier/status/1245390358848008192 (accessed April 17, 2020).

30 Draganfly Inc., "Draganfly selected to integrate breakthrough health diagnosis technology to detect & monitor COVID19," YouTube video, 1:26, March 26, 2020https://youtu.be/ot2jlr3d6ug (accessed April 17, 2020).

31 "Big Brother is watching you (from afar): US spies seek long-range facial recognition capabilities," *RT*, Sept. 18, 2019, https://www.rt.com/usa/469045-facial-recognition-height-surveillance-iarpa/.

32 Richard Hartley Parkinson, "Man jailed for visiting hospital with no good reason after Facebook boasts," *Metro UK*, April 3, 2020, https://metro.co.uk/2020/04/03/man-jailed-visiting-hospital-no-good-reason-facebook-boasts-12503535/.

Violating a quarantine order even cost several citizens their passports in Singapore.[33] The city-state adopted especially Orwellian measures to fight the epidemic, criminalizing "spreading rumors" about Covid-19, seizing vehicles found in quarantined areas, and threatening jail time to those who repeatedly violated social distancing guidelines. The latter measure popped up in the U.S., UK, and other "democratic" governments as well, even though processing social-distancing violators by sending them to already overcrowded jails is positively Kafkaesque in its absurdity. Some accounts of these arrests came with public-shaming-ready stories—a man running a speakeasy in south Brooklyn, a man holding a 60-person party in Charles County, Maryland—but never did they explain what purpose was to be solved by moving the offender from one overly-crowded circumstance of their own creation to another of the state's.

Mayors and prosecutors in several cities, including New York and San Francisco,[34] made a point of releasing hundreds of supposedly low-level offenders to reduce the risk of disease spreading behind bars.[35] Some municipalities, including Baltimore and Fort Worth, also announced they would no longer be arresting people for certain offenses. Philadelphia even released a list, which included "personal, retail, and vehicle theft," prostitution, and "all narcotics offenses."[36] Outbreaks of joyful looting in stores that hadn't yet been forced to close their doors were filmed and shared on social media for millions to watch in disbelief, as if the latest Purge film was unfolding in real life.

It may seem pointless to release low-level offenders only to fill the jails back up with different low-level offenders, but there was method to their madness—articles surfaced almost immediately from the Republican nemeses of these (largely Democratic) mayors, alerting the public to the sex offenders, violent criminals, and other fear-inducing types being released despite the governments' reassurances. The knowledge that such Bad People were roaming around served to encourage ordinary folks to not only remain indoors but to trust their local police force, even if its members had gone mad with the expanded power newly delegated to them

---

33 Special Correspondent, "Case against Singapore returnee for jumping quarantine," *The Hindu News,* updated March 29, 2020, https://www.thehindu.com/news/cities/Tiruchirapalli/case-against-singapore-returnee-for-jumping-quarantine/article31200556.ece.

34 Megan Cassidy, "Coronavirus: San Francisco, Contra Costa prosecutors join national call for jail releases," *San Francisco Chronicle,* March 18, 2020, https://www.sfchronicle.com/crime/article/Coronavirus-San-Francisco-Contra-Costa-15137291.php.

35 Alice Speri, "NYPD's aggressive policing risks spreading the Coronavirus," *The Intercept,* April 3, 2020, https://theintercept.com/2020/04/03/nypd-social-distancing-arrests-coronavirus/.

36 Danielle M. Outlaw, City of Philadelphia Memo, March 17, 2020, https://www.documentcloud.org/documents/6811943-Outlaw-Memo.html (accessed April 17, 2020).

by the state. Even when a veritable army of some two dozen police marched in formation on a little girl's birthday party in Los Angeles, commenters praised the show of force.[37]

This push to embrace Big Brother was concerted and deliberate. Every tightening of control on movement was accompanied by a hint that it was the people's own refusal to "behave"—to meekly stay indoors, waiting for orders from above before they dared stick their heads outside—that had made the crackdown necessary. *This is for your own good*, every order reminded them. The aim is to program the populace to think of the government as a stern, but loving parent, determined to use "tough love" to protect them from the mean nasty virus (and terrorists, and communists, and whatever other bogeyman happens along) outside.

The pandemic powerfully cemented the relationship between Big Brother and Big Tech. Government reached out to the tech platforms for help with enforcing quarantines and gathering restrictions, and Big Tech did not disappoint. Corporations like Google, Facebook, and Amazon have long operated hand-in-hand with the U.S. government (and to a lesser extent its allies), serving as a private-sector backchannel allowing agencies still theoretically subject to the restrictions set forth in the Constitution against suppressing free speech and warrantless search and seizure to circumvent those pesky protections. With coronavirus already in use in other areas of government to justify the detonation of all remaining civil rights, agencies didn't have to apply much pressure to gain access to mineable data on all citizens.

Just weeks after the western media excoriated China for the intrusive smartphone apps it was using to track coronavirus patients' quarantine compliance and possible exposure routes using cellphone location data, Israel publicly announced it was doing the same, enlisting its Shin Bet intelligence agency to surveil potentially infected individuals and trace their contacts over time in what PM Benjamin Netanyahu claimed was a method used to track terrorists that he'd never before turned on the civilian population.[38] Israelis, unused to being treated like Palestinians, were furious, gradually coming to realize they may be stuck with Netanyahu as dictator-for-life (the conveniently-timed outbreak had

37 Lauren Fruen, "Shocking moment huge line of police officers disperse 40 party-goers from one-year-old girl's birthday in LA after citywide shutdown amid coronavirus," *Daily Mail,* updated March 31, 2020, https://www.dailymail.co.uk/news/article-8169339/Shocking-moment-huge-line-police-officers-forced-disperse-girls-birthday-party-LA.html.

38 Noa Landau and Netael Bandel, "To Stop the Coronavirus, Shin Bet Can Now Track Cellphones Without Court Order," *Haaretz,* March 15, 2020, https://www.haaretz.com/israel-news/.premium-to-stop-coronavirus-spread-shin-bet-can-track-cellphones-without-court-order-1.8677696.

prevented his prosecution on multiple bribery and fraud counts).[39] Other countries went down the same technological path, albeit via the public-private partnership route. Finding themselves flush with money (the U.S. CDC got $500 million in the first coronavirus stimulus bill to build a "public health surveillance and data collection system"), health authorities were lured by the siren call of companies with expertise at building Orwellian surveillance systems. Police state cheerleader Peter Thiel's Palantir inserted itself into nascent coronavirus tracking systems in the U.S., UK,[40] France, Germany and Switzerland.[41] Facebook and Google met with the Trump administration to discuss drafting Americans' phone data into the fight against the virus. Google's sister company Verily built a coronavirus testing advisory platform in the U.S., while Amazon went one further and unveiled a program to deliver and test Seattle area residents (in partnership with the ubiquitous Bill Gates, who told anyone who'd listen that he wanted "digital certificates" attesting to the bearer's coronavirus—and vaccine—status for everyone).[42]

But location data isn't the only way the police state can surveil individuals within their homes. Amazon taught its AI voice assistant Alexa how to answer questions about the epidemic, announcing by the end of March that the device could now evaluate users' symptoms and advise them on whether or not they should get tested.[43] Whether or not it will report back to HQ on whether the user heeded its advice—and whether it has yet been trained to listen for the telltale "dry cough" that is supposed to be a hallmark of coronavirus—remain to be seen, but all "AI voice assistants" are likely to be pressed into service in the rush to surveil potential coronavirus patients. Israeli startup Vocalis Health was already

---

39 "'Slippery slope': Israel draws flak over coronavirus surveillance," *Aljazeera*, March 17, 2020, https://www.aljazeera.com/news/2020/03/slope-israel-draws-flak-coronavirus-surveillance-200317153457942.html/.

40 Matthew Gould, Dr Indra Joshi and Ming Tang, "The power of data in a pandemic," GOV.UK Blog: Technology in the NHS, March 28, 2020, https://healthtech.blog.gov.uk/2020/03/28/the-power-of-data-in-a-pandemic/.

41 Helene Fouquet and Albertina Torsoli, "Palantir in Talks With Germany, France for Virus-Fighting Tool," *Bloomberg Technology*, March 31, 2020, https://www.bloomberg.com/news/articles/2020-04-01/palantir-in-talks-with-germany-france-for-virus-fighting-tool.

42 Bill Gates, co-chair of the Bill & Melinda Gates Foundation (@thisisbillgates), Dr. Trevor Mundel (leader of the Gates Foundation's global health work), and Dr. Niranjan Bose (Bill Gates' chief scientific adviser), AMA about COVID-19, *Reddit,* March 18, 2020, https://www.reddit.com/r/Coronavirus/comments/fksnbf/ im_bill_gates_cochair_ of_the_bill_melinda_gates/ (accessed April 17, 2020).

43 "Alexa and Amazon Devices COVID-19 resources," Amazon Blog *Day One,* March 26, 2020, https://blog.aboutamazon.com/devices/alexa-and-amazon-devices-covid-19-resources (accessed April 17, 2020).

hard at work on such a system by April, announcing it was working on a program that would diagnose the disease based on vocal samples[44]—a technology that would allow the disease to be diagnosed over the phone, with or without the awareness of the individual on the other end of the line. Being ratted out as a coronavirus case by an overzealous AI practitioner of "telemedicine" is one thing, but the potential for worse abuses—say, a pharmaceutical company's robocalls "phishing" for coronavirus sufferers and profiting off their referrals to a local hospital—is huge. Given that legal experts have recommended that lawyers working from home bury their "smart" speakers deep in their backyards to avoid running afoul of confidentiality rules,[45] trusting Alexa, your phone, or any other electronic device not to report you to the authorities for coughing the wrong way is like trusting the government to safeguard your data.

The coronavirus-data gold rush eventually hit such a fever pitch that even the media establishment seemed to balk ("Today's Covid-19 data will be tomorrow's tools of oppression," warned the Daily Beast[46]). But their concern turned out to be mostly for those sad benighted people in "non-democratic countries" the U.S. would like to regime-change. In one breathtakingly naive piece, *The New York Times* lamented that "As coronavirus surveillance escalates, personal privacy plummets,"[47] earnestly suggesting that Americans "learned their lesson" from 9/11 about how temporarily "ratcheting up surveillance…could permanently open the doors to more invasive forms of snooping later." Apparently, the only Americans who have learned this lesson are those in the government who believe it's a grand idea.

Nothing says dystopian police state like a population outfitted with must-wear tracking armbands. Europe embraced the Chinese model of virus-tracking, though its Pan-European Privacy Preserving Proximity Testing (PEPP-PT) supposedly colors within the lines of EU privacy law by calling for "anonymous and

---

44 "Israel developing app to detect coronavirus by sound of an infected person's voice," *Deccan Chronicle,* March 31, 2020, https://www.deccanchronicle.com/technology/in-other-news/310320/israel-developing-app-to-detect-coronavirus-by-sound-of-an-infected-pe.html.

45 Chris Matyszczyk, "Working from home? Switch off Amazon's Alexa (say lawyers)," *ZDNet,* March 24, 2020, https://www.zdnet.com/article/working-from-home-switch-off-amazons-alexa-say-lawyers/.

46 Mona Sloane and Albert Fox Cahn, "Today's COVID-19 Data Will be Tomorrow's Tools of Oppression," *The Daily Beast,* updated April 2, 2020, https://www.thedailybeast.com/todays-covid-19-data-will-be-tomorrows-tools-of-oppression.

47 Natasha Singer and Choe Sang-Hun, "As Coronavirus Surveillance Escalates, Personal Privacy Plummets," *The New York Times,* updated April 17, 2020, https://www.nytimes.com/2020/03/23/technology/coronavirus-surveillance-tracking-privacy.html.

voluntary use" of Bluetooth instead of tracking citizens via their location data. Its creators admitted the app would require at least 60% of any country's population to install it in order to have an effect, but they had a shockingly tone-deaf solution: "Those without cell phones could wear Bluetooth-enabled armbands," as a wide-eyed Reuters report put it.[48] Given that the Germans least likely to have cell phones are also the oldest and most likely to remember the last time Germans habitually sported armbands, this seems like someone's idea of a sick joke, but it might be in the interest of a group conducting wide-scale behavioral reprogramming of a society to see how far it can push that society.

There was no mention made of what might happen if less than 60 percent of any given country were willing to download the app. The UK's National Health Service developed its own coronavirus-tracing app, assuring Britons the opt-in service would work just fine as long as more than half the population downloaded it. Users are supposed to upload their diagnostic information to the app, which then interacts with nearby phones via Bluetooth, alerting individuals when someone who has tested positive passes within the vicinity. Given the social stigma of sporting such a scarlet letter, it's difficult to imagine anyone voluntarily uploading a positive diagnosis. Coronavirus fraud will no doubt take off as a cottage industry among Britain's newly-unemployed should the quarantine ever end. Social shaming is powerful, but self-preservation is a difficult instinct to overcome. Google and Apple devised a similar collaboration for the U.S., announcing the contact-tracing function would eventually be integrated into both operating systems[49]—easily hacking a shortcut through the thorny issue of regaining customers' trust after violating their privacy again and again.[50]

Police-state tech need not be high-tech. Former New York mayor and billionaire failed presidential candidate Mike Bloomberg, who notoriously called the New York Police Department his own private army, apparently couldn't resist the urge to command another army, and invested $10 million in the hire of human contact-tracers to blanket the tri-state area (New York, New Jersey and Connecticut) and sniff out people who'd come into contact with infected individuals. Deputizing thousands of laid-off "citizen snitches" through the most densely populated parts

---

48 Douglas Busvine, "European experts ready smartphone technology to help halt coronavirus spread," *Thomson Reuters Foundation News,* April 1, 2020, https://news.trust. org/item/20200401131119-famq1.

49 "Apple and Google partner on COVID-19 contact tracing technology," Apple *Newsroom,* updated April 10, 2020, https://www.apple.com/newsroom/2020/04/apple-and-google-partner-on-covid-19-contact-tracing-technology/.

50 Glenn Greenwald and Ewen MacAskill, "NSA Prism program taps in to user data of Apple, Google and others," *The Guardian,* June 7, 2013, https://www.theguardian.com/world/2013/jun/06/us-tech-giants-nsa-data.

of the East Coast was bound to be unpopular, but owning a major media outlet to spin it positively no doubt helped, especially given that the Bloomberg-endowed School of Public Health hosted the Event 201 simulation[51] that seemed to spawn so much of the policy implemented in the wake of the pandemic.

Nor did low-tech enforcement even require such well-paid "private armies."Karnataka state in India issued an order requiring all individuals under home quarantine to send in selfies hourly to the government to prove they were staying at home.[52] The notice—simple, yet chilling—warned that attempting to fool the system with a doctored photo—photos taken with a smart phone include a bounty of identifying information, from geographical coordinates to date and time— would land the offender in "mass quarantine" and that government teams would be conducting random spot-checks to verify the quarantined individuals were in fact staying at home. The simple, elegant, yet wildly disturbing variants on house arrest make the quarantined subject complicit in their own imprison-ment, manufacturing consent by force in order to resolve an intense cognitive dissonance. Such a dynamic, however, is already present to some degree in any surveillance system that requires its "victim" to "voluntarily" download an app, the paradigm first set forth in Wuhan.

For those populations that won't accept technological solutions voluntarily, there's always force. Louisville, Kentucky outfitted some quarantine-violators with the type of geolocating ankle bracelet typically given to house-arrest pris-oners after one was spotted going shopping against court order.[53] Infrared "fever guns" became ubiquitous in China province, wielded by authorities at train sta-tions, markets, office buildings, and other public places; smaller versions were even installed at the entrance to apartment complexes, connected to alarms that

---

51 "Johns Hopkins Center for Health Security to host Event 201, a global pandemic exercise," Johns Hopkins Center for Health Security *Center News,* August 21, 2019, https://www.centerforhealthsecurity.org/newsroom/center-news/2019/2019-08-21-event201.html.

52 Bangalore Mirror (@BangaloreMirror), "JUST IN: All persons under home quarantine will have to send their selfies every hour to Karnataka government," Twitter, March 30, 2020, https://twitter.com/BangaloreMirror/status/1244618931806990337 (accessed April 17, 2020).

53 Andrea Ash and Shay McAlister, "Kentucky judges now putting defiant COVID-19 patients on house arrest," *KHOU-11,* updated March 30, 2020, https://www.khou.com/article/news/health/coronavirus/lou-judges-now-putting-defiant-covid-19-patients-on-house-arrest/285-e8c1ae19-84b6-423a-b210-90ce08b368e7.

would summon police if someone with a fever passed by.[54] It's easy to imagine this technology being integrated with a locking mechanism to confine repeat quarantine violators in the manner that someone convicted of drunk driving must blow into a breathalyzer before they can start their car. As technology advances—the Bill Gates-funded ID2020 project to outfit every individual with a "portable biometric identity" is already underway—the sky's the limit with regard to digitizing the ball and chain.

The international mobile phone industry may be one-upping even the most intrusive governments on surveillance, crafting a system that transcends national borders in the name of fighting the pandemic. Standards-setting body GSMA denied reports it is working on creating a *global* virus-tracking system, based on contact-tracing and location data sharing,[55] but rumors persisted. The supranational system would no doubt continue to be used long after the coronavirus was a distant memory, a key player in the post-pandemic "new normal."

Americans who try to hide from this Panopticon-on-steroids may find their usual technological disguises no longer apply. Capitalizing on the U.S.' distracted populace, Senators Lindsey Graham and Richard Blumenthal took aim at encryption—a technology the Five Eyes intelligence consortium declared Public Enemy Number One back in 2018[56]—with the EARN IT Act, which would effectively ban the technology without literally outlawing it. Introduced in March, the law would force tech platforms to adhere to a series of "best practices" drawn up in the service of "saving the children" from sexual exploitation, mostly focused on stepped-up policing of content. Platforms would be held liable for any exploitative content (or anything else the panel decided to declare off-limits, like political dissent) and potentially hauled into court, strongly incentivizing them to preemptively ban users considered likely to offend. Actual experts on child sexual exploitation saw through the ruse, panning the law as the "political theatre

---

54 Jamie L. LaReau, "US can learn how to beat coronavirus from China's best practices," *Omaha World Herald,* March 31, 2020, https://www.omaha.com/money/consumer/us-can-learn-how-to-beat-coronavirus-from-china-s-best-practices/article_e71258f1-d27d-592c-9f89-1dbcba232e94.html.

55 Stephanie Kirchgaessner, "Mobile phone industry explores worldwide tracking of users," *The Guardian,* March 25, 2020, https://www.theguardian.com/world/2020/mar/25/mobile-phone-industry-explores-worldwide-tracking-of-users-coronavirus.

56 Australian Government Department of Home Affairs, "Five Country Ministerial 2018: Statement of Principles on Access to Evidence and Encryption," *Internet Archive Wayback Machine,* accessed April 25, 2020, https://web.archive.org/web/20180925154820/https://www.homeaffairs.gov.au/about/national-security/five-country-ministerial-2018/access-evidence-encryption.

of child protection,"[57] and pointed out the futility of focusing on enforcement over protecting kids from being exploited in the first place. EARN IT constitutes a full frontal assault on the First Amendment that will hit independent journalists and any other political dissidents who do their work online particularly hard. The police state does not want to take any chances that some inconvenient truth might escape the cage it is building for the minds of its citizens.

It isn't just freedom of speech facing certain destruction at the hands of the "new normal"—freedom of religion is uniquely targeted by the pandemic police state. Churches, synagogues, and mosques were threatened with closure in some areas as their proprietors stubbornly persisted in holding services, reasoning (quite logically) that their flocks need God in the middle of the crisis more than ever. New York City mayor Bill de Blasio warned he would "permanently" shut down any church that insisted on holding in-person services after being told to disperse.[58] Megachurch pastor Rodney Howard-Browne was briefly detained and charged with breach of public health regulations for holding two massive Sunday services just days after Hillsborough County, Florida issued a "safer-at-home" (light lockdown) order.[59] The hallowed western tradition of separation of church and state, one of the founding principles of American jurisprudence and a fact of life even in many nations where it isn't expressly written into the constitution, was quietly shelved in favor of the pandemic society's new God: "flattening the curve."

The post-pandemic order preying on citizens' minds and souls hasn't forgotten about their bodies, of course. The social distancing diktat has had the effect of chilling existing protest movements out of existence, a rosy outcome for the Macronist government of France, which has struggled to keep the Yellow Vest movement (and the General Strike that followed on its heels in early 2020) from spiraling out of control. In the days following PM Emmanuel Macron's declaration

---

57 Prostasia Foundation, "EARN IT: The political theater of child protection," YouTube video, 20:48, March 2, 2020, https://prostasia.org/vodcast/earn-it-the-political-theater-of-child-protection/ (accessed April 17, 2020).

58 Matthew Schmitz (@matthewschmitz), "De Blasio: churches and synagogues that hold worship services may be closed permanently," Twitter, March 29, 2020, https://twitter.com/matthewschmitz/status/1244339404753289216 (accessed April 17, 2020).

59 Justin Schecker, "Coronavirus: Tampa pastor out on bond after allegedly violating safer-at-home order," *News Channel 8,* Tampa Bay, Florida, March 29, 2020, https://www.wfla.com/news/hillsborough-county/deputies-tampa-bay-church-violates-social-distancing-guidelines/.

of lockdown, the movement held one protest,[60] but there was little to no chatter about further demonstrations on social media. Less than a week after declaring the quarantine, almost 39,000 people had reportedly been fined for failing to produce their glorified permission-slips, a phenomenon that wasn't limited to France.[61] In the three days following Italy's similar declaration, its Department of the Interior revealed it had cited some 35,506 individuals for being outdoors without their "papers," which like France's constituted a sworn statement detailing their reasons for being outdoors.[62]

The military are joining the police on many countries' streets, absurdly deployed against a microscopic "enemy." While not every nation explicitly declared martial law, the psychological effect in western "liberal democracies" of seeing the streets and transit flooded with military assets is unnerving—perhaps deliberately so. Videos showing hundreds of tanks being shipped up the coast of California[63] and armored trucks rolling through the streets of Paris[64] were widely shared on social media, belying governments' insistence that the military activity planned for the coronavirus response merely constituted building field hospitals and delivering bag lunches for the quarantined elderly.

The U.S. has long been gradually reorienting its prodigious military resources toward training soldiers for urban warfare, with Pentagon-produced videos explaining how the notion of fighting wars against an enemy that has willingly separated itself from civilian populations is a thing of the past.[65] And military exercises have shifted accordingly, from something conducted in uninhabited areas

60 Alessandra Scotto di Santolo, "Coronavirus France fears: Yellow Vests protest despite Macron's ban on large gatherings," *Express,* March 15, 2020, https://www.express.co.uk/news/world/1255523/coronavirus-france-yellow-vests-protests-paris-emmanuel-macron-latest.

61 "Thousands of French citizens ignore quarantine as cops issue nearly 39,000 citations for violating lockdown," *RT,* March 21, 2020, https://www.rt.com/news/483722-france-fines-police-coronavirus-lockdown/.

62 "Plus de 35.000 cas de non-respect des règles de confinement en Italie," *7 Sur 7,* March 17, 2020, https://www.7sur7.be/monde/plus-de-35-000-cas-de-non-respect-des-regles-de-confinement-en-italie~ae5630c8/.

63 Washington News Line (@WashNewsLine), "Tanks have arrived in #SanDiego. This is not a scene from a movie. It's real," Twitter, March 28, 2020, https://twitter.com/WashNewsLine/status/1244136578529853441 (accessed April 17, 2020).

64 Alex Lantier and Jacques Valentin, "Army enters Paris as Macron announces coronavirus lockdown in France," *World Socialist Web Site,* March 17, 2020, https://www.wsws.org/en/articles/2020/03/17/fran-m17.html.

65 Fanatical Futurist, "Megacities Urban Future, the Emerging Complexity, Pentagon Video," YouTube video, 4:55, October 31, 2016, https://www.youtube.com/watch?v=iDxeKd_iR28 (accessed April 17, 2020).

to hiding in plain sight. North Carolinians were warned in February 2020 that they might catch a glimpse of an "unconventional warfare exercise" called Robin Sage, in which Special Forces troops dress up as "guerrilla freedom fighters" and engage with civilian volunteers across multiple counties.[66]

Conducting urban warfare drills during a period of de facto martial law is a remarkably unsubtle show of power. Such in-your-face flexing has been going on for years, but has recently intensified: Los Angeles residents were terrified in February 2019 by an unannounced military exercise that saw dozens of helicopters buzz the city, flying between buildings and in one case even landing in the middle of the street—without informing locals in advance.[67] A similar "classified" exercise planned for Washington, DC was inadvertently revealed in a Pentagon budget request to Congress just a few months later.[68]

The Robin Sage exercise strongly resembled Jade Helm, the controversial 2015 military exercise that so disturbed the Texas governor that he dispatched volunteer National Guardsmen to monitor it (a brouhaha that was retroactively written off as a product of "the alt-right and Russian bots"[69] by notorious perjurer[70] and former CIA director Michael Hayden). Jade Helm was an "unconventional warfare" exercise that featured military personnel (again, identifiable by armbands alone) descending on civilian areas to retake them from "hostile" militants—with Texas, Utah, and southern California mapped as enemy territory. While the military insists it has run both exercises for years, so little is known about either by civilians that a Special Forces soldier participating in Robin Sage was actually shot and killed in 2002 by a sheriff's deputy who thought his weapons were the real thing and believed he was acting "suspicious." Americans have a deep-seated distrust of even their own military operating on U.S. shores, as the

---

66 Mark Price, "Elaborate unconventional warfare exercise set for undisclosed sites in North Carolina," *The Charlotte Observer,* February 27, 2020, https://www.charlotteobserver.com/news/local/article240651992.html.

67 "'Nothing to see here'? Black helicopters swarm Los Angeles in surprise urban warfare drill (VIDEOS)," *RT,* February 5, 2019, https://www.rt.com/usa/450746-helicopters-blasts-los-angeles-drill/.

68 "Black helicopters over DC? Pentagon accidentally reveals 'classified' domestic Black Hawk mission," *RT,* July 23, 2019, https://www.rt.com/usa/464805-pentagon-reveals-black-hawk-dc/.

69 *The Texas Tribune,* "Hysteria over Jade Helm exercise in Texas was fueled by Russians, former CIA director says," YouTube video, 1:54, May 8, 2018, https://www.youtube.com/watch?v=t70Dv0es218 (accessed April 17, 2020).

70 Trevor Timm, "Stop treating former CIA chief Michael Hayden as an arbiter of truth," *Columbia Journalism Review,* April 4, 2017, https://www.cjr.org/first_person/cia_michael_hayden_expert.php.

frenzy over Jade Helm proved, and events like the coronavirus pandemic will have their hands full trying to reverse that feeling.

That would assume the goal was to endear the military to the population, of course. But the primary aim of flooding the streets with military personnel, as it has been ever since September 11 made M16-toting troops a common sight in train stations and even subways, was to instill fear. No doubt those American soldiers stationed in Europe after World War II, who took personal pride in the fact that their home streets were not under military occupation, are rolling over in their graves. And while the U.S. was not formally in a state of martial law as of the beginning of April, the president's order to authorize up to a million National Guard and Reserve troops for deployment by the Departments of Defense and Homeland Security[71] coupled with the various state-level emergency invocations meant Americans were now living under martial law in everything but name.

U.S. troops who served overseas might have felt a sinking sense of deja vu as they were pressed into service kicking in doors in the good ol' U.S. of A. In addition to the Rhode Island National Guardsmen deputized to sniff out refugees from New York, the Texas National Guard was detailed to go door-to-door coronavirus-hunting in the Dallas area in late March. The governor later tried to dispel "conspiracy theories" by insisting any military visitors would definitely be nurses on a "medical mission"—but still interrogating people about whether they'd had contact with any coronavirus patients.[72] The clarification wasn't particularly reassuring, given that Tarrant County, Texas' emergency orders permitted the government to "commandeer or use any private property" and "temporarily acquire, by lease or other means, sites required for temporary housing units or emergency shelters for evacuees"[73]—theoretically allowing a violation even of the rarely-mentioned Third Amendment forbidding the involuntary quartering of troops.

As the uniformed men with guns took to the streets, Congress was targeting civilians' own right to bear arms amid the largest surge in gun purchases since the U.S. started keeping track of background checks in 1998. Democratic congressman

---

71 Lara Seligman, "Trump authorizes call-ups of military reservists to fight virus," *Politico,* updated March 28, 2020, https://www.politico.com/news/2020/03/27/trump-dod-dhs-reserves-coronavirus-152513.

72 Billy Gates, "Texas National Guard troops could do door-to-door checkups around Dallas," *KXAN Austin,* updated March 27, 2020, https://www.kxan.com/news/coronavirus/texas-national-guard-troops-could-do-door-to-door-checkups-around-dallas/.

73 *Executive Order of County Judge B. Glen Whitley* (Amended by Commissioners Court action on March 24, 2020), Tarrant County, Texas, http://www.tarrantcounty.com/content/dam/main/global/Covid-19/covid-19-EO-stay-at-home-amended-signed03-24-20.pdf (accessed April 17, 2020).

Hank Johnson introduced a bill in March rolling together some of his party's favorite gun control restrictions, including a universal background-check measure that would require the identities of gun buyers who failed a background check to be turned over to local law enforcement. Congress would allow the government to arbitrarily deny citizens the right to a gun license—even in the absence of criminal convictions or mental health issues.[74] Adding insult to injury, the bill would slap a 50% tax on guns and 30% on bullets and prohibit the purchase of a gun by anyone who'd bought one in the preceding month. Some parts of the country weren't even willing to wait—as the state of California declared an emergency, Los Angeles County shut down gun stores as "nonessential businesses," landing the county sheriff in court.[75] Other states made their own, subtler incursions into Second Amendment territory, slow-walking background checks. Dick's Sporting Goods chose the middle of a pandemic to stop selling guns at 440 stores. It's clear many lawmakers are itching for an excuse to start confiscating firearms, and it won't require much of a trigger, especially with the military conducting door-to-door "wellness checks"—and hunting down those rogues who dare cross state borders.

Even before the coronavirus outbreak kicked off a cascade of state-level (and finally federal) emergency declarations, the U.S. Justice Department was quietly chipping away at habeas corpus in the name of stopping mass shootings. By December, Attorney General William Barr had rolled out a *Minority Report*-esque pair of initiatives that made the Patriot Act look positively restrained. One program, the Health Advanced Research Projects Agency (HARPA), would harvest data from an individual's electronic devices—including fitness trackers and AI voice assistants—to assemble a psychological profile with the help of machine learning, hunting for signs of mental illness that could be used to justify "pre-crime" intervention. The other, the Disruption and Early Engagement Program (DEEP), would intervene against individuals deemed to be "mobilizing toward violence," deploying "court ordered mental health treatment," electronic monitoring, and every other tool in the I-can't-believe-it's-not-detention toolbox against

---

74 Gun Violence Prevention and Community Safety Act of 2020, H.R.5717, 116th Congress, 2019-2020, https://www.congress.gov/bill/116th-congress/house-bill/5717.

75 Richard Winton, "Firearms activists sue California, L.A. County over gun shop closures tied to coronavirus," *Los Angeles Times,* March 27, 2020, https://www.msn.com/en-us/news/us/firearms-activists-sue-california-la-county-over-gun-shop-closures-tied-to-coronavirus/ar-BB11OomP.

individuals who've literally done nothing except worry law enforcement.[76] Given that all one has to do to be considered a dangerous extremist or "mentally ill" in the U.S. in 2020 is post what are regarded as "conspiracy theories" online (or cough in the wrong direction), political dissidents are uniquely at risk in the post-pandemic police state. "Pre-crime" algorithms are already a reality, and armed with all the data gleefully harvested from individuals' phones in the coronavirus gold rush, they are becoming much more powerful. Entire behavioral patterns will be criminalized if they can be said to resemble too closely those of "known subversives"—to say nothing of the guilt-by-association arrests that will be made through the enhanced contact tracing the new virus-tracker apps provide.

Since the Reagan years, the U.S. has kept a massive database of "unfriendly" citizens to be rounded up in case of ever-more-loosely-defined emergency, called Main Core. The list, which contained 8 million names by 2008, was reportedly a favorite of the Bush administration in deciding whom to target with its then-novel Patriot Act surveillance powers. While Main Core's capabilities include cutting-edge AI capability to predict targets' next move, allowing for "almost instantaneous" arrest of targets,[77] nationwide near-total lockdown places most Americans in their homes, meaning it's never been easier for authorities to "black-bag" inconvenient activists with no one being the wiser. Even when the quarantine is lifted, the powers seized under the cover of pandemic response set the stage for an appalling assault on dissent in the country that has the gall to still call itself the land of the free.

LOOSE LIPS SINK SHIPS

One of the highlight videos from the Event 201 pandemic response simulation focused solely on how to crack down on freedom of speech in response to the hypothetical outbreak; the seventh point of the group's "recommendations" urged public and private sectors to work together to stamp out "mis- and

---

76 U.S. Attorney William Barr to All U.S. Attorneys, All Heads of Department Components, All Law Enforcement Agencies, October 16, 2019, Office of the Attorney General, Washington, D.C., "Implementation of National Disruption and Early Engagement Programs to Counter the Threat of Mass Shootings," https://www.documentcloud. org/documents/6509496-Attorney-General-Memo-Implementation-of-National.html (accessed April 17, 2020).

77 Whitney Webb, "Coronavirus: What Newsweek Failed to Mention About 'Continuity of Government,'" *Mint Press News,* March 23, 2020, https://www. mintpressnews.com/coronavirus-what-newsweek-failed-mention-continuity-government/265954/.

disinformation."[78] More time is spent on the "threat" posed by non-approved narratives than on preparedness for or combatting the actual disease. The simulation has a detailed plan to address countervailing narratives that involves collaborating with "trusted sources" to put the message in their mouths as (it recognizes) popular distrust of authority figures will continue to grow.

And just as the simulation planned, the first patient cluster in Wuhan had barely coughed when the WHO's Emergencies Program director, Mike Ryan, was making the media rounds talking about the deadly "infodemic" riding the coattails of the virus itself. "We need a vaccine for misinformation," he said, setting the agenda for the pandemic to come:[79] "conspiracy theories" and other viewpoints unsanctioned by the establishment aren't just wrong—they're dangerous and must be stopped, by any means necessary, before they infect others.

Social media platforms rose to the occasion by broadly increasing the level of censorship, presumably as part of their publicly-declared partnership with the WHO. Facebook, Twitter and YouTube all published notices within a week of each other warning users that "because of coronavirus," automated systems would take up an increased share of content moderation, using algorithms which would necessarily make mistakes, resulting in some rule-abiding content being yanked. While YouTube initially demonetized all videos that even used the word coronavirus, forcing even the most mainstream-friendly users to come up with alternate terms for the only topic anyone was talking about, it "relaxed" its standards to allow a select few "authoritative" channels to opine on the epidemic. The same establishment lackeys were left throwing tantrums as a Facebook "glitch" marked all coronavirus-related news stories as "spam" for a few days.

The standards for what constitutes "harmful" shifted dramatically. Twitter warned users that any post that encouraged coronavirus-unsafe behavior would be removed, hinting that merely failing to comply with the official narrative (which had a nasty habit of constantly shifting, especially in the early weeks of the disease being publicized) could result in deplatforming. Facebook began confronting users who interacted with content it deemed "misinformation" with prominently-placed links to the WHO in their newsfeed, a subtle but firm step toward digital thought reform for those five percent of users who still clicked through the warning labels CEO Mark Zuckerberg claimed worked to deter 95%

---

78 "Public-private cooperation for pandemic preparedness and response: A Call to Action," *Event 201: A Global Pandemic Exercise,* Center for Health Security, accessed April 17, 2020, http://www.centerforhealthsecurity.org/event201/recommendations.html.

79 Malaka Gharib, "Fake Facts Are Flying About Coronavirus. Now There's A Plan To Debunk Them," *NPR,* February 21, 2020, https://www.npr.org/sections/goatsandsoda/2020/02/21/805287609/theres-a-flood-of-fake-news-about-coronavirus-and-a-plan-to-stop-it.

of users who saw them from reading articles the platform's "fact checkers" declared anathema.[80] It even deleted anti-lockdown protest events, with Zuckerberg going on TV[81] to denounce the demonstrations as "harmful misinformation" that must be destroyed—while the media rushed to demonize the protest organizers as gun nuts[82] and racists.[83]

It is highly unlikely any of these new standards will be restored to normal post-pandemic, even as the platforms' moderators return to work—*if* the moderators return to work. As third-party contractors, they were already the lowest on the totem pole, lacking job security or collective bargaining rights. After a few unsavory write-ups on its contractors in the Verge, Facebook may have decided they're not worth the trouble and opted to stick with algorithms instead.

The narrative managers were hard at work manufacturing consent for the permanent imposition of this new censor-heavy and privacy-free normal. "Data privacy is now gone from our hierarchy of needs," crowed a triumphant Bloomberg piece that warned "we can't just return to the status quo" after lockdown ends. Likening the various tech platforms to public utilities and social media to "sidewalks and parks," it demanded those spaces be "kept clean—virtually speaking—of misinformation and bad actors." E-commerce platforms are to ditch "fakes or quack cures"—a designation that, in the minds of the public health leaders who have been elevated to godlike status amid the pandemic, exiles naturopaths and other alternative medical practitioners to the dustbin of history.[84] The piece waited until the last line to acknowledge that "we don't know what the long-term effects will be of Big Tech making peace with Big Brother" and that "the mix could prove

---

80 Mark Zuckerberg (@zuck), "I want to share an update on the work we're doing to connect people with accurate information and limit the spread of misinformation about Covid-19..." Facebook, April 16, 2020, https://www.facebook.com/zuck/posts/10111806366438811.

81 ABC News, "Mark Zuckerberg on Facebook's plan to fight coronavirus: Full interview," Facebook video, 15:50, April 20, 2020, https://www.facebook.com/watch/?v=270128247486048.

82 Isaac Stanley-Becker and Tony Romm, "Pro-gun activists using Facebook groups to push anti-quarantine protests," *The Washington Post,* April 19, 2020, https://www.washingtonpost.com/technology/2020/04/19/pro-gun-activists-using-facebook-groups-push-anti-quarantine-protests/.

83 Jason Wilson, "The rightwing groups behind wave of protests against Covid-19 restrictions," *The Guardian,* April 17, 2020, https://www.theguardian.com/world/2020/apr/17/far-right-coronavirus-protests-restrictions.

84 Lionel Laurent, "Will Facebook and Amazon Need Quarantining After Covid-19?," *Yahoo! Finance,* March 30, 2020, https://finance.yahoo.com/news/tech-billionaires-making-friends-big-050050144.html.

toxic in the long run"— a fraudulent nod to dissent, covering their backsides in case the whole scenario doesn't play out as planned.

While the U.S. media establishment faithfully broadcast and published wall-to-wall fear porn about the coronavirus, the one fifth of Americans who get their news primarily from social media were seen as being insufficiently glued to their screens, with just 37% reporting that they were following the outbreak "very closely"—dismal results given the amount of work that was being put into churning out a compelling narrative.[85] One can only imagine what would have happened to public support for the disastrous invasion of Afghanistan if some segment of the population had been permitted to switch off the 24/7 replays of planes hitting buildings in the aftermath of 9/11. Worse—for the establishment, at least—fully 70% of the social media contingent agreed that the media was exaggerating the threat posed by the virus[86] and they were more likely than other groups to claim the virus had come out of a lab.

Meanwhile, the moribund U.S. journalism industry—already almost exclusively owned by a handful of massive conglomerates—wasn't spared by the nationwide shutdown, with some of the last independent local papers forced to furlough employees as ad revenue dried up. Given that these small local papers enjoyed a degree of trust their corporate peers could never dream of, their collapse presented a golden opportunity for those conglomerates, which could snap up a title or five at bargain-basement prices and ride their credibility into the ground as they'd done so many times before. However, with so many businesses kaput, the problem of who would fill the advertising void remained; some visionaries appear to have looked across the ocean to the UK, where state-owned outlets like the BBC weathered the storm unperturbed, their supervising governments always ready to pour out more cash to push the narrative.[87] *The Atlantic* proposed the government take up the slack, buying public health ads to go along with the census and military ads it already takes out (and presumably intensifying its conflict of interest with the publications in which it advertises). *The Columbia Journalism Review* was more ambitious, demanding a $2 billion stimulus program to beef up

---

85 Mark Jurkowitz and Amy Mitchell, "Americans who primarily get news through social media are least likely to follow COVID-19 coverage, most likely to report seeing made-up news," Pew Research Center, *Journalism & Media,* March 25, 2020, https://www. journalism.org/2020/03/25/americans-who-primarily-get-news-through-social-media-are-least-likely-to-follow-covid-19-coverage-most-likely-to-report-seeing-made-up-news/.

86 *Ibid.*

87 Kerry Flynn, "Hundreds of journalists are being laid off, right when the public needs them the most," *CNN,* March 27, 2020, https://www.msn.com/en-us/news/us/hundreds-of-journalists-are-being-laid-off-right-when-the-public-needs-them-the-most/ar-BB11O0sb.

funding of public outlets, supply cash infusions and sponsor individual positions at dying local outlets, and even supply loans to ailing newsrooms. Another $2 billion should go to creating a "First Amendment Fund," the writer suggested, presumably with a straight face,[88] to the same government currently trying to extradite publisher Julian Assange on espionage charges for publishing classified material. A *New York Times* piece even broached the possibility of a government bailout of individual journalists while letting the newspaper outlets themselves die,[89] an act which would make official the longstanding Operation Mockingbird relationship existing between the U.S. media establishment and the intelligence agencies that run it.

That establishment complained in its industry publications that "we are not seeing the "lift" for broadcast typically connected to a major story" in coronavirus-related ratings, observing that 61 percent of Americans blamed the media for inflating the coronavirus' importance. Even the pandemic couldn't jolt Americans out of their distrust of mainstream outlets, which has been at or near peak levels for years—over a third reported getting their news about the virus from social media, followed closely by local TV news. National channels lagged behind, making the post-pandemic crash a great time for the big networks to scoop up some now endangered local channels, and the cable networks (CNN, Fox, MSNBC) came in dead last, with just a fifth of poll respondents reporting they sought out the networks for coronavirus info.[90] Outlets like CBS didn't help their credibility by presenting footage of overwhelmed Italian hospitals as scenes from New York City.

The narrative managers' secret weapon seems to have been celebrities, a disproportionate number of whom turned up sick—but never looking sick—with the coronavirus. Those who didn't get "sick" made bizarre, tone-deaf videos about the virus being the "great equalizer" (Madonna, in a bathtub full of milk and rose petals) or sang literally tone-deaf covers of John Lennon songs (*Wonder Woman* actress and IDF war criminal Gal Gadot with a dozen of her closest friends). The idea was to create a sense of cross-class solidarity—convince the hoi polloi that their idols were suffering, too. Promotion of celebrity coronavirus content

---

88 Craig Aaron, "Journalism Needs a Stimulus. Here's What it Should Look Like," *Columbia Journalism Review,* March 24, 2020, https://www.cjr.org/analysis/journalism-stimulus.php.

89 Ben Smith, "Bail Out Journalists. Let Newspaper Chains Die.," *The New York Times,* March 29, 2020, https://www.nytimes.com/2020/03/29/business/coronavirus-journalists-newspapers.html.

90 Wayne Friedman, "Social Media, Local TV News Are Top COVID-19 Information Sources, Trust Issues Remain," *Media Post,* March 27, 2020, https://www.mediapost.com/publications/article/349137/social-media-local-news-are-top-covid-19-informat.html.

combined with stepped-up removal of dissenting opinions on social media created a powerful impression of a population content with being on house arrest that only upon closer examination revealed itself to be as inauthentic as it was imperfect.

Social media has never had a problem serving as a route for western governments to circumvent legal protections on freedom of speech, so its eagerness to serve as the foot soldiers of coronavirus narrative management was not unexpected. Twitter pledged to delete "content that increases the chance that someone contracts or transmits the virus," including "denial of expert guidance," support for "fake or ineffective treatments," and phony expert advice;[91] other platforms followed suit. But the stepped-up censorship wasn't enough for the UK government, which summoned reps from each platform for a scolding after they failed to squash rumors that the rollout of 5G technology was connected to the coronavirus epidemic, apparently unsatisfied with the shadow banning most 5G-critical content already received.[92]

Taking the extra step of crowning themselves the official arbiters of reality landed some platforms in hot water—the platforms, fully aware they were in many ways more powerful than the governments with whom they'd partnered, didn't always comply with governments' wishes. Twitter, like Facebook, previously promised it would not remove even untrue statements by prominent political figures. When a Chinese foreign ministry spokesman tweeted support for the theory that the U.S. brought coronavirus to Wuhan during the Military World Games in October, the anti-China faction of the U.S. Republican Party demanded Twitter remove the post; some even called for deplatforming the entire Chinese Communist Party.[93] Despite leaping to Washington's aid in quashing criticism of the 2019 Hong Kong protests (and wiping out dozens of official Venezuelan, Iranian, and even Russian accounts),[94] Twitter shied away from throwing China under the bus.

---

91 Vijaya Gadde and Matt Derella, "An update on our continuity strategy during COVID-19," Twitter Company Blog, March 16, 2020, https://blog.twitter.com/en_us/topics/company/2020/An-update-on-our-continuity-strategy-during-COVID-19.html.

92 Harriet Sherwood, "Call for social media platforms to act on 5G mast conspiracy theory," *The Guardian*, April 5, 2020, https://www.theguardian.com/technology/2020/apr/05/call-for-social-media-platforms-to-act-on-5g-mast-conspiracy-theory.

93 Chris Mills Rodrigo, "Twitter comes under fire over Chinese disinformation on coronavirus," *The Hill*, March 25, 2020, https://thehill.com/policy/technology/489363-twitter-comes-under-fire-over-chinese-disinformation-on-coronavirus.

94 Eva Bartlett, "After US killing of Iran's Soleimani, narrative control on social media is getting worse," *RT*, January 17, 2020, https://www.rt.com/op-ed/478241-narrative-control-social-media-soleimani-twitter/.

Shafting Brazil, apparently, was OK. President Jair Bolsonaro became the first pro-U.S. world leader to have a video removed under Twitter's new rules for "misinformation." The offending clip showed Bolsonaro endorsing the anti-malaria drug hydroxychloroquine, which had by the time of the posting racked up some positive trial results in China and elsewhere, saying it was "working in every place." Not exactly true, sure, but certainly not "misinformation that could lead to physical harm." Even then, the platform was gun-shy about censoring a politician—it required Bolsonaro to remove the tweet himself in order to unlock his account. (Facebook and Instagram apparently took the initiative and removed the message themselves.)

The ever-shrinking window of permissible discourse on social media risks taking root in the real world the longer societies are expected to use tech platforms to conduct their real-life business. Across-the-board lockdowns forced nearly every industry—plus services one doesn't typically think of as industries, like education, finance, and even some elements of medicine—online. This put unthinkable power in the hands of tech platforms and internet service providers, private companies now empowered to mediate the entirety of human interaction. Dissenters face a high risk of being shut out of a service as an act of political retaliation, with companies able to justify censorship by claiming an individual was spreading misinformation or otherwise endangering public health. ISPs can unilaterally block access to a particular website on one end, or bar a customer from accessing certain sites on another. Videoconferencing platform Zoom was caught sharing reams of user data with Facebook without users' knowledge, a violation that was no doubt only the tip of a huge surveillance iceberg. At the same time, the death of Net Neutrality means upsetting the wrong tech support person can result in a life sentence to the "slow lane" of the internet—and, in the post-pandemic digital world, of life itself. The threat of "limited internet shutdowns" described in the Event 201 pandemic simulation becomes much more ominous when one's entire life is conducted online. [95]

Dragging the entire human experience online opens people up to being packaged off and sold as "data" and brings societies one step closer to the social credit score many in the West still rightly revile in China. Even before coronavirus, political dissidents were losing access to social media platforms, online payment processors, and even their bank accounts for supposedly "hateful" speech. Tech platforms that have been caught selling users' data, building backdoors for the NSA's PRISM program and other intelligence agencies, and prioritizing the interests of large corporations over the customer have nevertheless become the kings

---

95 Center for Health Security, "Event 201 Pandemic Exercise: Segment 4, Communications Discussion and Epilogue Video," YouTube video, 36:09, Nov. 4, 2019, https://youtu.be/LBuP40H4Tko (accessed April 17, 2020).

of the post-coronavirus world, where there is no "real-world" recourse. Not participating in the system—and, when it comes online, not "opting in" to whatever form of biometric identity is pushed by one's government—excludes one from participation in society completely. When the quarantines are finally lifted, failing to "opt in" may stop one from being able to leave one's home.

PAY UP

> *"In developed countries, this heightened oversight took many forms: biometric IDs for all citizens, for example, and tighter regulation of key industries whose stability was deemed vital to national interests."*
> —*Lock Step*

The notion of government being empowered to declare which industries are "essential" and which are not would seem to be anathema in countries that worship at the feet of the "free market," but nations like the U.S. and UK have had de facto corporate socialism for decades even as they present themselves as good neoliberal acolytes. Given all the government subsidies quietly handed out to American industries from fracking to farming, it was only logical that government would finally come to exercise its ownership rights over everyone.

Once the state had its foot in the door of commerce, it was only a matter of time before it was no longer content with mere dispensation over who was allowed to operate and who had to close their doors and wait in the breadline. "Essential" big-box stores like Walmart were ordered to stop selling "non-essential" items, supposedly because people were breaking social distancing rules to stand around gawking at bathing suits,[96] but they were at least permitted to remain open. Amazon had already done the same, warning U.S. and UK customers that sellers would be unable to send non-essential items to its warehouses for weeks because the space was needed for high-priority goods—none of which, it must be noted, included books.[97] Nor would it even ship books to French and Italian customers—perhaps fearing they'd do the unthinkable and use their lockdown time

---

96 Jeanette DeForge, "Coronavirus prevention: Chicopee orders Walmart, BJ's, others to close areas that sell non-essential goods," *MassLive,* updated March 30, 2020, https://www.masslive.com/news/2020/03/coronavirus-prevention-chicopee-orders-walmart-bjs-others-to-close-areas-that-sell-non-essential-goods.html.

97 Joanna Partridge, "Amazon to suspend non-essential shipments to UK and US warehouses," *The Guardian,* March 17, 2020, https://www.theguardian.com/uk-news/2020/mar/17/amazon-to-suspend-all-non-essential-shipments-in-uk-and-us-until-april.

to read.[98] Michigan residents were prohibited from buying gardening supplies[99] like seeds, even as the threat of shortages made many consider growing their own food. However, medical marijuana was OK, just as individual states kept liquor stores open—a drugged populace is an obedient populace.

The post-coronavirus world order wouldn't be possible without a central component of the Shock Doctrine—what Nixon and the Chicago School acolytes after him fondly called "making the economy scream." Only by pulling the financial rug out from under society can sweeping economic changes be pushed through without opposition, forcing a desperate population to change their ways and embrace new forms of debt slavery. Just as the Chicago School shocks of late-20th-century Latin America forced those countries to take on impossible-to-repay IMF loans, then demanded devastating austerity cuts in order to pay for them, the "stimulus" money handed out to small businesses and individuals will not come without a price.

The sheer amount of money the Fed is pouring into the economy boggles the mind. Economic experts warned, as the trillions flowed, that the nation was entering uncharted territory. Detractors of Modern Monetary Theory (MMT), an alternate system popular among some progressive economists, complain it essentially calls for minting money as needed out of thin air, criticism that looks a bit absurd in light of the Fed's high-stakes game of make-believe; economists might expect MMT to be taken more seriously in "reputable" circles going forward.

Rep. Thomas Massie, a Republican congressman from Kentucky and the sole dissenter from the bloated stimulus coronavirus package pushed through the U.S. Congress on shame and guilt, referred to the $1,200 individual payments promised to individual Americans as "the cheese in the trap." It remains to be seen whether, like FEMA aid to disaster victims, the IRS will try to claw back any of the money, should it retrospectively find a recipient undeserving. But even if individuals are allowed to keep their pittance, by cashing the check, they bought in to a collapsing system, thereby allowing themselves to be ensnared in the same way as those countries pressured into taking IMF loans that they would never be able to pay back. There, accepting the payment was acceding to the serfdom the massive corporate bailouts would inflict upon future generations—if not this one.

---

98 Chris Smith, "Amazon will stop shipping nonessentials in Italy and France due to coronavirus," *BGR,* March 23, 2020, https://bgr.com/2020/03/23/coronavirus-update-amazon-stops-non-essential-deliveries-in-italy/.

99 The Office of Governor Gretchen Whitmer, Executive Order 2020-42, "COVID-19: Temporary requirement to suspend activities that are not necessary to sustain or protect life" (rescission of Executive Order 2020-21), *Michigan.gov,* accessed April 25, 2020, https://www.michigan.gov/whitmer/0,9309,7-387-90499_90705-525182--,00.html.

Americans should ask Argentina, or Peru, or the Congo about what it's like to live one's life in hock to vulture capitalists.

Massie correctly referred to March 2020's CARES Act—the coronavirus stimulus—as "the biggest wealth transfer from common folks to the super-rich (Wall Street and bankers) in the history of mankind."[100] While the $350 billion the package set aside for the small businesses employing half the country's workers under the Paycheck Protection Program sounded generous—at least compared to $1,200—it soon became clear that the banks and the government were on one side and the businesses scrambling to keep ahead of bankruptcy were on the other. Days before the banks were scheduled to begin taking loan applications, inside sources "leaked" to the media that an industry group representing many of the banks tasked with doling out the stimulus money was threatening to walk away from the project unless the Treasury increased the 0.5% interest rate on the loans to make it worth the lenders' while. According to the *Financial Times*, the banks got their wish; the jacked-up rates (as high as 5%) will allow them to make as much as $17.5 billion off distributing fiscal lifelines to dying American businesses.[101]

The day loan applications opened, Bank of America—the only large lender to get its site online close to schedule—shafted thousands of lifetime customers, revealing in terms posted to the portal that only businesses that had previously borrowed from Bank of America would be able to apply for the rescue package. The surprise caveat effectively sealed the fate of thousands of responsible business owners who'd never needed a line of credit because they had operated within their means. Certainly, the shunned entrepreneurs could try another bank, but with many more businesses seeking loans than there is money to go around, they'd have to get in line.

Just as the individual $1,200 checks were meant to soften Americans up to the notion of a Universal Basic Income—a supposedly progressive idea that was actually first proposed by uber-neoliberal Milton Friedman—the small business loans, which are essentially small business grants (they don't have to be repaid if they are spent on business expenses) were meant to generate positive feeling for the idea of having government as a silent partner in even the smallest American enterprises. Even though the "free market" has been little more than a beloved

---

100 Thomas Massie (@RepThomasMassie), "The stimulus package that just passed is the biggest wealth transfer from common folks to the super-rich (Wall Street and bankers) in the history of mankind. Done in the name of a virus with $1200 checks as the cheese in the trap. This will be obvious in short order." Twitter, March 29, 2020, https://twitter.com/RepThomasMassie/status/1244255601171054594 (accessed April 17, 2020).

101 Tyler Durden, "Banks To Make Billions On Small Business Bailout," *ZeroHedge,* April 1, 2020, https://www.zerohedge.com/economics/banks-make-billions-small-business-bailout.

American myth for generations, U.S. small business owners tend to be fiercely proud of having "made it" on their own, without government assistance. While some have no doubt been forced to turn to banks for loans over the years, the ones who don't—the most ruggedly individualistic—are also the least likely to accept the idea of government as an "investor"/co-owner. Rather than try to convert these types after giving them the money, the Treasury presumably figured it would be easier to just let them go bankrupt and bail out their more flexible competitors. Government has long provided hefty subsidies to high-dollar industries like oil and agriculture—it's only fair that such socialism-by-another-name should extend to the little guy.

The loans were an easy way for government to quietly play favorites, its preferences laundered through the banks doing the lending. Private equity firms who even during "normal" economic conditions were responsible for putting thousands out of work were rumored to be elbowing their way to the front of the gravy train. The president's sly reference to how Americans' "favorite restaurants" would still be around post-pandemic—just maybe under a different owner—foreshadowed the possibility that foreclosed-upon businesses might be doled out as rewards to cooperative institutions, perhaps bundled up and securitized in the same way Wall Street has packaged everything from mortgages to student loans.

The pandemic crystallized the reality that the elected U.S. government's power over the country's economy exists at the pleasure of the financial sector. The Fed has made its loyalties apparent, and they aren't with Trump. As president, he may be able to order companies like 3M to manufacture more masks under the Defense Production Act, but even hinting at wanting to see the country reopened for business met with sharp rebukes from "experts" like Bill Gates and AIDS profiteer Dr. Tony Fauci, who quickly became the face of the epidemic in the U.S. Only when he empaneled a group of big-business CEOs from some of the most hated companies in America to advise him, spitting in the face of his working-class supporters by putting Google, Goldman Sachs, JP Morgan, Walmart, and Lockheed Martin (among others) in charge[102] of when they'd be able to return to their jobs, did the media squeals relent—as the fat cats advised him to hit the brake pedal. At the same time, New York Governor Andrew Cuomo, who'd rapidly emerged as the leader of the Democratic "opposition," enlisted the services of elite management consultancies McKinsey & Co. and Deloitte, plus a pair of advisors from private equity giants Blackstone Group and MacAndrews & Forbes, to

---

102 John Fritze and David Jackson, "Trump taps US companies to advise on reopening economy amid coronavirus pandemic," *USA Today,* updated April 15, 2020, https://www.usatoday.com/story/news/politics/2020/04/14/coronavirus-trump-names-advisory-group-study-reopening-economy/2984793001/.

"Trump-proof" his own economic reopening plan,[103] guaranteeing a never-ending flood of business for all four companies' restructuring and turnaround divisions. A feeding frenzy for the vulture capitalists was all but guaranteed.

And the dominance of technocratic "consultants" was by no means limited to the U.S. UK PM Boris Johnson's attempts to manage his country's cases via "herd immunity" in an effort to avoid shutting down the entire country were also loudly condemned by the British intelligentsia as "Johnson wants your elderly relatives to get sick and die" and was quickly replaced with the usual shutdown—with Johnson himself getting a dose of the coronavirus for his trouble.

Nationwide lockdowns foisted a brutal economic Darwinism on nearly every sector of the economy, forcing small businesses to close their doors while larger ones were able to snap up their smaller competitors at bargain-basement prices. While other western countries were considerably more generous than the U.S. in the assistance they offered individual citizens, even the most robust social safety net measures could be seen as mere anti-riot insurance next to the gargantuan bailouts handed to financial institutions that provide no tangible value to the average person. Banks in the UK, which also dangled small-business rescue loans in front of shutdown-stricken enterprises, forced applicants to sign a personal guarantee that could see them lose everything in case of default.[104] Preying on the desperate was the rule, rather than the exception.

By cutting out small- and medium-sized businesses and leaving only those employed by mega-corporations and gig-work platforms on the job, the western economic shutdowns seemed carefully constructed to eviscerate workers' rights. Gig workers are independent contractors, meaning they rarely receive benefits and have no collective bargaining rights. Many gig workers have never even spoken to a human associated with the corporation that pays them—jobs, rides, or orders are served up on an automated platform, and there's no easy way to complain to a real person. Like the millions of freelancers who found themselves suddenly without work following the coronavirus crash, independent contractors are not eligible for unemployment benefits and have no safety net if they are laid off. The corporations that employ them—Amazon, Uber, Instacart—thus have no incentive to be responsive to grievances, with millions of newly-unemployed potential hires lined up behind them if they raise a fuss about working conditions. The career-based model of employment that suffered a crippling blow with the

---

103 Jarrett Renshaw, "New York forms team to develop 'Trump-proof' economic reopening plan," *Reuters,* April 15, 2020, https://www.reuters.com/article/us-health-coronavirus-usa-governors-excl-idUSKCN21Y01V.

104 Andy Verity, "Banks under fire for coronavirus loan tactics," *BBC,* March 30, 2020, https://www.bbc.com/news/business-52043896.

mass layoffs that followed the crash of 2008 was all but finished off by the coronavirus shutdowns.

Precarious employment aside, the psychological impact of being told—through Amazon and other employers' failure to provide basic protective items like gloves, masks, and hand sanitizer—that one's own life is less important than the delivery of the customer's dinner, toilet paper, or sex toys is demoralizing and dehumanizing. Delivery workers were classed with the "essential" occupations, but it's difficult to feel essential ping-ponging between holed-up bourgeois answering doors in their sweatpants and refusing to tip. With first Amazon and Instacart and then Whole Foods workers staging wildcat strikes for basic benefits, the epidemic brought the U.S. the closest it's been to a class war since Occupy—not that that's saying much.

But being employed at all was a luxury—workers were expected to be grateful, no matter how unpleasant their job. Imagine the psychological blow of being declared "non-essential"! Those who worked in non-essential industries didn't just lose their jobs—many stood poised to lose their homes. While the U.S. passed a three-month eviction moratorium, debts weren't cancelled—merely postponed. That $1,200 was a bandaid on a bullet wound in a country where two thirds of adults don't have $600 for an emergency expense and one fifth were living paycheck to paycheck *before* the collapse.

The mammoth consolidation of wealth coming out the other end of the coronavirus crisis will make the crash of 2008 look like a blip on the radar. The Federal Reserve's purchase of $250 billion in mortgage-backed securities in just two weeks, forcing down rates, detonated the mortgage industry—already moribund as millions of Americans found themselves out of work and unable to make payments. Certainly no one is *buying* houses. The Fed—and the too-big-to-fail banks—end up owning the lot.[105] Just as Blackstone Group snapped up hundreds of thousands of foreclosed homes in 2008, abusing the occupants of their new properties with practices so extortionate the UN had to step in,[106] a second wave of housing commodification is looming that will consign millions to glorified serfdom.

The Fed's ambitions are a lot bigger than a few doomed housing lenders or even weaponizing the need for shelter, however. In addition to the hefty stake it obtained by proxy in the American small businesses that received PPP loans, it

---

105 Ben Brown, "Did the Fed Just Accidentally Trigger a Housing Market Crash?" *CNN,* March 30, 2020, https://www.ccn.com/did-the-fed-just-accidentally-trigger-a-housing-market-crash/.

106 Patrick Butler and Dominic Rushe, "UN accuses Blackstone Group of contributing to global housing crisis," *The Guardian,* March 26, 2019, https://www.theguardian.com/us-news/2019/mar/26/blackstone-group-accused-global-housing-crisis-un.

also set up a "temporary repurchase agreement facility" to graciously offer foreign central banks the opportunity to unload their Treasury securities in exchange for cash—a sort of "sorry we tanked the value of your holdings, here's a consolation prize, now spend it while it's still worth something." Bloomberg sang the praises of the private corporation, quoting a former Fed official who described it as "playing central banker to the world."[107]

If anything, however, that was a distraction from the real consolidation of wealth taking place. The Fed hired BlackRock, the world's largest asset manager, to conduct the trades it couldn't legally run itself under a handful of other special purpose vehicles set up under the bailout legislation.[108] This handed even more power to one of the most preposterously-wealthy, insanely-powerful corporations on the planet. With $7.4 trillion assets under management, BlackRock was already one of the largest shareholders in nearly every megacorporation in the U.S., owning multi-billion-dollar stakes in...everything. Apple, Exxon, Lockheed Martin, Disney, Facebook, Boeing, Walmart, and so on (including the lion's share of the companies on Trump's economic reopening council). It is capable of setting the zeitgeist in a way few are, and ideally positioned to rebuild the American economy from the ground up in its image. BlackRock's CEO, Larry Fink, is a lifelong Democrat who recently reoriented his fund's investment strategy toward climate change, "predicting" with unsettling accuracy that "in the near future—and sooner than most expect—there will be a significant reallocation of capital."[109]

Fink's ambitions are global—BlackRock launched the Climate Finance Partnership in 2018 in conjunction with the governments of France and Germany and several private foundations in order to "nudge" institutional investors into "sustainable" industries in emerging markets, reasoning that—in the words of pro-war think tank the Atlantic Council—"there is simply not enough public money available globally to make a meaningful dent in our response to climate

---

107 Rich Miller, "Fed Takes on Role of World's Central Bank by Pumping Out Dollars," *Yahoo! Finance,* March 31, 2020, https://finance.yahoo.com/news/fed-takes-role-world-central-191339893.html (accessed April 17, 2020).

108 Jim Bianco, "The Fed's Cure Risks Being Worse Than the Disease," *Bloomberg,* March 27, 2020, https://www.bloomberg.com/opinion/articles/2020-03-27/federal-reserve-s-financial-cure-risks-being-worse-than-disease.

109 Laurel Wamsley, "World's Largest Asset Manager Puts Climate At The Center Of Its Investment Strategy," *NPR,* January 14, 2020, https://www.npr.org/2020/01/14/796252481/worlds-largest-asset-manager-puts-climate-at-the-center-of-its-investment-strate.

change."[110] And the CEO has warned companies that drag their feet on embracing the sustainability goals put forth in agreements like the Paris Climate Accord—to which the U.S. is not a signatory—that they may find themselves shut out from BlackRock's lucrative investments. Don't agree with his philosophy on climate, but still want to participate in any of the new Fed programs? Too bad—the U.S. economy belongs to him—and a handful of likeminded gatekeepers like him—now.

A *USA Today* piece added insult to injury, insisting the Fed was an "unsung hero" of the coronavirus crisis and that the world actually owes the predatory U.S. entity a debt of gratitude. In condescending language that portrayed the Fed as an almost godlike entity that works in mysterious ways—"its activities are arcane to most of us other than financial players, scholars and students," or otherwise put, "shut up and trust your betters, peon"—the writer warned that without the great Fed's benevolence, "we would be watching a chain reaction of bankruptcies and unemployment that would...exceed the depths of the Great Depression of the 1930s."[111] With 22 million Americans put out of work in the space of a month[112] and three quarters of the country's 30 million small businesses[113] reportedly in the red, the U.S. is already almost there—but the Fed apologist seems to hint that it can always get worse.

The veiled threat is all too apparent. As Orwell wrote, it is not enough to fear Big Brother—you must love him, as well. When "he"—or should we say "He"—becomes the source of one's paycheck, and His largesse permits one to continue occupying one's home, it's a lot easier to spare some space in one's heart—and a lot harder to defy Him by resisting the shackles of His police state.

110 John E. Morton, "The climate finance partnership: Mobilizing institutional capital to address the climate opportunity," *Atlantic Council,* November 8, 2018, https://atlanticcouncil.org/blogs/energysource/the-climate-finance-partnership-mobilizing-institutional-capital-to-address-the-climate-opportunity/.

111 Owen Ullmann, "An unsung hero of the coronavirus crisis: The Federal Reserve," *USA Today,* March 24, 2020, https://www.usatoday.com/story/opinion/2020/03/24/unsung-hero-coronavirus-crisis-federal-reserve/2902681001/.

112 Rebecca Rainey, "Jobless claims reach 22 million over four weeks," *Politico,* April 16, 2020, https://www.politico.com/news/2020/04/16/coronavirus-unemployment-claims-numbers-190026.

113 U.S. Small Business Administration, Office of Advocacy, *Small Business Profile,* 2017, https://www.sba.gov/sites/default/files/advocacy/All_States.pdf (accessed April 17, 2020).

Sell Out

The "wartime climate" enabled passage of seemingly unrelated legislation, especially in the U.S., where corporate lobbyists have long had an inside track to the most police-state-happy legislators. At least three U.S. state governments took advantage of the distracted populace to pass laws criminalizing protests against oil and gas pipelines. Kentucky, South Dakota, Alabama, and West Virginia passed nearly identical bills penned by the American Legislative Exchange Council, a federation of corporate lobbyists that cooks up boilerplate bills and hands them to its bought congressmen in various states for smooth passage. While the laws varied slightly—one elevated such protests to a felony, and tacked on a definition of "intentional use of force or violence by three or more persons" causing "any damage to property" as a felony "riot"—they had in common being completely, totally unrelated to any state-level coronavirus response.[114]

And the power grab on behalf of energy interests went even further. The Trump administration quietly paused enforcement of EPA pollution regulations and approved multiple mining and drilling initiatives—guaranteeing future increases in the same air pollution that some have blamed for causing so many deaths in Italy and China amid the epidemic. As oil prices plummeted toward an unthinkable $5 a barrel, Trump talked about bailing out the failing shale oil industry, a sector that has long been unprofitable but is essential to the U.S.' delusion of its own "energy independence." Thus even while the multi-billion-dollar climate change "industry" claimed the coronavirus "moment," the actual planet was getting shafted.

The corporate giveaways weren't limited to efforts to reverse the shale fail. The U.S. also tiptoed a few steps closer to the wildly controversial 5G rollout while everyone's back was turned, with a major 5G bill sailing through the Senate unanimously before being signed into law by Trump in March. Municipalities nation- and worldwide have made progress toward banning the dangerous technology, but the federal government has shown no interest in safety studies or the significant body of scientific knowledge that already exists showing 5G is

---

114 Alexander C. Kaufman, "States Quietly Pass Laws Criminalizing Fossil Fuel Protests Amid Coronavirus Chaos," *HuffPost,* updated March 31, 2020, https://www.huffpost.com/entry/pipeline-protest-laws-coronavirus_n_5e7e7570c5b6256a7a2aab41.

harmful.[115] Reports even surfaced on social media of surreptitious installation of 5G in schools shut down by the pandemic, though these were difficult to confirm.[116]

The big telecoms' fellow megacorporations went to the mat to defend 5G, heaping scorn upon skeptics of the technology and even booting some of them from social media platforms under a hastily-rolled-out YouTube policy banning any discussion of a potential link between 5G and the coronavirus, conflating all criticism of the technology with the unproven theory. A series of suspicious fires at 5G towers were held up as proof that 5G critics were encouraging violence, as if objecting to installing what is for all intents and purposes a weapons system in one's backyard was the equivalent of calling for attacks on one's fellow man. At the same time, consent was being manufactured for deplatforming all 5G skeptics, with tech publications complaining that YouTube was "only" suppressing the 5G-corona "conspiracy theorists."[117] Twitter vowed to remove all content that "could lead to the destruction or damage of critical 5G infrastructure" under its coronavirus content guidelines, incidentally (intentionally?) bolstering the claims of the same 5G-coronavirus conspiracy theorists they were supposedly trying to suppress by lumping the two together in a single policy.[118]

Such vociferous defense of 5G made it clear that the technology was more than just a faster telecoms network—it's the very operating system for the post-pandemic police state. 5G is a must for the 24/7 surveillance, the Internet of Things, the constant scanning and tracking and processing of all objects in space at all times. Massive bandwidth is required for processing the endless data streams through complex algorithms and using them to predict an individual's behavior before they themselves know what they will do. 5G isn't about being able to download movies faster. It's about the narrative managers gaining the power to turn people's lives into what are, in effect, movies—the actors unaware they lack

---

115 Joel M. Moskowitz, "We Have No Reason to Believe 5G Is Safe," *Scientific American,* Oct. 17, 2019, https://blogs.scientificamerican.com/observations/we-have-no-reason-to-believe-5g-is-safe/.

116 Take Back Your Power, "Are 5G / Biometric Systems Being Covertly Installed During the Lockdown, Where You Live?," *Global Research,* March 23, 2020, https://www.globalresearch.ca/are-5g-biometric-systems-being-covertly-installed-during-lockdown-where-you-live/5707159.

117 Jon Fingas, "YouTube will remove videos falsely linking COVID-19 to 5G," *Engadget,* April 5, 2020, https://www.engadget.com/2020-04-05-youtube-to-remove-5g-coronavirus-videos.html.

118 Twitter Safety (@TwitterSafety), "Since introducing our updated policies on March 18, we've removed over 2,230 Tweets containing misleading and potentially harmful content. Our automated systems have challenged more than 3.4 million accounts targeting manipulative discussions around COVID-19," Twitter, April 22, 2020, https://twitter.com/TwitterSafety/status/1253044659175034880.

free will and are merely following pre-determined character arcs. Criminalizing discussion of the negative health effects of 5G (and there are many[119]—electromagnetic radiation is a carcinogen,[120] and 5G is higher-intensity and higher-frequency than previous generations; with more towers needed to achieve the same level of coverage, the average person will receive a much higher dose, sending their likelihood of experiencing health problems through the roof) is necessary to manufacture consent for the rollout.

Western healthcare systems shed all pretense of prioritizing the health of the patient during the epidemic, instead swearing open fealty to the pharmaceutical industry and allowing medically-inept governments to oversee the practice of medicine. Despite clinical trials in China and elsewhere showing promising results for off-patent malaria drugs chloroquine and hydroxychloroquine, the governors of Nevada and Michigan banned doctors from prescribing them to treat Covid-19 even as President Trump sang the drug's praises and individual doctors were reported to be hoarding both drugs.[121] France saw its stockpiles of chloroquine "pillaged," while the drug itself was mysteriously banned as "poisonous" (after decades of uneventful usage to treat malaria) in January by a Health Minister uncomfortably close to PM Macron. One of the country's top doctors, Didier Raoult, was pilloried as a fraud in pro-Macron media (which subsequently was forced to retract its smears) for suggesting its usage, which the government finally allowed only in terminal cases (where, Raoult said, it would no longer be of any use).[122]

The banana-republic levels of corruption on display at UK and French hospitals, which while supposedly government-run have been stripped to the bone in preparation for privatization, exacerbated both nations' epidemics, even as European nations turned on one another to seize shipments of masks and protective

---

119 Small Cells, Mini Cell Towers, Wireless Facilities and Health: Letters From Scientists on the Health Risk of 5G: Scientific Appeals and Scientific Letters From Experts on The Impact of Wireless Antennas on Public Health," *Environmental Health Trust,* accessed April 25, 2020, https://ehtrust.org/small-cells-mini-cell-towers-health-letters-scientists-health-risk-5g/.

120 World Health Organization, International Agency for Research on Cancer, "IARC Classifies Radiofrequency Electromagnetic Fields as Possibly Carcinogenic to Humans," May 31, 2011, https://www.iarc.fr/wp-content/uploads/2018/07/pr208_E.pdf.

121 Topher Sanders, David Armstrong and Ava Kofman, "Doctors Are Hoarding Unproven Coronavirus Medicine by Writing Prescriptions for Themselves and Their Families," *ProPublica,* March 24, 2020, https://www.propublica.org/article/doctors-are-hoarding-unproven-coronavirus-medicine-by-writing-prescriptions-for-themselves-and-their-families.

122 Pepe Escobar, "Why France is hiding a cheap and tested virus cure," *Information Clearing House,* March 27, 2020, http://www.informationclearinghouse.info/54074.htm.

equipment. The U.S. got in on the *Lord of the Flies*-like behavior, snatching other countries' medical supplies off the tarmac and trying to bribe Germany to give it exclusive rights to a vaccine being developed. France perhaps won the booby prize for most flagrant disregard for humanity after a pair of elite doctors (from the world-renowned INSERM and Paris' Cochin Hospital) earnestly suggested testing coronavirus vaccines "in Africa where there are no masks, no treatment, no life-support"—even as Africa, for once, had been spared the brunt of an epidemic that may have had its origins with the colonial powers.[123] Meanwhile, even while western media sang the praises of doctors and nurses, hailing them as the coronavirus equivalent of 9/11's firefighters, hospitals across the U.S. were warning their staff that speaking to the media about their working conditions would get them fired.[124] If it is true that crises merely bring out an entity's true nature, the healthcare systems of the western world must be said to be rotten to the core.

MEDICAL MARTIAL LAW

A form of "medical martial law" actually predated coronavirus in the U.S., though it remained largely unexercised in the nearly two decades after its passage. Following the "anthrax attacks" on senators who opposed the draconian Patriot Act, presaged in Johns Hopkins' "Dark Winter" simulation, more than half of U.S. states passed the Model State Emergency Health Preparedness Act (written, in what is surely an innocent coincidence, by Professor Larry Gostin, Co-Director of the Center for Law and the Public Health at Johns Hopkins and Georgetown Universities[125]). This draconian slice of legislation allows government officials and public health officials to act in each other's roles in ways that go far beyond what a normal person would consider necessary to respond to a public health emergency: government officials may administer vaccines, public health officials can seize and destroy firearms and other property, parents who decline vaccines for their children can have them taken away and quarantined, martial law can be declared and the military placed under the direction of public health authorities. Intensely controversial when first proposed, even amid the cowed climate of

---

123 Julian Kossoff, "2 top French doctors said on live TV that coronavirus vaccines should be tested on poor Africans, leaving viewers horrified," *Business Insider,* April 3, 2020, https://www.businessinsider.com/coronavirus-vaccines-france-doctors-say-test-poor-africans-outrage-2020-4.

124 Olivia Carville, Emma Court and Kristen V Brown, "Hospitals Tell Doctors They'll Be Fired If They Speak Out About Lack of Gear," *Bloomberg,* March 31, 2020, https://www.bloomberg.com/news/articles/2020-03-31/hospitals-tell-doctors-they-ll-be-fired-if-they-talk-to-press.

125 "Model State Emergency Health Powers Act," ACLU, https://www.aclu.org/other/model-state-emergency-health-powers-act (accessed April 17, 2020).

post-9/11 America, the law has now aged safely enough to be put into practice without risk of legal challenge. And it's clear that states were itching to use these powers—many declared states of emergency with just a few cases of coronavirus, barely stopping to catch their breath before instituting lockdowns and calling up the National Guard to enforce quarantine and maybe kick in a few doors.

It isn't merely the right to be secure in one's home that is under threat in the pandemic world order, though. At a time when it had recorded just three corona-virus-associated deaths, Denmark passed legislation that will require its citizens to receive a yet-to-be-developed coronavirus vaccine—full stop. The law, which was unanimously approved by the Danish Parliament, gave health authorities (backed by police) the power to enforce quarantine, testing, and "treatment," specifically by a future vaccine. Individuals could be barred from public places, including public transit, and a provision that would have allowed authorities to enter private homes *without a court order* if coronavirus infection was suspected was only dropped at the last minute. No doubt, it is sitting on the shelf awaiting some future "health emergency."[126]

The notion of forced vaccination is not a conspiracy theory. No one thinks of Denmark as an authoritarian police-state, yet they passed a law that flagrantly vio-lates the Nuremberg Codes of 1947, specifically the notion of "informed consent" in medical experimentation.[127] Mandatory vaccination laws have been quietly passed in several U.S. states, though they were previously limited to children. A concentrated campaign has been under way to remove religious exemptions to vaccination mandates, and California has even done away with most medical exemptions—even as the U.S.' vaccine court, established when Washington in-demnified vaccine manufacturers from lawsuits in 1986, surpassed $4 billion in awards paid to the parents of vaccine-damaged children in 2018.[128] The profitable vista of potential vaccine targets opened up by the coronavirus pandemic is vast,

---

126 "Denmark rushes through emergency coronavirus law," *The Local,* March 13, 2020, https://www.thelocal.dk/20200313/denmark-passes-far-reaching-emergency-coronavirus-law.

127 Nuremberg Military Tribunal, "Nuremberg Code Establishes the Principle of Informed Consent," August 19, 1947 [Excerpt of the verdict in the case of U.S.A. v. Karl Brandt et al. ("Doctors Trial"), contained in Trials of War Criminals before the Nuremberg Military Tribunals under Control Council Law No. 10 (Washington, D.C., U.S. Government Printing Office, 1949), vol. 2, pp. 181-183] *Encyclopedia.com,* updated March 5, 2020, https://www.encyclopedia.com/science/medical-magazines/nuremberg-code-establishes-principle-informed-consent (accessed April 17, 2020).

128 "$4 Billion and Growing: U.S. Payouts for Vaccine Injuries and Deaths Keep Climbing," *Children's Health Defense,* November 19, 2018, https://childrenshealthdefense.org/news/4-billion-and-growing-u-s-payouts-for-vaccine-injuries-and-deaths-keep-climbing.

and while there will no doubt be a substantial contingent resisting the shots, they may find they are not just socially but physically compelled to take them.

Those who believe such a scenario will never unfold in their own country are fooling themselves. In 2019, New York City health authorities declared a state of emergency over a wildly-exaggerated "measles epidemic," designating three zip codes believed to contain an especially high portion of unvaccinated children and fining parents who refused to give their child the shot. The declaration targeted the city's large Hasidic Jewish population, who in the past have been able to secure religious exemptions to the increasingly heavy vaccine burden children must shoulder in order to enter public schools. City health commissioner Oxiris Barbot danced around the question of whether children would be forcibly vaccinated if their parents still—after fines and perhaps jail time—resisted, allowing only that holdouts would be dealt with on a "case-by-case basis."[129]

When coronavirus appeared in Britain, health authorities were ready mulling a law that would criminalize "anti-vaccine propaganda," which had previously been permitted so long as the individual posting it believed what they were posting to be true.[130] With prolonged campaigns underway in the UK and U.S. both to demonize "anti-vaxers," it will be no great stretch to criminalize expressing anti-vaccine sentiment, which already gets individuals booted off social media.

Governments that can't criminalize it outright may find it easier to declare vaccine criticism a form of mental illness, just as failing to follow orders has been classed as "oppositional defiant disorder." The UK made dramatic steps toward a Stalinesque weaponization of "mental health" during the pandemic, loosening requirements for sectioning troublesome citizens so that a single doctor's sayso became all that was necessary to detain someone in a mental health facility indefinitely. Previously, two doctors' approval had been required, and six months was the maximum length for involuntary detention.[131] Given the UK's ongoing efforts to criminalize "disinformation," it's very likely Britons will see proponents of "conspiracy theories" declared mentally ill and sectioned, where they are now merely socially shamed.

---

129 Jamie Ducharme, "New York City Is Requiring Some Residents to Get Vaccinated Against Measles. Is That Legal — And Ethical?" *Time,* April 10, 2019, https://time.com/5567422/mandatory-vaccination-legal-ethics/.

130 Mike Wright, "Posting anti-vaccine propaganda on social media could become criminal offence, Law Commissioner says," *The Telegraph,* Feb. 1, 2020, https://www.telegraph.co.uk/news/2020/02/01/posting-anti-vaccine-propaganda-social-media-could-become-criminal/.

131 U.K. Dept. of Health and Social Care, "What the Coronavirus Bill will do," updated March 26, 2020, https://www.gov.uk/government/publications/coronavirus-bill-what-it-will-do/what-the-coronavirus-bill-will-do.

The UK would not be alone in pathologizing political dissent—Germany and Switzerland both seized the epidemic as cause to begin locking up troublemakers in psych wards. German lawyer Beate Bahner, a medical law specialist, spent several days in a locked psychiatric ward after she called for Germans to take to the streets and protest, pointing out that the country's draconian lockdown was wholly out of proportion to the risks posed by the virus. Before she was violently apprehended at her home and carted off to the mental hospital, she attempted to sue the government and published a lengthy legal analysis explaining exactly how the lockdown was "the greatest legal scandal in the post-1940s history of Germany."[132] Her "crime"? "Incitement to criminal acts"—i.e., protesting.[133] Swiss doctor Thomas Binder was similarly carted off to a psych ward after a SWAT team raided his medical practice, accused of tweeting "threats against the authorities" and possessing a "presumably unstable psyche." Of course, one would have to be unstable to doubt the benevolent intentions of the pandemic police state.[134]

Alternately, dissenters from the medical police state could be criminally arrested—UK police have been arresting citizens for "offensive speech" for over a decade.[135] The U.S.' once-sanguine First Amendment protections won't prevent similar abuses across the Atlantic, either. The FBI had already linked "conspiracy theories" and "domestic extremism" before coronavirus hit, and "anti-vaccine conspiracy theories" will likely be conflated with terrorism against the public health and punished with jail time—just as the *Washington Post* demanded back in 2019.[136]

---

132 Beate Bahner, "Beate Bahner erklärt, warum der Shutdown verfassungswidrig ist und warum dies der größte Rechtsskandal ist, den die Bundesrepublik Deutschland je erlebt hat" ("Beate Bahner explains why the shutdown is unconstitutional and why this is the biggest legal scandal the Federal Republic of Germany has ever experienced"), April 7, 2020, http://beatebahner.de/lib.medien/Erklaerung%20Beate%20Bahner%207.4.2020.pdf.

133 Alex Thomson, "Coronavirus lockdown: German lawyer detained for opposition," *UK Column,* April 14, 2020, https://www.ukcolumn.org/article/coronavirus-lockdown-german-lawyer-detained-opposition.

134 "Polizei nimmt Arzt wegen Drohungen fest" ("Police arrest doctor for threats"), *20 Minuten,* April 13, 2020, https://www.20min.ch/schweiz/zuerich/story/Polizei-nimmt-corona-skeptischen-Arzt-fest-11735090.

135 Sadie Levy Gale, "Arrests for offensive Facebook and Twitter posts soar in London," *Independent,* June 4, 2016, https://www.independent.co.uk/news/uk/arrests-for-offensive-facebook-and-twitter-posts-soar-in-london-a7064246.html.

136 Juliette Kayyem, "Anti-vaxxers are dangerous. Make them face isolation, fines, arrests." *The Washington Post,* April 30, 2019, https://www.washingtonpost.com/opinions/2019/04/30/time-get-much-tougher-anti-vaccine-crowd/.

The U.S. CDC's own system for manufacturing vaccine consent, detailed in a PowerPoint titled "Recipe for Fostering High Vaccine Demand,"[137] consists of having medical experts and public health authorities play up the severity of the epidemic in the media, cautioning that it's worse than anything that came before and urging vaccination as the answer. Reports of mass death, preferably complete with photographs and sob stories from relatives, are a must, as are happy images of kids getting the shot and references to previous epidemics. The presentation laments the wide variety of information sources available to Americans, complaining that the CDC now has to get its message in front of people's faces 10 to 12 times before they're likely to seek out the jab.

Bill Gates, whom a sycophantic media has praised for his 2015 "prediction" of the coronavirus epidemic, demanded a total shutdown of society from day one, essentially echoing the Lock Step scenario. While the insanely-wealthy former programmer is not a medical expert, his billions have funded exploitative, harmful mass vaccination campaigns in India and Pakistan.[138] His goal of vaccinating the human race sounds benign enough to those without an understanding of the human immune system or the pharmaceutical industry's relationship with government. But the iron-fisted eugenicist inside the nerdy sweater-vest made itself felt as Gates did the talk-show circuit, suggesting Americans will all be walking around in face-masks soon: "we'll have a lot of unusual measures until we get the world vaccinated," he told the Daily Show's Trevor Noah, clarifying that he did indeed mean "7 billion people"—and that they wouldn't have a choice in the matter.[139]

Even if the vaccine certificate, microchip, or other identifier is not made mandatory in a particular country's population, the idea is being normalized rapidly, with Gates and other technocrats funding research into how to make the eventual universal biometric ID as unobtrusive as possible. In the same way that Facebook CEO Mark Zuckerberg has long sought to make an individual's login on the platform a sort of "internet driver's license," Gates' biometric identifier may become an all-purpose user-ID that gives the bearer access to a "fast lane" for travel and

---

137 Glen Nowak, "Increasing Awareness and Uptake of Influenza Immunization," CDC, archived November 26, 2017 at *Wayback Machine,* https://web.archive.org/web/20200206004032/https://www.nationalacademies.org/hmd/~/media/Files/Activity%20Files/PublicHealth/MicrobialThreats/Nowak.pdf (accessed April 17, 2020).

138 Christina Sarich, "Bill Gates Faces Trial in India for Illegally Testing Tribal Children with Vaccines," *Natural Society,* October 13, 2014, https://naturalsociety.com/bill-gates-faces-trial-india-illegally-testing-tribal-children-vaccines/.

139 The Daily Show with Trevor Noah, "Bill Gates on Fighting Coronavirus | The Daily Social Distancing Show," YouTube video, 22:07, April 2, 2020, https://www.youtube.com/watch?v=iyFT8qXcOrM (accessed April 17, 2020).

other perks (the ability to skip the "social distancing" line at the supermarket, perhaps?). The UK floated the idea of making a coronavirus antibody test—an "immune passport"—mandatory to return to work post-quarantine, despite concern about the test's accuracy.[140] Italy also considered the idea.[141]

MIT Technology Review's Gideon Lichfield expanded on how even a non-mandatory vaccination might be forced on people, explaining that unless "we" want to spend half the year trapped under house arrest due to recurrent outbreaks of coronavirus, "we" will have to get used to a privacy-free world in which "proof of immunity" in the form of a vaccine certificate or documentation confirming that one has had and recovered from the virus is required to enter public spaces, travel, work, and socialize in person.[142] "The intrusive surveillance," he wrote, "will be considered a small price to pay for the basic freedom to be with other people."

And lest individuals believe they are safe at home, the WHO poured cold water on that idea early on. After achieving the lockdown of more than half the planet, Mike Ryan, the group's director of emergency response, lamented that the only way to *really* beat the disease was to go door to door, removing the infected from their families. The medical police state does not stop at the door to one's home. If they do not respect your bodily integrity with regard to vaccines, do you really think they will respect private property?[143]

---

140 Rowena Mason, Rajeev Syal and Dan Sabbagh, "No 10 seeks to end coronavirus lockdown with 'immunity passports,'" *The Guardian,* April 2, 2020, https://www.theguardian.com/politics/2020/apr/02/no-10-seeks-to-end-covid-19-lockdown-with-immunity-passports.

141 "In Italy, Going Back to Work May Depend on Having the Right Antibodies," *DNYUZ,* April 4, 2020, https://dnyuz.com/2020/04/04/in-italy-going-back-to-work-may-depend-on-having-the-right-antibodies/.

142 Gideon Lichfield, "We're not going back to normal," *MIT Technology Review,* March 17, 2020, https://www.technologyreview.com/s/615370/coronavirus-pandemic-social-distancing-18-months/.

143 World Health Organization (WHO), "Live from WHO Headquarters—coronavirus—COVID-19 daily press briefing 30 March 2020," YouTube video, 1:05:12, Streamed live on March 30, 2020, https://youtu.be/2v3vlw14NbM (accessed April 17, 2020).

PSYCHOLOGICAL REPERCUSSIONS

> *"We can only win here if you and I are able to surrender the 'me' to the 'we.'"* —Chris Cuomo, CNN

Just as putting a country on a war footing predisposes its people to expect sacrifices—of luxuries, of liberties, even of basic needs—so too does it elicit a predictable and easily manageable form of reactionary patriotism. With two generations of Americans now having spent their entire adult lives in a country that was technically "at war," the effect won't be as pronounced stateside as when the U.S. kicked off the War on Terror. Nevertheless, a spike in fear will manifest in xenophobia (already unprovoked attacks on Chinese and other Asians are reported to be on the rise) and suspicion of outsiders, even if the "outsiders" are just from across state lines. When one's world has shrunk to the boundaries of one's home over months of quarantine and "social distancing," everyone is an outsider. In the UK, where cultural memory of having to "do without" during wartime is stronger, alerts from the National Grid that blackouts may occur (because of a *virus*?) lend verisimilitude to their leaders' wartime rhetoric.[144]

Social Distancing is just another term for alienation, and alienation has long been the means by which control of the individual is achieved. A person who has been alienated from the land, from society, from his family, and finally from himself is putty in the hands of his controllers, defenseless against any kind of psychological operation from totalitarian thought-reform down to the lowliest advertisement. Separated from their communities and forced to interact via artificial means, individuals under lockdown lose touch with their very humanity. There's a reason why solitary confinement has been banned in many countries and considered a form of torture in many more.

Isolation's negative effects on the individual are not merely psychological, either. Just a year ago, thought-pieces pondering the central role of loneliness in many common health problems were a dime a dozen. Social isolation, study upon study has found, is as deadly as smoking or obesity, with multiple studies finding it causes weakening of the immune system, inflammation, and several other ailments that would work synergistically with the coronavirus to greatly increase

---

144 Levi Winchester, "Lights Out: Energy firms warn of blackouts plunging coronavirus lockdown Brits into darkness," *The Sun,* updated April 1, 2020, https://www.thesun.co.uk/money/11292200/coronavirus-energy-electricity-blackout/.

the likelihood of death.[145] In fact, loneliness is most lethal to the elderly—the population most at risk for coronavirus. Social distancing not only does not save these lives—it actively helps end them.

An individual cut off from other human beings and the outside world loses touch with reality, becoming reliant on a media that has proven itself to lie as often as it tells the truth. Only by enforced isolation could the ruling power structure begin to rebuild the trust it has steadily lost over the past several decades, immersing the individual in a sort of epistemological sensory deprivation chamber and offering only the establishment narrative as an alternative to darkness.

Questioning authority became more rare, as it always does in times of war—as western countries inched closer than ever to criminalizing it. It's fitting that the Espionage & Sedition Acts the U.S. passed during World War I, which criminalized speaking out against the war (among other things), resurfaced in the public consciousness in 2019—while the Sedition Act was struck down as unconstitutional, the Espionage Act was used to charge Julian Assange, a non-U.S. citizen who was not under U.S. jurisdiction at the time he committed the "crime" of publishing classified information leaked by a Defense Department insider (a "crime" American news outlets have received journalistic awards for committing). Certainly, the average American was only too willing to scrap their constitutional rights in exchange for a vague promise of safety from a virus, just as they'd been quick to invite the government into their private lives in return for the promise of no more 9/11s. Given the prevailing narrative that "conspiracy theories" about coronavirus are a public health hazard,[146] questioning the vaccine, when it arrives, will likely prove the camel's nose under the tent of scrapping the First Amendment entirely.

"Authority" now definitively includes medical authorities. As the foot soldiers on the front lines of the "war" on coronavirus, doctors and public health

---

145 U.S. Dept. of Health & Human Services, National Institute on Aging, "Social isolation, loneliness in older people pose health risks," April 23, 2019, https://www.nia. nih.gov/news/social-isolation-loneliness-older-people-pose-health-risks; Anthony D. Ong, Bert N. Uchino and Elaine Wethington, "Loneliness and Health in Older Adults: A Mini-Review and Synthesis," *Gerontology,* 2016; 62(4): 443–449, National Institutes of Health Archive, PubMed Central, Nov. 6, 2015, https://www.ncbi.nlm.nih.gov/pmc/articles/PMC6162046/; and Carla Perissinotto, "Loneliness in older persons: a predictor of functional decline and death," *Archives of Internal Medicine,* National Institutes of Health Archive, PubMed Central, July 23, 2012, https://www.ncbi.nlm.nih.gov/pubmed/22710744 (all accessed April 17, 2020).

146 Emma Grey Ellis, "Coronavirus Conspiracy Theories Are a Public Health Hazard," *Wired,* March 27, 2020, https://www.wired.com/story/coronavirus-covid-19-misinformation-campaigns/.

professionals became above reproach. The bizarre "balcony applause videos" heavily pushed on establishment media channels became the yellow ribbons and ubiquitous post-9/11 flag stickers of their day.[147] As physicist Neil deGrasse Tyson quipped on late-night TV in what was not quite a joke, the coronavirus epidemic was in one sense a behavioral experiment regarding whether people can be made to listen to scientists—but it goes without saying that only the practice of allopathic (pharmaceutical) medicine conferred this authority. If it didn't require a prescription, it was declared anathema, even tried-and-true herbal remedies like elderberry, echinacea, and astragalus whose immune-boosting properties were scientifically established. Products containing colloidal silver, famous for its antibacterial and antiviral properties, were temporarily yanked from Amazon, supposedly because televangelist Jim Bakker and conservative political performance artist Alex Jones had claimed their own silver-containing products could cure coronavirus.

Medical authorities wouldn't be true police-state authority figures if they didn't come armed, and coronavirus' shock troops also came strapped with the infrared fever guns that had become an early visual symbol of the epidemic in China. While western media initially dismissed the guns as "notoriously not accurate,"[148] Western governments soon realized that their value is not in their accuracy—after all, individuals infected with coronavirus may walk around spreading the virus for two weeks with no symptoms. Instead, they're marvelously efficient at instilling fear. Having a gun of any sort pointed at you by a uniformed stranger is unnerving, and the sense of having no place to hide—*is my body giving me away? I don't feel sick, but what if I have a fever?*—is unnerving.

Even the nigh-omniscient new tech-enabled Big Brother comes attended by legions of busybodying Little Brothers, unhinged by cabin fever and eager to refashion themselves as quarantine crusaders Doing Their Part for what front-line propagandists like CNN's Chris Cuomo called "our 9/11" (apparently the original 9/11 no longer belongs to "us"). Several countries took advantage of the void left in citizens' identities by newfound unemployment to draft them into service as junior members of the coronavirus Stasi. New Zealand's website for ratting out quarantine violators was so overwhelmed with "Covid-19 L4 breach

---

147 *The Corbett Report,* "The Totally Spontaneous Health Worker Balcony Applause Phenomenon—#PropagandaWatch," YouTube video,19:10, March 30, 2020, https://www.youtube.com/watch?v=_dslfuSBY2U (accessed April 17, 2020).

148 David Yaffe-Bellany, "'Thermometer Guns' on Coronavirus Front Lines Are 'Notoriously Not Accurate,'" *The New York Times,* February 14, 2020, https://www.nytimes.com/2020/02/14/business/coronavirus-temperature-sensor-guns.html.

reports" on its first day that it crashed, according to police chief Mike Bush.[149] Bellevue, Washington whipped up a similar app in an effort to discourage citizens from clogging 911 emergency lines with calls about social distancing violations, though Police Chief Steve Mylett insisted responding officers were "not going to arrest people."[150] Los Angeles Mayor Eric Garcetti went even further, encouraging citizens to rat out construction sites that failed to follow the rules by praising "snitches," quipping during a press conference: "You know the old expression about snitches, well in this case snitches get rewards."[151] It wasn't immediately clear what those rewards would be, but it's easy to imagine special privileges rolled out for the extra-obedient equivalent to an extra square of chocolate in our 21st-century *1984.*

Hand in hand with the promotion of tattletale psychology came acceptance of the idea of collective punishment—putting all the kindergarten class in "time out" because a few kids got in a fight. The UK tightened its lockdown and banned gatherings of more than two people, PM Boris Johnson stated, because *some* Britons hadn't heeded the previous stay-indoors order, instead taking advantage of a warm weekend to revel in nature.[152] Reuters and other establishment media encouraged this conceptualization, spreading videos that appeared to show right-thinking New Yorkers leaning out their windows and shouting insults at "irresponsible" people who dared to walk outside. Hashtags like #StayHome (and its more profane cousin, #StayTheFuckHome) trended relentlessly on Twitter, while anti-lockdown protesters were portrayed on the news and social media as selfish and unthinking pigs putting their own comfort above the lives of the vulnerable—instead of impoverished and increasingly desperate people concerned about how they were supposed to feed their families if they weren't allowed to work. Such claustrophobic groupthink seeped into every corner of the fear-paralyzed psyche,

---

149 Eleanor Ainge Roy, "New Zealand site to report Covid-19 rule-breakers crashes amid spike in lockdown anger," *The Guardian,* March 30, 2020, https://www.msn.com/en-nz/news/national/new-zealand-site-to-report-covid-19-rule-breakers-crashes-amid-spike-in-lockdown-anger/ar-BB11TlMR.

150 KIRO 7 News Staff, "Bellevue police launch new tool to report 'stay home, stay healthy' violations," *KIRO-7,* Bellevue, Washington, March 26, 2020, https://www.kiro7.com/news/local/bellevue-police-launch-new-tool-report-stay-home-stay-healthy-violations/Q7XV53TB4FHTTPFJMRLJFKMSPA/.

151 "'Snitches Get Rewards': Garcetti Issues New Rules For Construction Sites, Encourages Community To Report Safer At Home Violators," *CBSN Los Angeles,* March 31, 2020, https://losangeles.cbslocal.com/2020/03/31/coronavirus-los-angeles-eric-garcetti-snitches-get-rewards/.

152 Naman Ramachandran, "U.K. Declares Partial Coronavirus Lockdown, Bans Gatherings of More Than Two People," *Yahoo! Entertainment,* March 23, 2020, https://www.yahoo.com/entertainment/u-k-declares-partial-coronavirus-204715201.html.

to the point where an open-mic organizer was found to be preemptively censoring poets, warning them against including any "conspiracy stuff" in their art.[153] When the Thought Police are no longer wearing the uniforms of corporations and governments, a people can be said to have well and truly lost its soul.

Public shaming became an epidemic in itself, almost as if the fear-stricken public believed that by ratting out rule-breakers they could gain some degree of protection from the virus. Magical thinking like this thrives in isolation, bolstered by viral, dubiously-true "I-told-you-so" stories about girls who pooh-poohed social distancing testing positive for coronavirus and defiant spring breakers coming home from Cabo only to find that they were all infected. A strong link between obedience and health was encouraged. UK police even went above and beyond their expanded powers under medical martial law by scolding shopkeepers for selling "non-essential goods"—items like chocolate eggs which hardly hamper dealing in critical items but have the undesirable side effect of bringing joy to the purchaser.[154] The threat of being ratted out for not maintaining "social distancing" in one's place of business led even fully-stocked supermarkets to force "excess" customers to line up outside, getting even those citizens who hadn't been driven to bankruptcy in the wave of layoffs used to "queuing for essentials" while their less fortunate peers waited in actual breadlines that sometimes stretched for miles.

CNN's Chris Cuomo, who—as the brother of self-styled Coronavirus Commissar Andrew Cuomo—held a critical propaganda role for Americans, laid it on thick with the wartime sacrifice shtick. Channeling JFK and Rosie the Riveter, he implored the cable network's geriatric audience, with equal parts guilt and shame: "You are being asked to stay on the couch." At the same time, he poured on the fear: "Any of us could get it. Any of us could spread it, suffer. Maybe it doesn't end."[155] When he supposedly tested positive weeks later, the narrative was sealed. Cuomo had made his sacrifice—*will you?*

Such sacrifice was taken literally, with the crisis used to accustom societies to the notion that the old and sick are disposable, even a nuisance. Terminally ill and elderly patients in the UK were shocked to be presented with "do not resuscitate" orders, asked to put aside their lives for "the greater good" in this Brave New World of "healthcare rationing." While Llynfi Surgery, which sent out the

---

153 Janet Phelan, "Book Burnings in the Digital Age: Facebook, Twitter, YouTube and now….Poetry?" *Activist Post,* April 10, 2020, https://www.activistpost.com/2020/04/book-burnings-in-the-digital-age-facebook-twitter-youtube-and-now-poetry.html.

154 "Coronavirus: Easter egg crackdown over essential status 'wrong,'" *BBC,* March 30, 2020, https://www.bbc.com/news/business-52090441 (accessed April 17, 2020).

155 CNN, "Chris Cuomo gets personal: Coronavirus scares me as a parent," YouTube video, 5:42, March 16, 2020, https://www.youtube.com/watch?v=tXKmsbYAsP8 (accessed April 17, 2020).

forms, subsequently apologized and claimed the forms didn't constitute "official guidance,"[156] Sir David King, the one-time scientific adviser to former UK PM Tony Blair, pleaded with the oldsters for compliance anyway, urging those over 90 years old to skip hospital treatment should they fall ill to avoid overburdening the NHS his erstwhile boss had gutted while in power.[157] A column from the *Telegraph*'s assistant editor, Jeremy Warner, confirmed that Social Darwinism had returned triumphantly to mainstream thought, reasoning that "from an entirely disinterested economic perspective, the COVID-19 might even prove mildly beneficial in the long term by disproportionately culling elderly dependents."[158] The situation was not too different across the pond, with several U.S. states' emergency plans explicitly deeming even mentally-disabled patients without a terminal illness to be "poor candidates" for lifesaving care. Other states' rules were more vague, leading some patient advocates to fear these might be broadly interpreted by mercenary hospital administrators to deny otherwise-viable patients care.[159]

Coronavirus patients in the U.S. weren't even given the option to sign away their future—hospital administrators were said to be "consulting" with ethicists to figure out if there was a way to impose (on a case-by-case basis, of course) DNRs *against the will of the patient and their family*. Northwestern Memorial Hospital intensive care director Richard Wunderink modeled the desired behavior for hospital staff when he expressed relief to the *Washington Post* that his coronavirus patients had experienced a slow and steady decline that gave him time to work their families for that vital DNR, rather than a sudden crash that would have required him to resolve some tricky ethical dilemmas on the fly.[160] Such

---

156 Rachel Wearmouth, "Age UK Calls Pushing People To Sign 'Do Not Resuscitate' Forms 'Morally Repugnant,'" *HuffPost*, updated April 3, 2020, https://www.huffingtonpost.co.uk/entry/do-not-resuscitate-age-uk-coronavirus_uk_5e877643c5b609ebfff0b746.

157 Olivia Tobin, "Over-90s should 'rethink hospital treatment' during coronavirus," *Echo*, March 27, 2020, https://www.liverpoolecho.co.uk/news/liverpool-news/over-90s-should-rethink-hospital-17990300.

158 Joe Roberts, "Telegraph journalist says coronavirus 'cull' of elderly could benefit economy," *Metro News*, March 11, 2020, https://metro.co.uk/2020/03/11/telegraph-journalist-says-coronavirus-cull-elderly-benefit-economy-12383907/.

159 Amy Silverman, "People With Intellectual Disabilities May Be Denied Lifesaving Care Under These Plans as Coronavirus Spreads," *Arizona Daily Star*, updated April 11, 2020, https://tucson.com/news/local/people-with-intellectual-disabilities-may-be-denied-lifesaving-care-under-these-plans-as-coronavirus-spreads/article_8c8b430c-ea41-52d5-9f4c-5a89c51e8bb0.html.

160 Ariana Eunjung Cha, "Hospitals across U.S. consider universal do-not-resuscitate orders for coronavirus patients," *Anchorage Daily News*, March 25, 2020, https://www.adn.com/nation-world/2020/03/25/hospitals-across-us-consider-universal-do-not-resuscitate-orders-for-coronavirus-patients/.

circumstances were unthinkable in medical ethics pre-coronavirus, but in a time of scarcity, one has to be, as the *Post* put it, "pragmatic." New York, the epicenter of the U.S. epidemic, ordered paramedics to forego attempts at resuscitating patients in cardiac arrest, weeks after forbidding them to bring flatlining patients to the hospital.[161] With U.S. healthcare facilities receiving a premium from Washington for every coronavirus patient treated,[162] it's not difficult to imagine ambulances eventually being forbidden from going out at all—unless the dispatcher suspects there's corona cash at the end of the rainbow.

Certainly, if the coronavirus was mowing down thousands of healthy young individuals with no existing health issues, such upheavals in societal values could be understood as regrettable but unavoidable, and the climate of fear understandable. But statistics released by Italy's national health authority in mid-March revealed that 99 percent of the country's coronavirus deaths were in patients with serious comorbidities, usually more than one,[163] a pattern that resurfaced again and again in other countries as "confirmed" infection numbers continued to soar. A small but vocal group of experts tried to draw attention to the testing kits' inaccuracy—antibody tests didn't imply someone was sick, but that their immune system had fought (and possibly beaten) the virus; coronavirus tests merely meant the person had *a* coronavirus, not COVID-19 (the common cold is a type of coronavirus). Municipalities like New York frankly admitted they were no longer making an effort to distinguish between coronavirus and other respiratory conditions as they continued pumping out disturbing numbers,[164] and the U.S. decision to financially incentivize coronavirus diagnosis likely contributed to immense inflation.[165] Giving that respiratory conditions are the fourth leading killer of Americans normally, conflating the two permitted the epidemic-pushers to claim truly stratospheric body counts—and justify draconian interventions.

---

161 Carl Campanile and Kate Sheehy, "NY issues do-not-resuscitate guideline for cardiac patients amid coronavirus," *New York Post,* April 21, 2020, https://nypost.com/2020/04/21/ny-issues-do-not-resuscitate-guideline-for-cardiac-patients/.

162 Rich Daly, "Coronavirus bill provides hospitals with $100 billion, other policy wins," *HFMA,* March 25, 2020, https://www.hfma.org/topics/news/2020/03/coronavirus-bill-provides-hospitals-with--100-billion--other-pol.html.

163 Tommaso Ebhardt, Chiara Remondini and Marco Bertacche, "99% of Those Who Died from Virus had Other Illness, Italy Says," *Bloomberg,* March 18, 2020 https://www.bloomberg.com/news/articles/2020-03-18/99-of-those-who-died-from-virus-had-other-illness-italy-says.

164 Larry Buchanan, Jugal K. Patel, Brian M. Rosenthal and Anjali Singhvi, "A Month of Coronavirus in New York City: See the Hardest-Hit Areas," *The New York Times,* April 1, 2020, https://www.nytimes.com/interactive/2020/04/01/nyregion/nyc-coronavirus-cases-map.html.

165 Rich Daly, *op cit.*

Other COVID-19 tests actually arrived contaminated, as if to further unbalance the population: *nothing is safe*. The lengthy incubation period of the virus—as long as two weeks before symptoms appear—added to the atmosphere of paranoia and justified social distancing even from loved ones, as everyone came to be seen as a potential carrier. Thus the nuclear-strength fearmongering which began subtly, with comparisons of the epidemic which was then still largely confined to China to the deadly "Spanish Flu" influenza pandemic of 1918 (a virus that was not, in fact, Spanish in origin, but American[166]) coming out of the WHO and bolstered by a mysterious cadre of Wikipedia editors, had risen to a fever pitch by the time the virus arrived on western shores. By the time New York City mounted an emergency siren on the spire of the Empire State Building, citizens were too exhausted to take a critical look at the narratives of death and panic they were being sold, and they willingly retreated into the perceived safety of their homes and the comfort of following orders.

The CDC did its part to gaslight Americans, telling them for months that face masks offered little by way of protection—unless one was a healthcare worker, in which case they could mean the difference between life and death. Despite the obviously flawed logic, desperate Americans put their faith in the "experts"— only to watch their story change halfway through the epidemic. By April, the U.S. media establishment was already floating the idea of the masks as the "new normal," churning out heart-warming stories of newly-laid-off millennials whipping up hundreds of DIY face masks on their own to fill the supply gap it had helped create by stoking panic.[167] Laredo, Texas even threatened residents with a $1,000 fine if they ventured outdoors without one. Hiding half the face from view has the effect of muting social cues, compounding the difficulty of readjustment as individuals emerge from weeks of enforced isolation with blunted ability to recognize emotion in their fellow humans.

To encourage this subservient psychology, the narrative managers tried to gamify it. Data-mining company Unacast.com created a tool to encourage competition between American municipalities, allowing local governments to pit communities against each other in "obedience contests" after locking them down.

------

166 John M. Barry, "The site of origin of the 1918 influenza pandemic and its public health implications," *Journal of Translational Medicine,* National Institutes of Health Archive, PubMed Central, Jan. 20, 2004, https://www.ncbi.nlm.nih.gov/pmc/articles/ PMC340389/ (accessed April 17, 2020).

167 Ruben Vives, "Coronavirus could leave U.S. with a lasting imprint: Masks as normal part of life," *Los Angeles Times,* April 3, 2020, https://www.latimes.com/california/ story/2020-04-03/coronavirus-could-leave-u-s-with-a-lasting-imprint-masks-as-normal-part-of-life.

The company's "social distancing scoreboard,"[168] updated in real-time as states pass new restrictions on movement, shows how well each community is obeying stay-at-home orders. This Orwellian delight uses cell-phone GPS data to track individuals and gauge their obedience, an apparent privacy intrusion that has gone utterly unremarked-upon in local coverage.[169]

When even a libertarian outlet like Reason is singing the praises of a location-tracking app that turns an individual's phone into a pocket-snitch recording the identity of every other phone it has been within six feet of, we're not in Kansas anymore.[170] Indeed, the coronavirus epidemic has seen surprisingly large swathes of the government-skeptical Right and Left uncritically embrace authoritarian measures like lockdowns and increased surveillance, even when the circumstances do not justify their adoption. Such surrender of dissident political identity is one of the main goals of externally-imposed alienation of this nature. The narrative-managers might congratulate themselves for a job well done.

AGENDA 2030

Agenda 2030 is an ambitious plan to unite humanity under a technocratic global regime under the guise of "eliminating poverty" and "promoting sustainable development." Adopted by the United Nations in 2015, its 17 "sustainable development goals" and 169 targets sound quite benign on the surface, even noble—who doesn't want to end poverty and save the planet?—but viewed from another angle form the scaffolding for an unprecedented and inescapable control grid that will leave no one behind.[171] The police state emerging from the coronavirus pandemic fulfills a staggering number of these goals, and not in the warm fuzzy way the plan was presented at the UN.

The moneyed elite who tirelessly promote Agenda 2030 and related initiatives have seen in coronavirus a flashing bat-signal (irony alert!) from the international

---

168 "Social Distancing Scoreboard," *Covid-19 Toolkit,* Unacast, https://www. unacast.com/covid19/social-distancing-scoreboard (accessed April 17, 2020).

169 Kelsey Sunderland, "Grading social distancing in Tampa Bay: Residents still mobile, terrible at staying home," *News Channel 8,* Tampa Bay, Florida, updated March 31, 2020, https://www.wfla.com/community/health/coronavirus/coronavirus-in-florida-most-tampa-bay-counties-terrible-at-social-distancing-study-says/.

170 Stewart Baker, The Volokh Conspiracy, "The Singapore location app that could elect a President," *Reason,* March 30, 2020, https://reason.com/2020/03/30/the-singapore-location-app-that-could-elect-a-president/.

171 United Nations General Assembly, "Transforming our world: the 2030 Agenda for Sustainable Development," Resolution adopted by the General Assembly on 25 September 2015 at UN General Assembly Seventieth session (Agenda items 15 and 116), https://www.un.org/ga/search/view_doc.asp?symbol=A/RES/70/1&Lang=E.

community, crying out for global governance. Former UK PM Gordon Brown called for a "coordinated global response" merging G20 and the UN Security Council, forming an entity that would wield the twin economic guns of a beefed-up World Bank and International Monetary Fund.[172]

Others pointed to those countries, like Sweden and Belarus, that refused to participate in wholesale panic-induced shutdowns as proof that a stepped-up form of global governance was needed. Clearly, nations couldn't be trusted to responsibly police their own pandemic response; Bill Gates even hinted that those countries that refuse to comply with his vaccine regime would forever see their citizens quarantined by "enlightened" countries.[173] As globalist mouthpiece Emmanuel Macron reminded the world, "the virus has no passport."

Even as international cooperation collapsed among NATO allies, with the U.S. fighting tooth and nail with France and Germany to appropriate deliveries of medical equipment, the UN was unveiling a "multi-partner Trust Fund for COVID19 Response and Recovery," scrambling to put together what even their press release referred to as an Agenda-2030-friendly remedy to "the socio-economic shock."[174]

"With the right actions, the COVID-19 pandemic can mark the beginning of a new type of global and societal cooperation," UN Secretary-General Antonio Guterres declared, stating that only international "solidarity" in the form of "a multilateral response that amounts to at least 10 per cent of global GDP" could defeat the pandemic. That fund would be in addition to the UN's $2 billion "humanitarian response plan," scheduled to run through the end of 2020 and provide testing kits, "handwashing stations," lab equipment, and "airbridges and hubs across Africa, Asia and Latin America" for moving humanitarian workers and supplies.

It's not clear how the crashed economies of the West are supposed to come up with those funds—or why, when the virus has done comparatively little health damage in Africa and most of Latin America, billions should be prioritized to fight it there while other nations are dealing with tens if not hundreds of thousands more cases—but that program's head, Mark Lowcock, repeated a favorite

---

172 Larry Elliott, "Gordon Brown calls for global government to tackle coronavirus," *The Guardian,* March 26, 2020, https://www.theguardian.com/politics/2020/mar/26/gordon-brown-calls-for-global-government-to-tackle-coronavirus.

173 *The Daily Show with Trevor Noah,* "Bill Gates on Fighting Coronavirus | The Daily Social Distancing Show," YouTube video, 22:07, April 2, 2020, https://www.youtube.com/watch?v=iyFT8qXcOrM (accessed April 17, 2020).

174 United Nations, "UN launches COVID-19 plan that could 'defeat the virus and build a better world,'" *UN News,* March 31, 2020, https://news.un.org/en/story/2020/03/1060702.

globalist talking point that has become a rallying cry for coronavirus do-gooders: "nobody will be safe until everybody is safe."[175] The UN could hardly repurpose the funding from current initiatives, he argued—if aid agencies are distracted even for a moment from their existing fight against cholera and other diseases of poor sanitation in the world's most destitute places, coronavirus could settle in for the long haul, periodically emerging from the slums to menace western liberal democracies.[176]

Despite the apparent broad appeal of its "Global Goals," Agenda 2030 has long been controversial among those who read the fine print, and with the coronavirus crisis, the mask has come off. A piece titled "The coronavirus crisis shows it's time to abolish the family" appeared on OpenDemocracy.net[177] in late March, complaining that the nuclear family model "genders, nationalizes and races us" and "norms us for productive work." It promotes homeownership and private property—two major no-nos—but worst of all, "it makes us believe we are individuals." OpenDemocracy isn't some antifa kid's Tumblr—it's an NGO funded by George Soros' Open Society Foundations, among other globalist bigwigs. Such an open declaration of war on the fundamental building-block of society means Big Money has big plans for the post-pandemic restructuring.

The cashless society is a critical stepping stone to the globalist utopia presented in Agenda 2030, and its proponents seized on coronavirus early on to push their pet project. As the epidemic intensified in early March, a WHO spokesman urged the world to use contactless payment systems wherever possible because cash carries disease, a sentiment echoed by the Bank of England—whose former director, Mark Carney, recently waxed poetic about creating a digital "synthetic hegemonic currency" backed by a "basket" of other currencies including the euro and ruble[178] and modeled after Facebook's Libra. Another WHO spokesperson

---

175 Megan Rowling, "UN aid chief on coronavirus: 'No one is safe until everyone is safe,'" *Thomson Reuters Foundation News,* March 25, 2020, https://news.trust.org/item/20200325144228-it6cy/.

176 "UN issues $2 billion appeal to combat COVID-19," United Nations Office for the Coordination of Humanitarian Affairs, March 25, 2020, https://www.unocha.org/story/un-issues-2-billion-appeal-combat-covid-19.

177 Sophie Lewis, "The coronavirus crisis shows it's time to abolish the family," *Open Democracy,* March 24, 2020, https://www.opendemocracy.net/en/oureconomy/coronavirus-crisis-shows-its-time-abolish-family/.

178 Kalila Sangster, "Banknotes may be spreading coronavirus, World Health Organisation warns," *Yahoo! Finance,* March 3, 2020, https://www.msn.com/en-gb/news/uknews/banknotes-may-be-spreading-coronavirus-world-health-organisation-warns/ar-BB10GafV.

had to walk the claim back less than a week later,[179] replacing the fatwa on cash with yet another reminder to wash one's hands. While actual microbiologists cast doubt on the notion that cash is an especially virulent viral vector,[180] cashless cheerleaders didn't miss a beat, shifting to championing the efficiency of electronic money—wouldn't you rather get your stimulus check in weeks than months? And the news media kept up the drumbeat that cash = dirty, spurred by "experts" like Deutsche Bank macro strategist Marion Laboure, who predicted that central banks would rush to develop their own digital currencies as touching money became a "risk factor."[181]

Many countries, as well as the UN, were already in various stages of developing central bank digital currencies (CBDC) before coronavirus struck. The U.S. has been quietly researching a means of "modernizing the U.S. payments infrastructure" since 2015, with the help of blockchain company Ripple.[182] The UN integrated blockchain into its Sustainable Development Goals and has used the technology to track some 106,000 refugees from Syria alongside pigs and cocoa.[183] While Bitcoin was introduced to the world as a subversive way to anonymously conduct transactions online, its descendants may end up locking down the market beyond what was previously thought possible.

Going cashless is key to adopting another central element of Agenda 2030—digital identity. Amid the height of the pandemic, with international travel at rock-bottom levels, the World Economic Forum unveiled the Known Traveler Digital Identity, an RFID chip that in its current form would be embedded in a traveler's passport and hold a wealth of biometric data, immigration and border crossing records, and a detailed record of all financial transactions, hotel stays,

179 Meera Jagannathan, "World Health Organization: 'We did NOT say that cash was transmitting coronavirus,'" *Market Watch,* March 9, 2020, https://www.marketwatch.com/story/who-we-did-not-say-that-cash-was-transmitting-coronavirus-2020-03-06.

180 Mike Orcutt, "No, coronavirus is not a good argument for quitting cash," *MIT Technology Review,* March 12, 2020, https://www.technologyreview.com/s/615356/coronavirus-contaminated-cash-quarantine/.

181 Deutsche Bank (@DeutscheBank), "The COVID-19 pandemic is accelerating the rise of central bank #digitalcurrencies as many governments see the handling of cash as a potential risk factor. This will likely add to calls to move towards #digitalcash according to our #dbresearch colleague," Twitter, April 3, 2020, https://twitter.com/DeutscheBank/status/1245986930455691264 (accessed April 17, 2020).

182 Team Ripple, "Federal Reserve Task Force: Ripple Improves Speed and Transparency of Global Payments," *Ripple,* July 21, 2017, https://ripple.com/insights/federal-reserve-task-force-ripple-improves-speed-transparency-global-payments/.

183 Bit Coin News Network, "United Nations Adopts Blockchain to Meet its Sustainable Development Goals," *BTCNN,* updated February 29, 2020, https://www.btcnn.com/united-nations-adopts-blockchain-to-meet-its-sustainable-development-goals/.

immunization records, and other movements, all stored on the blockchain. Additionally, it would feature a *Minority Report*-esque "risk assessment" that would tip authorities off to the bearer's likelihood of committing a crime or otherwise causing trouble, pre-assigning a "risk level" based on unspecified "biographical information" supplied to authorities at border checkpoints. Travelers supposedly decide what information to share ahead of a trip, becoming a participant in their own oppression in the same way as residents of Wuhan or Singapore downloaded the app meant to keep them obedient under quarantine.

KTDI is essentially a social credit score: "The more approved digital verification stamps a traveler acquires, the more credibility that individual will have in their next journey," a chipper voiceover explains in a WEF-produced video.[184] Once again, the victim of an oppressive system is incentivized to participate in their own oppression—who wouldn't want to accumulate "credibility" if it helps their trip go smoothly, even if the only way to do so is to subject oneself to repeated and invasive surveillance of one's activities? A white paper outlines a system with echoes of the Black Mirror episode "Nosedive," in which positive interactions increase one's credibility score (and presumably negative interactions decrease it—the paper mentions an exit-point assessment of whether an individual "acted appropriately" while in a country, though it's unclear how this would be determined or by whom). While KTDI would begin life as a beefed-up passport, the WEF admits it "shows great potential for use beyond travel, such as in healthcare, education, banking, humanitarian aid, and voting" and stresses that "broad adoption is crucial for the success of the concept."[185] The paper also hints at developing a "framework" that "takes into consideration the digital identities of people as well as inanimate objects and entities," whatever that means.

The continued existence of cash has long irked the technocratic elite because it's difficult to surveil and control—individuals can use it to dodge taxes, to buy black-market goods, or simply to maintain their privacy. If the coronavirus crisis is harnessed to do away with paper money entirely, individuals can only buy and sell with the permission of the financial institution that holds their money. That's bad enough—JP Morgan Chase has forced people to close their accounts over wrongthink online—but after lockdowns forced most of the world's economic transactions online, the additional consent of both the online store (i.e. Amazon or eBay) and the payment processor (i.e. Paypal or Stripe) are needed—both of

184 World Economic Forum, "Known Traveller Digital Identity: Advancing secure and seamless travel," https://www.weforum.org/projects/shaping-the-future-of-security-in-travel (accessed April 17, 2020).

185 World Economic Forum, *The Known Traveller: Unlocking the potential of digital identity for secure and seamless travel,* January 2018, http://www3.weforum.org/docs/WEF_The_Known_Traveller_Digital_Identity_Concept.pdf (accessed April 17, 2020).

which have the power to decline transactions for those whose social credit (or "credibility") scores are too low.

There will be ways to get one's score up, of course, should one find oneself relegated to the digital ghetto. Reporting your neighbors for social-distancing violations will be an easy way to bolster even the lowest score. But there will be no cheating the blockchain.

Agenda 2030 won't be content with a digital identity that is physically separate from its owner for too much longer. Bill Gates' money is hard at work at Massachusetts Institute of Technology and other research facilities developing ways to get that information into the actual population, buoyed by feigned concern for the "unbanked" and the extreme poor, without cellphones to serve as digital wallets. The Gates-funded ID2020 program unveiled an initiative in October 2019 to implant a biometric identity in babies born in Bangladesh, hinting in the accompanying press release that such a project was already underway among the homeless in Austin, Texas. An MIT team developed a technology for storing vaccination history in a patient's skin using a specially-designed dye, creating a pattern that can be read with a souped-up smartphone.[186]

Once the psychological barrier of bodily integrity has been breached, the sky's the limit regarding how the bodies of worker-bees might be put to use by their social betters. In March, Microsoft filed a patent for a cryptocurrency mining system that uses sensors to detect a person's body activity and generates crypto if that activity "satisfies one or more conditions set by the cryptocurrency system."[187] The sensors can be simple, monitoring heart-rate, temperature, or blood-pressure, or complex in the manner of Elon Musk's Neuralink—a network of minuscule fibers woven over the brain to chips that connect with as many as 1,000 brain cells each. While Musk's invention, due to begin human testing in 2020, was initially touted as a route for humanity to merge with AI (rather than be "left behind" in the slow lane of the information superhighway), he later reframed it as a benign invention to help the paralyzed and the Parkinson-stricken—or perhaps the depressed, anxious, and otherwise emotionally-dysfunctional. Hooking Microsoft's system into Musk's neural net would allow the operator to specify in minute detail what brain functions are to be rewarded with crypto generation—perhaps a user would be rewarded for getting a warm, fuzzy feeling in response to an advertisement,

---

186 Anne Trafton, "Storing medical information below the skin's surface," *MIT News*, December 18, 2019, https://news.mit.edu/2019/storing-vaccine-history-skin-1218 (accessed April 17, 2020).

187 "1. WO2020060606 – Cryptocurrency System Using Body Activity Data," MicroSoft application (abstract), *PatentScope*, March 26, 2020, https://patentscope.wipo.int/search/en/detail.jsf?docId=WO2020060606&tab=PCTBIBLIO (accessed April 17, 2020).

but not if the ad left them cold. Perhaps the emotional stimulus could even be artificially-induced—via a Clockwork-Orange-esque form of conditioning, or by mere application of electrical stimuli in the right places. The only guarantee is that one's "self" is no longer one's own when wires and chips are deployed to alter the functioning of one's brain.

Days after its patent was filed, the WHO debuted a "COVID-19 information highway" called MiPasa on the blockchain, built in collaboration with Microsoft, IBM, Oracle, and Hacera. The platform purports to be able to "help monitor and foresee local and global epidemiological trends. And detect likely asymptomatic carriers. By feeding big data on infection routes and occurrences to powerful AI processors around the world." The initiative is backed by the U.S., European, and Chinese Centers for Disease Control, as well as the Canadian government and (who else?) Johns Hopkins University.[188] Once humans are outfitted with sensors tracking their vital signs—the equivalent of a built-in Fitbit, hooked up to Microsoft's human-crypto blockchain—epidemiology becomes nearly an exact science, and the medical police state becomes impossible to fool. One still hears of concerned parents faking their child's vaccination certificates, desperate to enroll them in school but terrified of subjecting them to a chemical Russian roulette—but in Agenda 2030's future, brought to you by the blockchain, this will be impossible.

The program's boosters have sought to seize the moment created by the total economic collapse and rebuild the financial system "sustainably." By now, it should be clear that the planet pimps are merely taking the Shock Doctrine approach, throwing everything at the wall and see what sticks during a period of chaos—any crisis could have triggered this outpouring of Agenda 2030–adjacent "plans," and coronavirus has nothing to do with climate change. But the idea of sustainability represented by Agenda 2030 and its environmental "brands," including the New Deal for Nature, is less about saving the planet than it is about monetizing it. With a straight face, the green grifters sell nuclear energy as the answer to fossil fuels, indulgence-like carbon offsets as the answer to carbon emissions, and greenwashing buzzwords as the answer to years of pollution and environmental devastation. It's a twisted system under which deep-pocketed Bayer-Monsanto can hire a former German Green Party wunderkind as its star lobbyist to present the company as a saint of sustainability because its carcinogenic glyphosate-based herbicide Roundup allows farmers to grow more crops on less land. Any company that can afford to pay through the nose to hire a green consulting firm and sponsor a few photogenic sustainability initiatives is welcome

---

188 Daniel Abel, "WHO to Start Blockchain COVID-19 Data Hub," *Altcoin Buzz,* April 1, 2020, https://www.altcoinbuzz.io/cryptocurrency-news/blockchain-technology/who-to-start-blockchain-covid-19-data-hub/.

in the New Green Future, represented by the acronym ESG (environmental, social and governance). But those corporations that can't afford specialists to navigate a dense thicket of sustainability ratings—one such consulting firm, SustainAbility, remarked in its 2020 Rate the Raters report that keeping abreast of all the different types of sustainability investment ratings "can require hundreds of hours and multiple dedicated staff"[189]—will increasingly find themselves exiled from the marketplace.

This is not an idle threat. In the same way that BlackRock, which now controls a substantial part of the trading activity of the U.S. Federal Reserve and has declared war on those companies that don't divest from fossil fuels fast enough, has made a point of shoehorning climate change into the asset management sector, the Task Force on Climate-Related Financial Disclosures was established to force "sustainability" into the corporate mainstream. Chaired by New York ex-mayor plutocrat Michael Bloomberg, TCFD is an international oversight body that purports to determine what risk a company poses to the environment and then communicate that to other financial institutions, which can then decide whether or not to do business with that entity. Unlike the other ESG-related ratings, however, the TCFD has teeth: it is partnered with nearly all the major banks and central banks, as well as many governments, and Carney (who founded it with Bloomberg) has threatened to force reluctant companies to adopt a set of climate risk disclosure rules if they do not do so voluntarily. An analogous body, the Network for Greening the Financial System, aims to integrate climate risk into the very fabric of the global financial system. Failure to play the sustainability game would thus not merely force one to look for a new bank—it would force one to give up on the global monetary system entirely. Adopting the blockchain to service such a system is merely placing a state-of-the-art security system on their gated community.

There's something to be said for using the coronavirus crisis as an opportunity to let the grotesquely wasteful, destructive process of fracking die and investing that money in geothermal, wave power, and other truly sustainable forms of energy—certainly those with nefarious motives should not be the only ones permitted to "not let a crisis go to waste"—but that isn't what's happening here. The "net zero carbon emissions" demanded by Agenda 2030 are to be accomplished by balance-sheet trickery—"offsetting" the continued use of fossil fuels to wage war and power private jets with the purchase of carbon credits whose distribution will be controlled by the UN's Intergovernmental Panel on Climate Change, operating like a sort of central bank for this new carbon currency. The IPCC is controlled

---

189 Christina Wong and Erika Petroy, *Rate the Raters 2020: Investor Survey and Interview Results*, SustainAbility, March 2020, https://sustainability.com/wp-content/uploads/2020/03/sustainability-ratetheraters2020-report.pdf (accessed April 17, 2020).

by the same interests that are behind the fossil fuel infrastructure that has supposedly brought the planet to the brink of destruction—a conflict of interest if ever there was one. An artificial superstructure of emissions buck-passing will grow up around fundamentally unsustainable industries, all of whom will be able to claim they're doing good even when not a single tree is planted.

Agenda 2030 is also obsessed with land use, namely dictating the ever-dwindling areas in which human activity is permitted. The New Deal for Nature, which glommed onto coronavirus as a cause célèbre early on, wants humanity kicked off 30% of the earth's surface—land currently inhabited by indigenous peoples in the global South. Reasoning that the corona crisis has proved humanity can change dramatically in a very short time, groups like the Club of Rome—who've been singing the same songs of depopulation for close to half a century—are rushing to accustom Western societies to a fossil-fuel-free future, while politically-correct rhetoric hides the same paternalistic racism and classism that has always seen the poorest nations of Africa selected for the dubious "privilege" of receiving "free" (experimental) vaccinations from the benevolent hands of Bill Gates.

Climate change is the pandemic's spiritual forebear in that it is held up as a reason for humanity to unite under a global government. "This is too big for any one country to solve" has been the recurring refrain. The same billionaires fronting the "cause" of saving the planet—the descendants of the robber barons whose fossil fuel empires trashed the planet in the first place—claim to be intent on saving humanity, even though their own words betray their loathing for the species.

THE NEW NEW NORMAL

The shifts set in motion by the coronavirus pandemic have fundamentally reoriented society along draconian lines that were once unthinkable in the "liberal democracies" of the West. Humanity's fundamental adaptability is typically considered an asset, but there are some circumstances one should actively fight against "getting used to." As lockdowns drag on for weeks, with some nations threatening months more indoors, memories of the vibrant, people-filled Life Before the Plague will begin to fade, replaced with a sense of fatalism: it has always been like this, therefore it will always be like this. A sort of inertia will set in, accompanied by an emotional numbness to each new horror as it is unveiled.

The narrative managers, unsurprisingly, encourage this view. "Life will never be the same" was the line taken by War on Terror mythmaker Bill Kristol—whose publication *The Bulwark* couldn't even wait until U.S. coronavirus deaths exceeded the 9/11 body count to publish a "COVID-19 Has Killed More Americans Than

9/11" think piece.[190] Just as the 9/11 fearmongers warned Americans that failing to go to war in Iraq would guarantee that the smoking gun would be a mushroom cloud, *MIT Technology Review* editor-in-chief Gideon Lichfield warned the world that if they did not "go to war" against their own way of life, recurrent coronavirus outbreaks could force societies to re-adopt social distancing cyclically, spending half the year on house arrest.[191] The only alternative, according to these leading lights of the ruling class intelligentsia, is to submit to endless surveillance including bodily intrusion, listen to bought-and-paid-for "experts," and "sacrifice the me to the we," in the words of ruling class toady Chris Cuomo.

In the new technocratic future, everything is measured, tracked, and monitored. Smart meters gauge electricity use (and throttle an individual's consumption if some distant manager decides they're getting too greedy); smart streetlights monitor a city's residents as they walk through the streets, constantly scanning for rule-violators (have *you* gotten your flu shot this year? good luck entering *this* neighborhood); smart, self-driving cars move people from place to place, within limits of course (don't even try driving after curfew, and remember that all your conversations inside the car are being monitored for disinformation—there's an infodemic on the loose); smart chips implanted in every individual track their whereabouts at all times and interact with every other object in the 5G-enabled "smart" cities of the future. This is not science fiction—"smart cities" are in the process of rolling out in Toronto and China. The only elements that aren't smart are the people. Why bother to use your brain, when your environment does the thinking for you?

Even Henry Kissinger, the *eminence grise* of the U.S. empire, emerged from the shadows to weigh in on the opportunity represented by coronavirus with a *Wall Street Journal* op-ed about how "the coronavirus pandemic will forever alter the World Order."[192] Personally responsible for millions of deaths and unable to travel to several countries for fear of being arrested for war crimes, Kissinger clearly wasn't content to rest on his laurels—he demanded all national recovery

---

190 Bill Kristol (@BillKristol), "This pandemic will be more consequential than 9/11. It probably already is. People just don't realize it, because they still think—still feel—that once this is all over we'll go back to the way things used to be. We won't." Twitter, March 30, 2020, https://twitter.com/BillKristol/status/1244757942538289155 (accessed April 17, 2020).

191 Gideon Lichfield, "We're not going back to normal," *MIT Technology Review,* March 17, 2020, https://www.technologyreview.com/s/615370/coronavirus-pandemic-social-distancing-18-months/.

192 Henry A. Kissinger, "The Coronavirus Pandemic Will Forever Alter the World Order," *The Wall Street Journal,* April 3, 2020, https://www.wsj.com/articles/the-coronavirus-pandemic-will-forever-alter-the-world-order-11585953005.

programs be coupled with a "global collaborative vision and program," warning that failing to heed his advice will result in untold suffering for humanity. Kissinger can perhaps consider himself a godfather of this pandemic—it was he who wrote the infamous 1974 report that called for the imposition of strict population-control measures on the Third World, to ensure its resources would be easily plundered for decades to come. Listening to Kissinger and his fellow oligarchs, who see humans as speed bumps on the road to power, was what got the U.S. into this mess. Continuing down that path—embracing the police state ever more tightly, giving away ever more liberty in the name of ever more hollow security-theatre—will only compound our suffering.

Those who lived through 9/11 and saw the destruction it wrought upon the U.S.' national character can see it happening again on an international scale. It is our duty to warn the world and avert that outcome. One country falling under the thrall of a totalitarian technocratic police state is a tragedy; the entire world falling under an authoritarian global government is a nightmare from which humanity might never wake up.

April 2020

CHAPTER FOURTEEN

THE POST-COVID WORLD
NEEDS A NEW SOCIAL CONTRACT[*]

Alfred de Zayas

The COVID-19 pandemic is a game-changer and offers a historic opportunity to radically rethink the prevailing financial and economic system characterized by its boom-and-bust cycles, widespread unemployment, demonstrably unjust distribution of wealth and unwise allocation of national budgets, which have left societies inadequately prepared to deal effectively with disasters including pandemics, hurricanes, earthquakes and volcanic eruptions.[1]

This is a propitious moment for the Members of the United Nations (UN) to take the initiative to reform the dysfunctional paradigm of globalization, which has been accompanied by extreme poverty and endemic social injustice.

This is the time to replace the outdated Bretton Woods system[2] and to reorganize economic and trade priorities so as to achieve the Sustainable Development

---

1 See UN Press Release, "'We Are Only as Strong as the Weakest', Secretary-General Stresses, at Launch of Economic Report on COVID-19 Pandemic," March 31, 2020, https://www.un.org/press/en/2020/sgsm20029.doc.htm; "UN chief says mankind 'so unprepared' for COVID-19, world lacks solidarity," *CGTN,* May 15, 2020, https://news.cgtn.com/news/2020-05-15/UN-chief-says-mankind-so-unprepared-for-COVID-19-Qvi8tVla2k/index.html; "The Secretary-General's UN COVID-19 Response and Recovery Fund (April 2020)," UN report, April 26, 2020, posted by *reliefweb,* May 4, 2020, https://reliefweb.int/report/world/secretary-generals-un-covid-19-response-and-recovery-fund-april-2020; and UN Secretary General, "Launch of Global Humanitarian Response Plan for COVID-19," *United Nations,* March 25, 2020, https://www.un.org/sg/en/content/sg/press-encounter/2020-03-25/launch-of-global-humanitarian-response-plan-for-covid-19.

2 My July 20, 2017 report to the UN Human Rights Council (https://ap.ohchr.org/documents/dpage_e.aspx?si=A/HRC/36/40), and my July 21, 2017 report to the UN General Assembly (https://www.un.org/en/ga/search/view_doc.asp?symbol=A/72/187), formulate concrete proposals on how to reform the World Bank and the International Monetary Fund so that they are no longer "human rights free zones" and make their activities more compatible with the UN Charter.

---

*First published by The South Centre in *SouthViews,* No. 197, May 22, 2020.

Goals (SDGs) and give practical meaning to the right of self-determination of all peoples and their right to development.

This is the time for António Guterres to confer with economic advisors including Jeffrey Sachs, Joseph Stiglitz and Thomas Piketty and make concrete proposals to world leaders on how best to reform the system in conformity with the Purposes and Principles of the UN Charter, taking due account of General Assembly Resolutions 2625 and 3314.[3] In this context, it may be appropriate to convene a World Conference on Post-Covid Recovery, with a mandate to revive multilateralism, reject unilateral coercive measures and ensure the proper funding of all UN agencies and establish mechanisms to enhance their coordination and efficiency. But the conference, if it is going to have any added value, would have to go beyond cosmetic adjustments and a return to the broken status quo ante. Without amending the UN Charter under Article 108, the Conference should issue a pledge, a good faith statement recognizing the Purposes and Principles of the United Nations as the best hope of humanity, and committing to applying the UN Charter as a world constitution, and respecting the judgments and advisory opinions of the International Court of Justice as the authoritative statements of a world constitutional court. This would entail the progressive incorporation of UN Charter provisions into the domestic legislation of UN member States.

A world conference could revisit the Four Freedoms of Franklin Delanao Roosevelt and It should rediscover the spirituality of the Universal Declaration of Human Rights and revive the legacy of Eleanor Roosevelt, René Cassin, Charles Malik and John Humphrey.

The paradigm shift will entail a change in national budgetary priorities, away from the arms race, war, military bases, procurement, drones and missiles. What is urgent and feasible is a gradual, step by step conversion of military-first budgets into human-security budgets. The new mantra must be "Disarmament for Development." Indeed, a significant reduction in military expenditures will liberate the necessary funds to achieve the SDGs and ensure the enjoyment of all human rights by all, including and most importantly the right to health, food, water, etc. Taxpayers' money that has been wasted in Orwellian "mass surveillance" activities, such as those revealed by Edward Snowden,[4] must be redirected to social services.[5] World Conference on Post-Covid Recovery should address

---

3 See the 23 Principles of International Order formulated in my January 25, 2018 report to the Human Rights Council, paragraph 14, available at https://ap.ohchr.org/documents/dpage_e.aspx?si=A/HRC/37/63.

4 Edward Snowden, *Permanent Record* (Macmillan, 2019).

5 In my July 17, 2014 report to the UN Human Rights Council I called for the military establishment to be gradually converted into peacetime industries at all levels,

measures to abolish tax havens and ensure the payment of taxes by investors and transnational corporations without phoney registrations or "sweetheart deals."[6]

The failures of the neo-liberal ideology, the systematic exploitation of peoples worldwide, the destruction of the environment and the constant threat posed by the arms race, stockpiling of weapons of mass destruction, research and development programs into lethal autonomous weapon systems and other aberrations have become all too evident. Surely the gravity of the COVID-19 pandemic would have been considerably less lethal if governments had implemented human-rights centered economies in which the right to life and the right to health had enjoyed priority over market speculation, the drive to make short-term profits and continue the ecocide that plagues the world today.

A NEW FUNCTIONAL PARADIGM FOR HUMAN RIGHTS

Civil society in all countries should now demand from their governments a new social contract based on the implementation of the ten core UN human rights treaties. Admittedly, the task of standard-setting has not been completed, since codification of human rights is never definitive and never exhaustive but constitutes an evolutionary *mode d'emploi* for the exercise of civil, cultural, economic, political and social rights. Alas, the interpretation and application of human rights has been hindered by wrong priorities, sterile positivism and a regrettable tendency to focus only on individual rights while forgetting collective rights. It is all too obvious that many in the "human rights industry" show little or no interest for the social responsibilities that accompany the exercise of rights, and fail to see the necessary symbiosis of rights and obligations as formulated in article 29 of the Universal Declaration of Human Rights.

The time has come to change the human rights paradigm away from narrow positivism toward a broader understanding of human rights norms in the context of an emerging customary international law of human rights. Law is neither physics nor mathematics, but a dynamic human institution that day by day addresses the needs and aspirations of society, adjusting here, filling lacunae there. Every human rights lawyer knows that the spirit of the law (Montesquieu) transcends the limitations of the letter of the law, and hence codified norms should always be interpreted in the light of those general principles of law that inform all legal systems, such as good faith, proportionality and *ex injuria non oritur jus*.

---

creating many more jobs in education, healthcare, housing, environmental protection and other social services. See https://ap.ohchr.org/documents/dpage_e.aspx?si=A/HRC/27/51.

6 My August 4, 2016 report to the General Assembly was devoted specifically to the criminalization of tax fraud and tax evasion. See https://ap.ohchr.org/documents/dpage_e.aspx?si=A/71/286.

A World Conference on Post-Covid Recovery could propose discarding the obsolete and artificial division of human rights into those of the falsely called first generation (civil and political), second (economic, social and cultural) and third generation (environment, peace, development) rights –with its obvious predisposition to favour civil and political rights. This generational divide is part of a structure that perpetuates a world order that much too often appears to allow injustice. I propose instead a functional paradigm that would consider rights in the light of their function within a coherent system—not of competing rights and aspirations, but of interrelated, mutually reinforcing rights which should be applied in their interdependence and understood in the context of a coordinated strategy to serve the ultimate goal of achieving human dignity in all of its manifestations. Four categories would replace the skewed narrative of three generations of rights.

First we would recognize **enabling rights,** among which I would list the rights to health, food, water, shelter, development, homeland–but also the right to peace, since one cannot enjoy human rights unless there is an environment conducive to the exercise of those rights. Article 28 of the Universal Declaration of Human Rights postulates the right of every human being "to a social and international order in which the rights and freedoms set forth in this Declaration can be fully realized." This entails the basic necessities of life and the right to a level playing field.

Secondly, I would propose a category of inherent or **immanent** rights, such as the right to equality, the right to non-arbitrariness; indeed, every right necessarily contains in itself the element of equality, the self-evident requirement that it be applied equally and equitably, that there be uniformity and predictability (in German *Rechtssicherheit*). Immanent rights also encompass the rights to life, integrity, liberty and security of person, in the light of which other rights must be interpreted and applied. There are also inherent limitations to the exercise of rights. The general principle of law prohibiting abuse of rights (*sic utere tuo ut alienum non laeda*—use your right without harming others, a principle advocated by Sir Hersch Lauterpacht as an overarching norm prohibiting the egoistic exercise of rights to achieve anti-social results or unjust enrichment) means that every right, also a human right, must be exercised in the context of other rights and not instrumentalized to destroy other rights or harm others. There is no right to intransigence as we know from Shylock in the Merchant of Venice. The letter of the law must never be used against the spirit of the law.

Third, I would propose a category of procedural or **instrumental** rights, such as the rights to due process, access to information, freedom of expression and peaceful assembly, work, education, social security, leisure—rights that we need to achieve our potential, to complete our personalities, to engage in the pursuit of happiness. Also in this category I would include the right to international solidarity as formulated by UN Independent Expert Virginia Dandan in her 2017 report to the Human Rights Council.[7]

Finally, I would postulate the category of end rights or **outcome** rights, that is, the concrete exercise of human dignity, that condition of life that allows each human being to be himself or herself. This ultimate right is the right to our identity, to our privacy, the right to be ourselves, to think by ourselves and express our humanity without indoctrination, without intimidation, without pressures of political correctness, without "mass surveillance" from governments or private enterprises, without having to sell ourselves, without having to engage in self-censorship. The absence of this outcome right to identity and self-respect is reflected in much of the strife we see in the world today. It is through the consciousness and exercise of the right to our identity and the respect of the identity of others that we will enjoy the individual and collective right to peace.[8]

A World Conference on Post-Covid Recovery should urge all States to enhance cooperation with the UN Human Rights Treaty Bodies and with the UN Human Rights Council, and to implement the recommendations emanating from the Universal Periodic Review. The United Nations Human Rights Council should become the international arena where governments compete to show how best to implement human rights, how to strengthen the rule of law, how to achieve social justice, where they display best practices and give life to this new functional paradigm of human rights. This kind of competition in human rights performance is the noblest goal and challenge for civilization.

The Human Rights Council should become the preeminent forum where governments elucidate what they themselves have done and are doing to deliver on human rights, in good-faith implementation of pledges, in adherence to a daily culture of human rights characterized by generous interpretation of human rights treaties and a commitment to the inclusion of all stakeholders. What the Council must not be is a politicized arena where gladiators use human rights as weapons to defeat their political adversaries and where human rights are undermined through "side shows," the "flavor of the month" or "legal black holes." The civilization model of the globalized world must not be one of positivism, legalisms and loopholes, but one of ethics, direct democracy, respect for the environment, international solidarity and human dignity.

While the Human Rights Council is subordinated to the UN General Assembly, the UN Security Council is in the better position to support the implementation of

---

7 See "Report of the Independent Expert on human rights and international solidarity," *United Nations Human Rights,* April 25, 2017, https://ap.ohchr.org/documents/dpage_e. aspx?si=A/HRC/35/35.

8 See my August 7, 2013 report to the UN General Assembly, paras. 67–68, available at https://www.un.org/en/ga/search/view_doc.asp?symbol=A/68/284.

Human Rights Council decisions and resolutions, which hitherto are considered "soft law" and for which no enforcement mechanisms have been established.

A World Conference on Post-Covid Recovery should enhance the faculties of the Human Rights Council to ensure that it has greater structural impact on the UN Security Council.

Contributors

Gary D. Barnett is a writer and a retired investment professional with over 30 years experience. While his main career was in finance, his college background was in biology and zoology. He has also owned several additional businesses and has over 1,000 published posts and articles to his credit. He is a voluntaryist, is anti-war, anti-state, believes in non-aggression, and promotes the natural rights of man. His publications, especially concerning real history, the dishonesty and evil nature of the state, the heinous nature of war and aggression, and corruption at every level of power, have been widely read in the U.S. and in many countries around the world. He has published articles for Lew Rockwell, The Future of Freedom Foundation, The Foundation for Economic Education, and many others.

Jeff J. Brown is Editor-in-Chief of China Rising Radio Sinoland (https://www.chinarising.puntopress.com), producer of *China Tech News Flash!* (http://www.chinatechnewsflash.com), author of *The China Trilogy* and Curator of the Bioweapon Truth Commission Global Online Library (BWTC-GOL—https://www.bioweapontruth.com). He grew up on a family livestock and orchard farm, where he lived and worked with microbiology up close and personal. Jeff has a B.S. and M.S. in Animal Sciences and is a U.S. state certified science teacher.

Helen Buyniski is an American journalist and political commentator based in Brooklyn. She has written for and appeared on *RT, PressTV, Global Research, Ghion Journal, Progressive Radio Network,* and *Activist Post,* among others. Helen has a BA from New School University and also studied at Columbia University and New York University. Her work is collected at http://helenofdestroy.com. She is also an accomplished violinist and photographer.

Alfred de Zayas is an American lawyer, writer, historian, expert in the field of human rights and international law and retired high-ranking United Nations official. From 1 May 2012 to 30 April 2018 he served as the first UN Independent Expert on the Promotion of a Democratic and Equitable International Order (appointed by the United Nations Human Rights Council). He holds a J.D. from Harvard University and a doctorate of philosophy in modern history from the University of Göttingen (Germany). He was also a research fellow at the Max Planck Institute for Comparative Public Law and International Law in Heidelberg, Germany. He worked with the United Nations from 1981 to 2003 as a senior lawyer with the Office of the UN High Commissioner for Human Rights and the Chief of Petitions.

Michael Hudson is an American economist, Professor of Economics at the University of Missouri, Kansas City and a researcher at the Levy Economics Institute at Bard College. He is a former Wall Street analyst, political consultant, commentator and journalist, and worked as a balance of payment economist Chase Manhattan Bank. He was assistant professor of economics at the New School for Social Research and worked for various governmental and non-governmental organizations as an economic consultant. He holds a Ph.D. from New York University. His latest book is *Forgive Them Their Debts: Lending, Foreclosure and Redemption from Bronze Age Finance to the Jubilee Year.*

Peter Koenig is an economist and geopolitical analyst. He is also a water resources and environmental specialist. He worked for over 30 years with the World Bank and the World Health Organization around the world in the fields of environment and water. He lectures at universities in the U.S., Europe and South America. He writes regularly for *Global Research; Information Clearing House* (ICH); *New Eastern Outlook* (NEO); *RT,* the China-focused *21st Century* and other online journals. He is the author of *Implosion: An Economic Thriller about War, Environmental Destruction and Corporate Greed*—fiction based on facts and on 30 years of World Bank experience around the globe.

Cynthia McKinney was the 2008 Green Party Candidate for President and a former U.S. Congresswoman. She is the author of *Ain't Nothing Like Freedom* and editor of *The Illegal War On Libya* and *How the U.S. Creates "Sh*thole" Countries.* She holds a B.A. from the University of Southern California, an M.A.L.D. from The Fletcher School of Law and Diplomacy and a Ph.D. from Antioch University. She is an international peace and human rights activist, noted for her inconvenient truth-telling about the U.S. war machine.

Claudio Peretti is an Aerospace engineer, presently working as a freelance consultant in the business of high tech, where deep capabilities of problem-solving and creativity are requested. He has worked as design director in many aircraft manufacturing companies. He is a former NATO expert for anti-aircraft missile systems and expert adviser to the European Commission for the evaluation of funding requests by aeronautic companies for new development projects.

Jack Rasmus currently teaches economics at St. Marys College in Moraga, California. Prior to teaching and publishing, he was an economist and strategic market analyst for various global tech and market research companies for twenty years. Before that, for more than a decade, he was a local union president, contract negotiator, strike coordinator, and organizer for various unions. He holds an M.A. and Ph.D. from the University of Toronto, Canada in Political Economy. A Chinese edition of his latest book, *The Scourge of Neoliberalism,* will shortly be forthcoming. He blogs regularly at *Znet* and *Counterpunch* (USA), *Global Research* (Canada), and *Telesur* (Caracas).

William I. Robinson is a distinguished professor of sociology, global studies, and Latin American studies at the University of California at Santa Barbara. His latest book is *The Global Police State* (Pluto Press, 2020).

Larry Romanoff is a retired management consultant and businessman. He has held senior executive positions in international consulting firms, and owned an international import-export business. He has been a visiting professor at Shanghai's Fudan University, presenting case studies in international affairs to senior EMBA classes. Mr. Romanoff lives in Shanghai and is currently writing a series of ten books generally related to China and the West.

Whitney Webb is a professional writer, researcher and journalist, and is the co-founder and editor of Unlimited Hangout. She currently writes for *The Last American Vagabond,* and from 2017 to 2020, was a staff writer and senior investigative reporter for *Mint Press News.* She has contributed to several independent media outlets and her work has been featured by *The Real News Network, The Ron Paul Institute, The Zero Hour,* and *The Jimmy Dore Show,* among others. She has made several radio and television appearances and is the 2019 winner of the Serena Shim Award for Uncompromised Integrity in Journalism.

INDEX